CORNEAL TOPOGRAPHY
The State of the Art

CORNEAL TOPOGRAPHY
The State of the Art

James P. Gills, MD
Clinical Professor
University of South Florida
Tampa, Florida
St. Luke's Cataract and Laser Institute
Tarpon Springs, Florida

Donald R. Sanders, MD, PhD
Associate Professor of Ophthalmology
University of Illinois at Chicago Eye Center
Director, Center for Clinical Research
Chicago, Illinois

Spencer P. Thornton, MD, FACS
Director, Thornton Eye Surgery Center
Nashville, Tennessee

Robert G. Martin, MD
Director, Medical Care International
Ophthalmic Research and Training Institute
Founder, Carolina Eye Associates
Southern Pines, North Carolina

Johnny L. Gayton, MD
EyeSight Associates of Middle Georgia
Warner Robins, Georgia

Jack T. Holladay, MD, FACS
Houston Eye Associates
Houston, Texas

Michelle Van Der Karr
Project Coordinator
Medical Editor
Evanston, Illinois

SLACK Incorporated, 6900 Grove Road, Thorofare, NJ 08086-9447

Acquisitions Editor: Amy E. Drummond
Publisher: John H. Bond
Production Editor: Debra L. Clarke
Associate Editor: Jennifer J. Dyer

Corneal topography: the state of the art/edited by James P. Gills...[et al.].
    p. cm.
  Includes bibliographical references and index.
  ISBN 1-55642-268-7 (hard cover)
  1. Corneal topography. I. Gills, James P. [DNLM: 1. Cornea—anatomy & histology.
  2. Cornea—surgery. WW 220 C8139 1995]
RE336.C695 1995
617.7'19—dc20
DNLM/DLC

for Library of Congress   95-1080

Printed in the United States of America

Published by: SLACK Incorporated
               6900 Grove Road
               Thorofare, NJ 08086-9447

Last digit is print number: 10 9 8 7 6 5 4 3 2 1

Dedication

To Spencer Thornton,
   a beloved friend,
   an accomplished teacher,
   and a trusted colleague,
   who every day shows how to triumph in adversity.
   We love you.
   JPG, DRS, RGM, JLG, JTH

Contents

Dedication v

Acknowledgments xi

Contributing Authors xiii

Other Books by the Authors xvii

Preface xix

Section I: Overview of Corneal Topography

Chapter 1   Introduction to Corneal Topography   3
               Douglas D. Koch, MD
               Elizabeth A. Haft, BS

Chapter 2   Alignment of Videokeratographs   17
               Robert B. Mandell, OD, PhD
               Douglas Horner, OD, PhD

Chapter 3   Characterizing Astigmatism: Keratometric Measurements
               Do Not Always Accurately Reflect Corneal Topography   25
               Donald R. Sanders, MD, PhD
               James P. Gills, MD
               Robert G. Martin, MD

Section II: Current Technology

Chapter 4   Corneal Topography as Measured by the EyeMap EH-270   37
               Sami G. El Hage, OD, PhD, DSc
               James J. Salz, MD
               Michael W. Belin, MD
               John A. Costin, MD
               Michael G. Gressel, MD

Chapter 5   The EyeSys 2000 Corneal Analysis System   55
               Spencer P. Thornton, MD, FACS
               Joseph Wakil, MD, MEE

Chapter 6   MasterVue Topography Systems   77
               Glenda G. Anderson

Chapter 7   Pachymetry and True Topography Using the ORBSCAN System   89
               Richard K. Snook

Chapter 8 PAR Corneal Topography System   105
Michael W. Belin, MD
James L. Cambier, PhD
John R. Nabors, MS

Chapter 9 The Tomey Technology/Computed Anatomy TMS-1 Videokeratoscope   123
Michael K. Smolek, PhD
Stephen D. Klyce, PhD

Chapter 10 The TOPCON Computerized Mapping System CM-1000   151
Kazuo Nunokawa

Section III: Clinical Applications

Chapter 11 Corneal Topography to Detect and Characterize Corneal Pathology   159
Douglas D. Koch, MD
Syed E. Husain, MD

Chapter 12 The Contribution of Corneal Topography to the
Evaluation of Cataract Surgery   171
Robert G. Martin, MD
James P. Gills, MD
Johnny L. Gayton, MD

Chapter 13 Corneal Topography in Refractive Surgical Procedures   195
Johnny L. Gayton, MD
David Dulaney, MD
Spencer P. Thornton, MD, FACS
Robert G. Martin, MD

Chapter 14 Cataract Surgery Combined with Astigmatic Keratotomy   215
James P. Gills, MD
Robert G. Martin, MD

Chapter 15 Corneal Relaxing Incisions, Multifocal Corneas, and "Omnimmetropia"   225
James P. Gills, MD

Chapter 16 Evaluating Excimer Laser Procedures   241
Daniel S. Durrie, MD
Donald R. Sanders, MD, PhD
D. James Schumer, MD
Manus C. Kraff, MD
Robert T. Spector, MD
David Gubman, OD

Chapter 17   Corneal Topography in Lamellar Refractive Surgery   263
            Stephen A. Updegraff, MD
            Luis A. Ruiz, MD
            Stephen G. Slade, MD

Chapter 18   Corneal Topography in the Evaluation of the Corneal Transplant Patient   287
            Roger Steinert, MD
            Johnny L. Gayton, MD
            Robert G. Martin, MD

Chapter 19   The Holladay Diagnostic Summary   309
            Jack T. Holladay, MD, FACS

Index   325

Acknowledgments

The editors wish to expressly thank the following individuals for their kind assistance:

Robert Anello
Lynda Antman
Mark Findahl
Thomas Wiener

Contributing Authors

Glenda G. Anderson
Humphrey Instruments, Inc.,
Azusa, CA

Michael W. Belin, MD
Albany Medical College,
Ophthalmology Department,
Albany, NY

James L. Cambier, PhD
PAR Vision Systems Corporation,
New Hartford, NY

John A. Costin, MD
Lakeland Eye Surgeons and Consultants, Inc.,
Lorain, OH

David Dulaney, MD
Dulaney Eye Clinic,
Phoenix, AZ

Daniel S. Durrie, MD
Hunkeler Eye Clinic,
Kansas City, MO

Sami G. El Hage, OD, PhD, DSc
Alcon Surgical Inc.,
Fort Worth, TX

Johnny L. Gayton, MD
EyeSight Associates of Middle Georgia,
Warner Robins, GA

James P. Gills, MD
Clinical Professor,
University of South Florida,
Tampa, FL
St. Luke's Cataract and Laser Institute,
Tarpon Springs, FL

Michael G. Gressel, MD
Lakeland Eye Surgeons and Consultants, Inc.,
Lorain, OH

David Gubman, OD
Pennsylvania College of Optometry,
Philadelphia, PA

Elizabeth A. Haft, BS
Cincinnati Eye Institute
Cincinnati, OH

Jack T. Holladay, MD, FACS
Houston Eye Associates,
Houston, TX

Douglas Horner, OD, PhD
School of Optometry,
Indiana University,
Bloomington, IN

Syed E. Husain, MD
Clinical Instructor,
Cullen Eye Institute,
Baylor College of Medicine,
Houston, TX

Stephen D. Klyce, PhD
Professor of Ophthalmology,
LSU Eye Center,
Adjunct Professor of Biomedical Engineering,
Tulane University,
New Orleans, LA

Douglas D. Koch, MD
Associate Professor of Ophthalmology,
Cullen Eye Institute,
Baylor College of Medicine,
Houston, TX

Manus C. Kraff, MD
Professor of Clinical Ophthalmology,
Northwestern University,
Chicago, IL

Robert B. Mandell, OD, PhD
School of Optometry,
University of California,
Berkeley, CA

Robert G. Martin, MD
Director, Medical Care International
Ophthalmic Research and Training Institute,
Founder, Carolina Eye Associates,
Southern Pines, NC

John R. Nabors, MS
PAR Vision Systems Corporation,
New Hartford, NY

Kazuo Nunokawa
TOPCON America,
Paramus, NJ

Luis A. Ruiz, MD
Barraquer Institute
Bogata, Colombia

James J. Salz, MD
Clinical Professor of Ophthalmology,
University of Southern California,
Los Angeles, CA

Donald R. Sanders, MD, PhD
Associate Professor of Ophthalmology,
University of Illinois at Chicago Eye Center,
Director, Center for Clinical Research,
Chicago, IL

D. James Schumer, MD
Ohio Eye Associates,
Mansfield, OH

Stephen G. Slade, MD
Hermann Eye Center, Clinical Faculty,
University of Texas,
Houston, TX

Michael K. Smolek, PhD
Research Associate, LSU Eye Center,
New Orleans, LA

Richard K. Snook
Vice President of Engineering, Orbtek, Inc.,
Tucson, AZ

Robert T. Spector, MD
Sight Foundation,
Fort Lauderdale, FL

Roger Steinert, MD
Harvard Medical School,
Center for Eye Research,
Ophthalmic Consultants of Boston,
Boston, MA

Spencer P. Thornton, MD, FACS
Director, Thornton Eye Surgery Center,
Nashville, TN

Stephen A. Updegraff, MD
Hermann Eye Center, Cornea Fellow,
University of Texas,
Houston, TX

Joseph Wakil, MD, MEE
EyeSys Technologies,
Houston, TX

Other Books by the Authors

Surgical Treatment of Astigmatism
James P. Gills, MD,
Robert G. Martin, MD,
Spencer P. Thornton, MD, FACS,
Donald R. Sanders, MD, PhD

Ophthalmic Anesthesia
Robert F. Hustead, MD,
James P. Gills, MD,
Donald R. Sanders, MD, PhD

Foldable Intraocular Lenses
Robert G. Martin, MD,
James P. Gills, MD,
Donald R. Sanders, MD, PhD

Radial and Astigmatic Keratotomy:
The American System of Precise,
Predictable Refractive Surgery
Spencer P. Thornton, MD, FACS

Small-Incision Cataract Surgery:
Foldable Lenses, One-Stitch Surgery,
Sutureless Surgery, Astigmatic Keratotomy
James P. Gills, MD,
Donald R. Sanders, MD, PhD

Sutureless Cataract Surgery: An Evolution
Toward Minimally Invasive Technique
James P. Gills, MD,
Robert G. Martin, MD,
Donald R. Sanders, MD, PhD

An Atlas of Corneal Topography
Donald R. Sanders, MD, PhD,
Douglas D. Koch, MD

Lens Implant Power Calculation:
A Manual for Ophthalmologists and
Biometrists, Third Edition
John Retzlaff, MD,
Donald R. Sanders, MD, PhD,
Manus Kraff, MD

Preface

Since computerized videokeratography was introduced several years ago, providing for the first time both qualitative and quantitative information about the entire corneal contour, there has been an explosion of new technology and a wealth of new information on the clinical applications and research possibilities. In this book, we explore seven different corneal topography systems, all employing new and unique designs for improving accuracy and repeatability. New clinical applications of this technology are also represented here, from combined cataract and refractive surgery to lamellar and excimer procedures, as well as its use in screening for, evaluating, and tracking corneal pathology. New software that provides not only topographical information about the cornea but also true refractive power, sphericity, and optical quality is also introduced here. We hope that this book will not only prove informative about the current state-of-the-art, but will provide an impetus toward even more refinements and advancements in this technology.

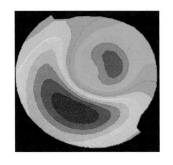
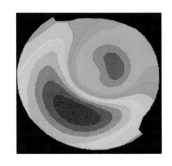
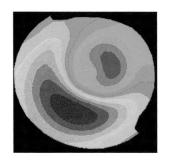
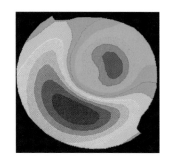

OVERVIEW
OF
CORNEAL
TOPOGRAPHY

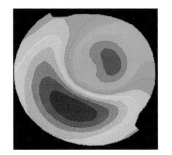
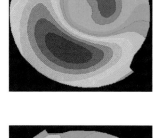
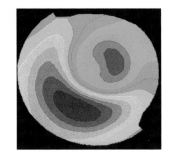
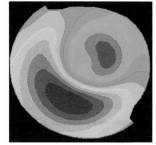
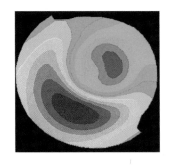
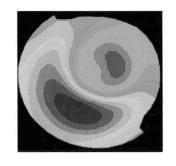
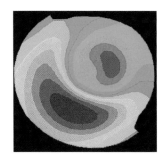
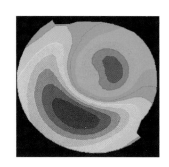
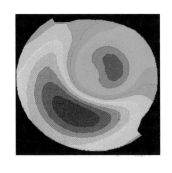
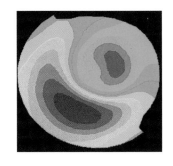
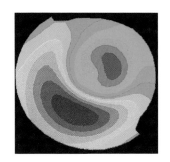
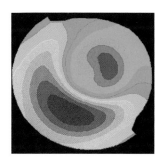

INTRODUCTION TO CORNEAL TOPOGRAPHY

Douglas D. Koch, MD
Elizabeth A. Haft, BS

In refractive surgery the surgeon must be able to measure precisely and modify predictably. The cornea, lens, and axial length are the key refractive elements of the eye. Of these three factors, the cornea is by far the most accessible for both clinical measurement and modification. Measurement of lens power is problematic, and lens power can only be modified by lens extraction, intraocular lens implantation, or both. Axial length can be measured, but refractive surgical modification is not possible. At this time, the cornea offers the greatest opportunities for surgical correction of refractive errors.

EVALUATING TOPOGRAPHICAL MAPS

Since we will be illustrating a number of the points in this chapter with examples of corneal topographic maps, it is appropriate to discuss how to interpret them. Figure 1-1 is a typical color contour map of a normal, essentially non-astigmatic cornea. In interpreting these maps, it is important to recognize that the so-called "hot" colors—red, orange, and yellow—are steeper portions of the cornea. Green is intermediate, and cool colors—light and dark blue—are flatter portions. It is essential when looking at these maps to check the color scale to see which colors correspond to which dioptric powers and to determine the dioptric interval between color changes. In this case the color changes are in .5 D increments, and since 15 distinct colors are represented on the scale to the right, the entire range represents 7.5 D. In this map the power of the central cornea is in the 46.5 to 47 D range. The white circle in the center of the image represents the pupil outline.

The cursor, which is represented by a " + ", is initially located at the point that represents the center of the corneoscopic rings. This center point is referred to as the videokeratographic (or VK) axis or as the vertex normal. When viewing the topographical map on the color monitor of the system, the cursor can be moved around the color map with the computer mouse. The information box, which in this figure is in the lower right corner, reports the radius of curvature (mm) and dioptric power at the location of the mouse cursor (see Figure 1-1). The position with respect to the center of the rings is displayed in radial degrees and millimeters. This and most of the other maps shown have a grid pattern superimposed upon the image. Each square is 1 mm by 1 mm, which allows one to quickly determine how far from the corneal center an abnormality occurs. Also note the peripheral circle marking the axes for 360,° which is especially helpful in assessing astigmatism.

The sensitivity of the map can be decreased by using larger increments on the dioptric scaling to screen for gross pathology. Conversely, the sensitivity can be increased for detecting much smaller and more subtle corneal topographic changes by decreasing the increments between color changes. Figure 1-2 demonstrates the same eye displayed with four different dioptric intervals or sensitivities. Keep in mind that when you "zoom in" for a closer look at the corneal curvature it is essential to be aware of the magnification (that is, the dioptric power scale) or you may become confused by clinically insignificant corneal changes. The color changes in the central pupillary area in the lower right image of Figure 1-2 are clinically insignificant in this essentially spherical central cornea.

In addition to the highly flexible "normalized" scale where the dioptric intervals and colors can be individualized, many systems also generate an absolute scale with preset minimum and maximum values and dioptric steps. Figure 1-3 shows an image in the EyeSys absolute scale, ranging from 35 to 52 D in .5 D steps, effectively producing a 17 D range with 34 intervals. While often not as dramatic in appearance

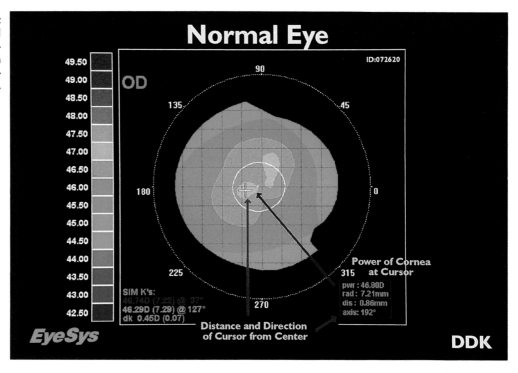

as the normalized scale, the value of an absolute scale is that the same color and pattern always represent a specific dioptric range, eliminating the confusion that may occur if the user fails to pay attention to the color scale. Its value, especially in pathological corneas, will be demonstrated.

NORMAL CORNEAL CURVATURE AND POWER

The normal cornea is aspheric and is typically steepest centrally with progressive flattening towards the periphery (see Figures 1-1 through 1-3). The nasal cornea is often flatter than the temporal cornea. This aspheric curvature is similar to the curvature of the long end of an ellipse. A wide variety of different corneal shape patterns can be seen in some virgin corneas and in great frequency in corneas that have been extrinsically modified. For example, following radial keratotomy, the cornea typically flattens centrally and steepens toward the periphery.

Corneal refractive power is determined by both its anterior and posterior curvatures. The power of the anterior surface of normal corneas is approximately 49 D, and that of the posterior surface is approximately -6 D. Since we can presently measure only the anterior curvature of the cornea, and since clinically we wish to know the true corneal refractive power, a modified value for corneal refractive index is used for calculating corneal power. For most corneal measuring devices the value 1.3375 is used instead of 1.376,

which is the true refractive index (n) of the cornea. For example, for a radius of curvature of 8.00 mm, the actual anterior corneal curvature is 47.00 (using n = 1.376), but from a clinical device we would obtain the value of 42.19 for net corneal power (using n = 1.3375).

Limitations of the Keratometer

For decades, the keratometer was the standard for measuring corneal curvature, and until recently, keratometric data were sufficient for most clinical situations. The keratometer projects a single mire on the cornea, and the separation of two points on the mire is used to determine corneal curvature. The zone measured depends upon corneal curvature; the steeper the cornea, the smaller the zone. For a 36 D cornea, the keratometer measures a 4 mm zone; for a 50 D cornea, the size of this zone is 2.88 mm.

The keratometer has several positive features:
1. Accuracy and reproducibility for measuring regular corneas within the normal range of curvatures (40 to 46 D)
2. Speed
3. Ease of use
4. Low cost
5. Minimal maintenance requirements.

Unfortunately, however, the keratometer has several major inherent limitations:
1. The keratometer measures only a small region of the cornea; central and peripheral regions are ignored.

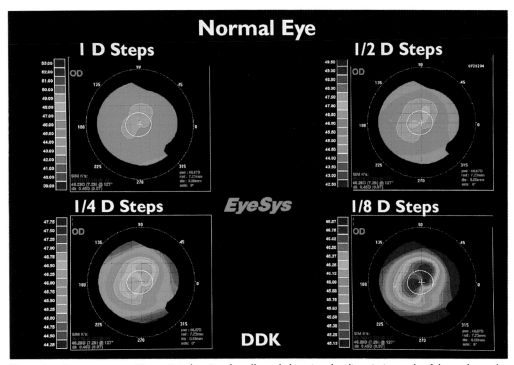

Figure 1-2. Same cornea as Figure 1-1 showing the effect of changing the dioptric intervals of the scale on the appearance of the topographic map. Upper left, 1 D intervals; upper right, ½ D intervals; lower left, ¼ D intervals; lower right, ⅛ D intervals.

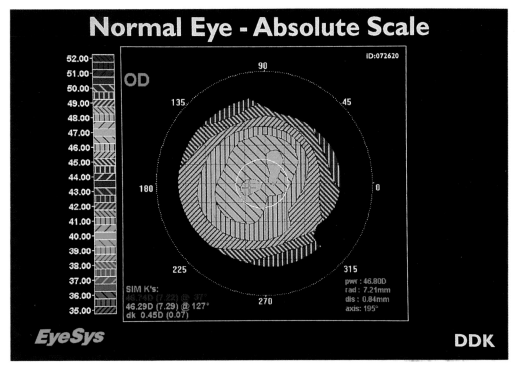

Figure 1-3. Same cornea as Figures 1-1 and 1-2 using the EyeSys absolute scale.

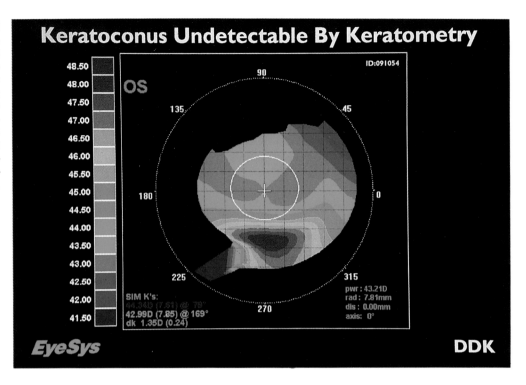

2. The keratometer assumes that the cornea is symmetrical; it therefore averages the two semi-meridians of any given meridian.
3. For corneas of different powers, the keratometer measures different regions.
4. The keratometer loses accuracy when measuring very flat or very steep corneas, particularly those in excess of 50 D.

With these limitations in mind, the keratometer gives a reasonable estimate of central corneal curvature for normal regular corneas. However, many cases with undetected pathology (Figure 1-5) and virgin corneas (i.e., no previous surgery or contact lens wear) are not regular, and corneas that have sustained some form of trauma typically demonstrate some degree of topographical irregularity. As a result, keratometric readings are subject to at least four types of clinically important errors:
1. Inaccurate reading for central corneal curvature (Figure 1-5)
2. Incorrect or misleading dioptric assessment of 3 mm zone
3. Incorrect reading for orientation of steep and flat meridians (Figure 1-6)
4. Omission of critical information regarding the topography of the corneal periphery.

To understand corneal topography, one must be able to evaluate central and peripheral corneal curvature. The central 3 to 5 mm region of the cornea refracts the light that provides central vision; the precise regions of the cornea responsible for this refraction are determined by pupil size and the Stiles-Crawford effect.[1] The corneal periphery also has an important refractive function, since its refraction of off-axis light affects contrast sensitivity and glare, again as a function of pupil size. More importantly, the topography of the corneal periphery is a major determinant of central corneal curvature. With the need for this information in mind, it is apparent that the keratometer has become outmoded as the primary means of evaluating corneal curvature.

QUALITATIVE MEASUREMENT OF CORNEAL TOPOGRAPHY

Several devices have been developed for qualitative measurement of corneal topography. These include the von Loehnan keratoscope (JedMed) (Figure 1-7), the Klein keratoscope (Keeler Instruments), and the Placido image that Rowsey and colleagues provided in their classic article[2] (Figure 1-8). These devices offer the advantages of low cost and rapid use, and they facilitate analysis of large regional differences in corneal curvature, such as high astigmatism following penetrating keratoplasty. However, detection of small but clinically important topographic features and quantitative measurements are not possible.

The CorneaScope (KERA Corporation) provides photographic images of Placido rings projected onto the cornea[2] (Figure 1-9). The introduction of this unit in the early 1980s was an important catalyst in the explosive progress in this field.

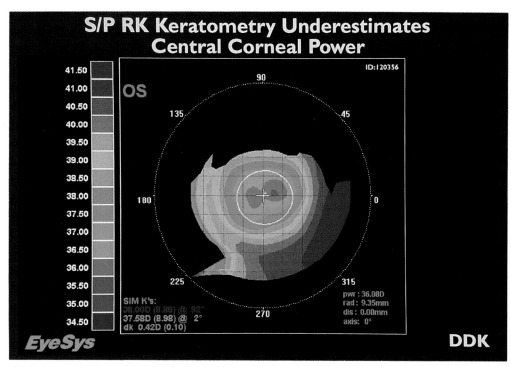

Figure 1-5. Marked central corneal flattening 2 weeks following eight-incision RK. Keratometry was 37/37.5 at 80,° but central corneal power by topography is 36.08 D, consistent with +2.00 D refraction.

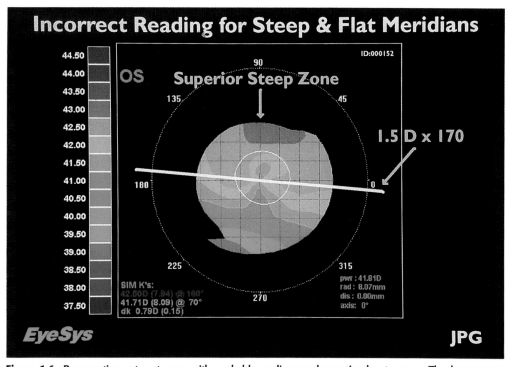

Figure 1-6. Preoperative cataract case with probable undiagnosed superior keratoconus. The keratometer localized the astigmatism axis at 170.° Topography shows the steepest portion of the cornea to be superiorly at 90.°

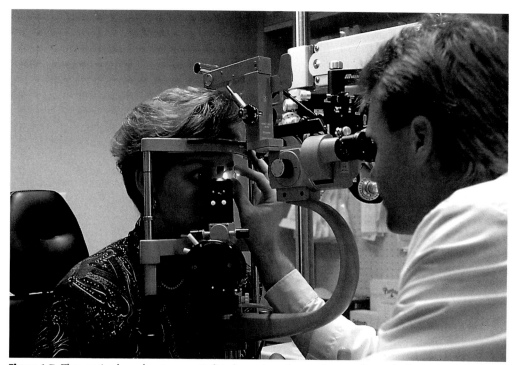

Figure 1-7. The von Loehnan keratoscope (JedMed) consists of a translucent white cylinder with Placido rings lining its inner surface. The device is held close to the patient's cornea and is illuminated by a bright oblique slit beam, thereby projecting the Placido rings onto the cornea.

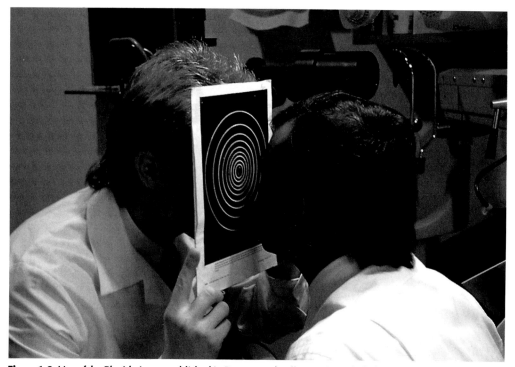

Figure 1-8. Use of the Placido image published in Rowsey and colleagues' article.[2] The spacing of the rings on the curved face plate of the CorneaScope (KERA Corporation) has been preserved by transposition onto a flat plane. A 15 to 20 D lens is taped behind a small hole made in the center of the rings, and the reflected image is used for qualitative keratoscopy.

CorneaScope photographs permit qualitative analysis of corneal topography (Figures 1-10 and 1-11) but quantitative analysis is cumbersome and accuracy is limited to ± 1 to 2 D.

Computerized Videokeratography: The Breakthrough in Corneal Topographic Analysis

The introduction of the Corneal Modeling System ushered in the new era of corneal topographic analysis.[3] This instrument and its successors have completely changed our ability to measure and modify corneal curvature. The remainder of this book is devoted to the burgeoning contributions of these instruments to our understanding of the cornea and vision.

Computerized videokeratographs (CVKs) share certain common features:
1. Some form of light is projected onto the cornea
2. The modification of this light by the cornea is captured by a video camera
3. This information is analyzed by computer software
4. The data are displayed in a variety of formats.

There are numerous ways to measure corneal curvature, and several have been utilized in currently available and prototype devices.

Computerized Videokeratographs: Placido-Based Devices

The prevalent approach in these new devices is the use of Placido disk imaging, which is an extension of the single mire used in the keratometer. This type of imaging has the potential for excellent accuracy and reproducibility.[4] A series of rings is projected onto the cornea, and the reflected images are detected by a video camera. (The virtual image of these reflected rings is located just anterior to the iris.) Curvature data are derived from the measured distances between rings. Standard algorithms for this analysis assume that the cornea is spherical, and small errors are introduced as a result.

Other algorithms for analyzing ring data are now available in some devices. These new algorithms may provide unique advantages in interpreting curvature data in certain clinical and research settings. One of these is based on the instantaneous radius of curvature along a particular meridian and essentially utilizes local changes in curvature to generate topography maps. This type of map can be particularly useful in looking at small changes in curvature at specific points on the cornea. Another new algorithm is based on the posterior focal power of the cornea and is calculated using Snell's law.[5] It therefore incorporates the element of spherical aberration and more likely reflects the true *refractive* power of the cornea. This algorithm is discussed in detail in Chapter 19.

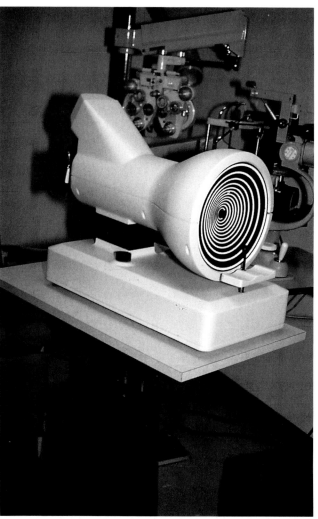

Figure 1-9. The CorneaScope provides Polaroid photographic images of Placido rings projected onto the cornea.

Computerized Videokeratographs: Other Technologies

A variety of other technologies are being utilized in devices that are currently either available or under development. These present new possibilities and limitations in the design of clinically useful devices.

The PAR Corneal Topography System (CTS) (PAR Technology Corporation) uses rasterphotogrammetry, in which a two-dimensional grid pattern is projected onto the cornea and then imaged from a different orientation.[6] This technology is fully described in Chapter 8. Another method, offered by ORBTEK and described fully in Chapter 7, uses slit projection rather than Placido rings. Other technologies under investigation include laser holography and Moiré fringe detection, and undoubtedly new technologies will emerge.

Figure 1-10. CorneaScope photograph of a cornea with against-the-rule astigmatism following cataract surgery. Note the vertically oval shape of the rings.

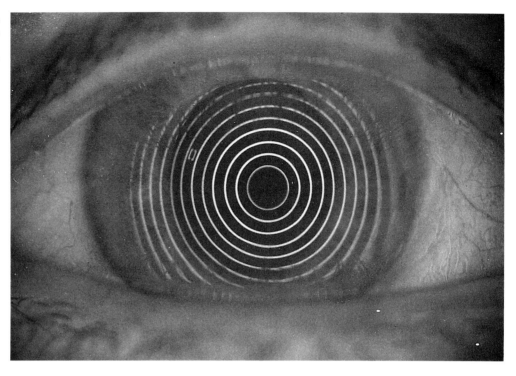

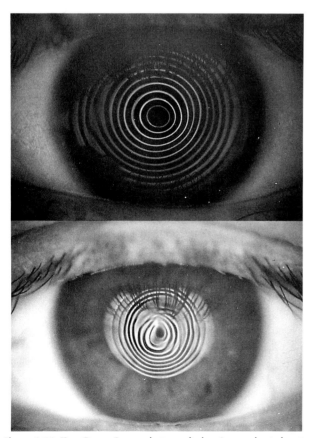

Figure 1-11. Top, CorneaScope photograph showing moderate keratoconus, with inferotemporal steepening. Bottom, CorneaScope photograph of advanced keratoconus, showing marked central steepening (compare ring sizes to those in Figure 1-10) and distortion of the ring pattern.

Applications of Computerized Videokeratography

In subsequent chapters, this book will describe at length various applications of computerized videokeratography in different clinical settings. As our understanding of these devices and the interpretation of their data have advanced, the range of uses has multiplied, particularly in surgical patients. Two fundamental applications have been the elucidation of normal corneal topography, described below, and the detection of corneal topographic abnormalities, discussed in further chapters in this book.

Normal Corneal Topography

Using the Corneal Modeling System, Bogan and colleagues provided the first classification of CVK patterns of normal corneal topography.[7] These patterns are:

1. Round—22.6%
2. Oval—20.8%
3. Symmetric bowtie—17.5% (Figure 1-12)
4. Asymmetric bowtie—32.1% (Figure 1-13)
5. Irregular—7.1% (Figure 1-14).

As the authors point out, this classification represents positions along a spectrum of topographic patterns. Corneas classified as "irregular" undoubtedly include anomalies that have previously not been detected and can only now be evaluated using topographic images (Figure 1-15). Our own experience with the EyeSys device suggests that fewer corneas have round or oval patterns than Bogan reported, which is most likely attributable to hardware and software

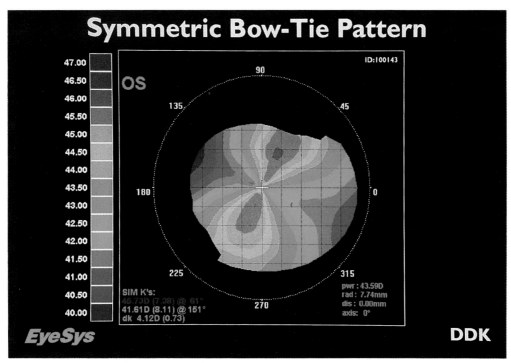

Figure 1-12. Symmetrical bowtie pattern of astigmatism.

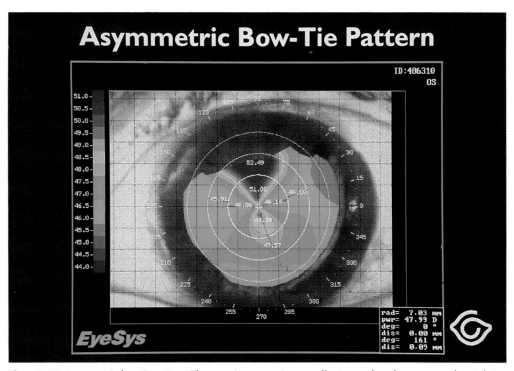

Figure 1-13. Asymmetric bowtie pattern. The superior cornea is generally steeper than the corresponding inferior regions.

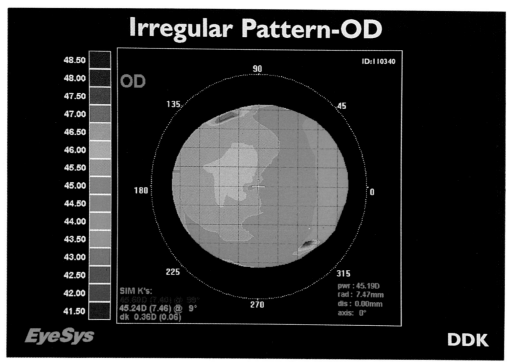

Figure 1-14. Irregular pattern. Note the greater steepness of the temporal cornea. For example, at corresponding points along the horizontal meridian 1.5 mm from the corneal center, corneal curvature is 46 D temporally and 44.6 D nasally.

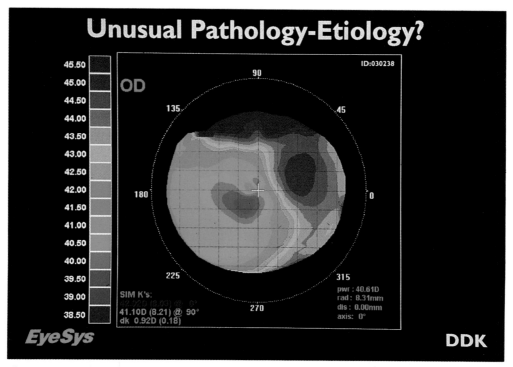

Figure 1-15. Unusual irregular topographic pattern in right eye of a 53-year-old male who presented complaining of blurred vision OD. Refraction 1 year earlier had been +1.00 D OU; new refraction was +4.00 D OD and +1.00 D OS, giving 20/20 OU. Note the large flat zone inferotemporally, extending into the central cornea. The etiology of these refractive changes and topographic findings is unknown.

advances in the newer Placido-based devices. Section III in this book will be dedicated to documenting in a very visual fashion the uses of corneal topography in present clinical practice.

IMAGE ACCURACY

Accuracy of computerized topographic data depends upon proper acquisition of good images. Poor focusing, decentration, and shadows can all adversely affect the image. Many systems employ hardware and software strategies for improving image quality by making acquisition easier and more forgiving of slightly off-axis placement or defocus. Since the human brain is markedly superior to a computer as a pattern recognition system, some systems allow editing of the Placido rings to eliminate anomalies such as artifacts caused by shadows.

Figure 1-16 demonstrates a grossly decentered image. Simply viewing a color map would not expose this problem and could lead to misinterpretation of the image. Even

smaller decentrations can lead to inaccurate color maps. To verify proper centration the user can overlay the color map on the eye image as in Figure 1-16.

Figure 1-17A demonstrates a large artifact caused by a computer detecting the limbus as a ring edge. This artifact can be ignored, or the image retaken. Alternatively, in systems that permit editing, the incorrect ring edge can be eliminated (Figure 1-17B).

SUMMARY

Since the introduction of computer-assisted videokeratography, there has been an explosion of technology to improve accuracy and simplify operation. Likewise, through clinical applications of corneal topography, we now have an improved understanding in a number of ophthalmic fields, from refractive surgery to cataract surgery to corneal pathology. The remainder of this book will document the current state of videokeratographic technology and its clinical application.

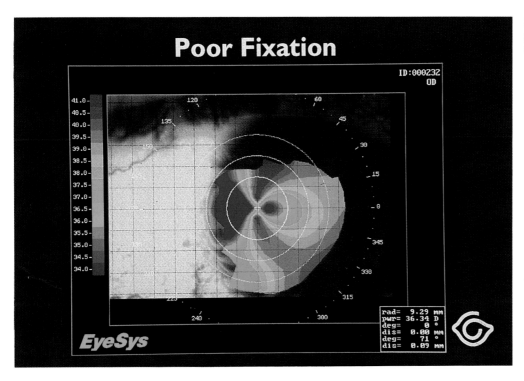

Figure 1-16. Incorrect color map generated from a grossly decentered image.

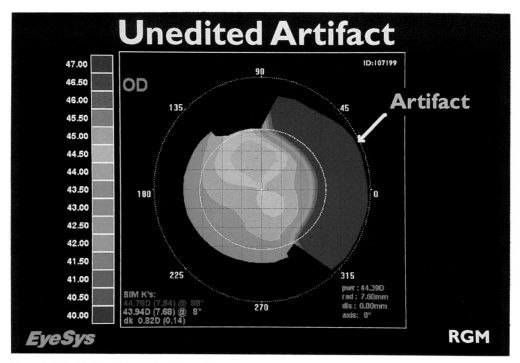

Figure 1-17A. The large blue region is an artifact.

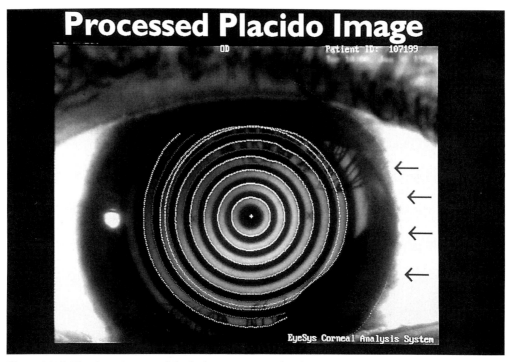

Figure 1-17B. The ring edge around the limbus (arrows) can be eliminated in many systems, correcting the image.

REFERENCES

1. Moon P, Spencer DE. On the Stiles-Crawford effect. *J Optical Society America.* 1944;34:319-329.
2. Rowsey JJ, Reynolds AE, Brown R. Corneal topography. *Arch Ophthalmol.* 1981;99:1093-1100.
3. Gormely DJ, Gersten M, Koplin RS, Lubkin V. Corneal modeling. *Cornea.* 1988;7:30-35.
4. Heit LE, Franco CM, Graham KT, Koch DD. Corneal topographical measurements of spheric, aspheric and bicurved surfaces. *Invest Ophthalmol Vis Sci.* 1992;33/4(suppl):996.
5. Roberts C. The accuracy of "power" maps to display curvature data in corneal topography systems. *Invest Ophthalmol Vis Sci.* 1994;35(9):3525-3532.
6. Koch DD, Wakil JS, Samuelson SW, Haft EA. A comparison of the EyeSys Corneal Modeling System with standard keratometry. *J Cataract Refract Surg.* In press.
7. Wilson SE, Verity SM, Conger DL. Accuracy and precision of the corneal analysis system and the topographic modeling system. *Cornea.* 1992;11:28-35.
8. El Hage SG. Computerized corneal topographer. *Contact Lens Spectrum.* 1989;45-50.
9. Belin MW, Litoff D, Strods SJ, Winn SS, Smith RS. The PAR technology corneal topography system. *Ref & Corn Surg.* 1992;8:88-96.
10. Bogan SJ, Waring GO, Ibrahim O. Classification of normal corneal topography based on computer-assisted videokeratography. *Arch Ophthalmol.* 1990;108:945-949.

ALIGNMENT OF VIDEOKERATOGRAPHS

Robert B. Mandell, OD, PhD
Douglas Horner, OD, PhD

The correct alignment for videokeratography is a critical requirement for high accuracy and precision, although its importance is frequently underestimated in a clinical setting. The ideal corneal alignment position for vision purposes is the point where the line of sight intersects the corneal surface, the corneal sighting center (CSC). The CSC is the corneal surface point about which light rays are centered as they enter the eye, are refracted by the ocular interfaces and ultimately form the foveal image. It is the primary reference point for refractive surgery in that it usually represents the center of the area to be ablated in photorefractive keratectomy, and the center of the area to be spared in radial keratotomy (RK).[1,2]

Unfortunately, in order to simplify their design, present videokeratographs do not align on the CSC,[3] which is usually of little clinical consequence except for special applications. However, a knowledge of the alignment process is necessary in order to properly interpret more complex corneas. Understanding the alignment system requires a knowledge of some basic principles for ocular reference points and lines. These principles are made complex by the fact that the human eye is an imperfect optical system. Both the cornea and crystalline lens have aspherical surfaces of irregular shape that are not radially symmetrical. Unlike a schematic eye, the real eye has no single optical axis and its aperture, the pupil, may change in diameter and position.[4-6] Hence it is necessary to identify reference points and lines that can be located and measured in the real eye without resorting to the theoretical constructs of schematic eyes, which fortunately is possible if the appropriate ocular angles, lines, and points are selected.

The bundle of light rays from the point of fixation that passes through the corneal surface is limited by the real pupil serving as the aperture stop of the eye's optical system (Figure 2-1). The intersection of this light bundle with the corneal surface can be determined by using the concept of the entrance pupil. The entrance pupil is the image of the real pupil formed by the optics in front it, consisting of the anterior chamber and cornea (tears can be ignored because their minimal thickness has negligible effect). When observing a patient's eye we cannot actually see the real pupil but only its virtual image, which fortunately has a predictable relationship to the real pupil in that the diameter and position of the entrance pupil always have a constant ratio to the diameter and position of the real pupil. It is not necessary to know the position or dimensions of the real pupil in order to precisely locate the bundle of light rays entering the eye that actually travel through the eye's optical system. All of the information needed can be determined from only the entrance pupil.

Basic optics dictates that a light ray from a point of fixation that is directed towards a point on the entrance pupil will, after refraction by the cornea and aqueous, pass through the corresponding point on the real pupil and eventually reach the retina (see Figure 2-1). If the light ray from the point of fixation is directed towards the center of the entrance pupil, then it will pass through the center of the real pupil and strike the retina at the foveal position, which in a symmetrical eye system is the chief, or central, ray about which the total ray bundle from the object point is dispersed, and determines the line of sight (see Figure 2-1).[7] It is important to recognize that the line of sight accurately specifies only the straight-line beginning segment of the real light path that is refracted as it passes through the eye to the fovea, but is sufficient to locate where the ray intersects the corneal surface. The actual path of the light ray within the eye is not needed.

The pupillary axis has been defined in several ways but

Figure 2-1. Reference points and lines for the eye. Line of sight intersects the cornea at the CSC, S, and continues to the center of the entrance pupil, E. The exit pupil is ignored. The visual axis passes through the nodal point, which is near to the center of curvature of the cornea, C.

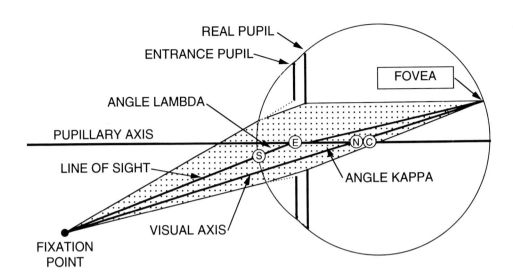

is usually considered to be the line from the center of the real pupil that is perpendicular to the corneal surface (see Figure 2-1). Hence, it must also pass through the center of curvature of the corneal surface and is thus unique. This principle is most easily understood by considering the cornea as a simple sphere (only a small difference occurs for the real cornea of aspherical shape). As with the line of sight, the pupillary axis can be located in a real eye using clinical test methods, as follows. If the clinician holds a penlight in front of his own eye and views the corneal light reflex (first Purkinje image) in a patient's eye, that light reflex will always be on a line from the penlight to the center of curvature of the patient's cornea. The clinician will find that as he moves his eye back and forth there is only one position where the corneal light reflex appears to be centered with respect to the pupil, which locates the pupillary axis (Figure 2-2).

Since the line of sight and the pupillary axis both pass through the center of the entrance pupil, they form an angle which can be accurately measured in a real eye, known as angle lambda (see Figure 2-1). Angle lambda must be distinguished from the more commonly used angle kappa which is defined as the angle between the visual axis and the pupillary (or sometimes optic) axis. In a clinical setting it is angle lambda that is actually measured even though it is commonly called angle kappa, which by definition cannot be located in a real eye. It is important to clearly distinguish the

definitions of these angles because their differences are clinically significant.

VIDEOKERATOGRAPH ALIGNMENT

Regardless of their apparent differences, all currently available videokeratographs utilize the same alignment principle.[8] On the optic axis of the videokeratograph is a luminous fixation point that is surrounded by a series of concentric rings comprising the object target. When the videokeratograph is aligned so that the reflected corneal image of the luminous fixation point is seen in the center of the display monitor, then the videokeratograph optic axis is normal to the cornea (the reflected corneal image of the videokeratograph target rings may be used instead of the fixation point for the same purpose, and the center of the monitor is indicated by various reference patterns). Alignment is accomplished by the operator making transverse movements of the videokeratograph until the image of the fixation point (or the target rings) is centered with respect to a reference pattern on the monitor, which is also coaxial with the videokeratograph optic axis. The patient follows the moving fixation point while the examiner carries out alignment and focusing, which, when achieved, gives a unique solution for the position of the line of sight, the optic axis of the videokeratograph, and its distance from the cornea (Figure 2-3). The reference pattern on the monitor may vary

(EyeSys broken square, Tomey TMS cross within square, Alcon EH-270 not seen and internal, Humphrey MasterVue square) and the focusing systems differ, but the alignment principle is exactly the same.

Currently, videokeratographs are aligned along an axis which is near to, but significantly displaced from, the line of sight.[8] The optic axis of the videokeratograph is aligned perpendicular to the cornea and is thus directed towards the instantaneous center of curvature rather than the center of the entrance pupil, a corneal position that is more peripheral than the CSC (see Figure 2-3). The corneal position intersected by the optic axis of the videokeratograph is sometimes called the vertex normal and has the relationship of being approximately twice the distance from the pupillary axis as the CSC (see Figure 2-3). The term vertex normal is confusing and should be replaced with a term such as the videokeratograph (VK) axis point because the vertex normal has no special relationship to the corneal topography and because the corneal vertex is defined in at least two other ways—the corneal point of maximum height from the pupillary plane or the point of maximum curvature. The VK axis point on the cornea varies in distance from the line of sight for each eye and is determined primarily by angle lambda.

Redirecting the videokeratograph so that its optic axis is aligned on the line of sight could be accomplished by centering the monitor reference pattern with respect to the

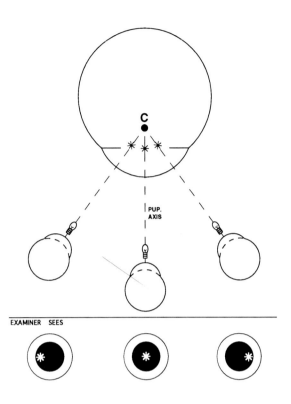

Figure 2-2. Locating the pupillary axis with a penlight below the examiner's eye and being moved with the eye until the light reflex is seen in the center of the pupil.

Figure 2-3. Standard alignment method for all videokeratographs directs the optic axis of the videokeratograph (VK) towards the center of curvature of the cornea, C, and perpendicular to the corneal surface. The center for the ring target image and the corneal map is on the optic axis of the videokeratograph and only coincides with the line of sight and the CSC if angle lambda is zero.

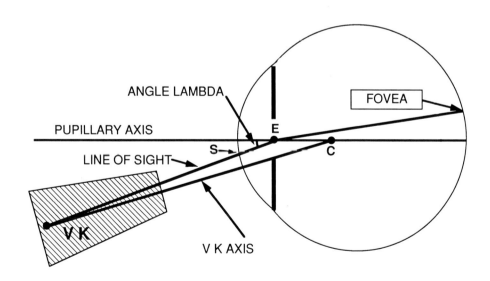

patient's entrance pupil, as viewed in the monitor. Theoretically, this alignment could also be accomplished by utilizing a second fixation point at a different position on the optic axis of the videokeratograph and allowing the patient to self-align the two points by moving his head until the two points are superimposed in the manner of a gunsight. With this adjustment, however, the videokeratograph would not be aligned normal to the cornea, the target image in the monitor would not be centered, and the radius reconstruction algorithm would no longer be valid. The magnitude of this error is yet to be determined. A correct alignment along the line of sight with the videokeratograph normal to the cornea can be accomplished by having the subject view an eccentric fixation point on the videokeratograph target, but the correct position to place the fixation point must be determined for each eye.[3]

The corneal position for which the videokeratograph is aligned is directly related to angle lambda, which can be illustrated by a model eye in which a spherical cornea and circular pupil are centered on the optic axis. If the eye has zero angle lambda, the videokeratograph optic axis would be aligned directly on the line of sight, and the image of the entrance pupil in the monitor display would appear in the center of the target rings. The position of the pupil in the corneal map would also be centered. However, if angle lambda is any value except zero, the image of the pupil in the monitor will be decentered from the target ring. The relationship of the videokeratograph image to the center of the

entrance pupil position is shown diagrammatically in Figure 2-4, with the angles exaggerated for clarity. The line of sight, LE, forms angle lambda with the pupillary axis, PEC. The fixation point, L, lies on the optic axis of the videokeratograph, LA, which is aligned normal to the corneal surface and ensures that the optic axis also passes through the center of curvature of the cornea, C. The apparent lateral displacement of the center of the entrance pupil, E, from the optic axis of the videokeratograph is EA.

The solution for EA can be found from the geometry as:

$$EA = EC \sin \alpha$$

The displacement of the entrance pupil in videokeratography is due primarily to angle lambda and the real pupil position, with only a minor contribution from other corneal parameters. This displacement is determined from the videokeratograph and displayed on the corneal topography map.

MEASUREMENT OF ALIGNMENT ERROR

The videokeratograph provides a convenient and simple means for finding the alignment error, based on the displacement of the pupil image from the optic axis of the videokeratograph when alignment is accomplished. A subprogram detects the outline of the pupil and locates its center. The distance of the pupil center from the optic axis of the videokeratograph is then used in the computer to determine the distance of the CSC from the VK axis.

Figure 2-4. The location of the CSC may be found directly from the videokeratograph, which measures the distance, EA, from the center of the entrance pupil to the optic axis of the video-keratograph.

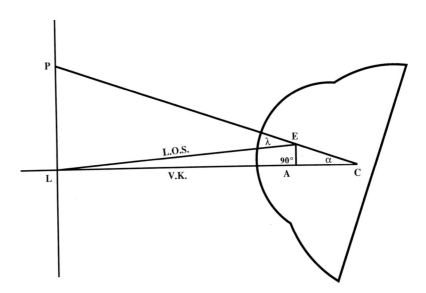

REPEATABILITY OF ALIGNMENT

The ability of the operator to repeat measurements with the videokeratograph and achieve consistent results depends upon minimizing the focusing and alignment errors. The instruments are inherently capable of achieving repeatability of < 0.25 D, but this precision is rarely achieved in practice due to operator error. Many experienced operators are found to minimize the importance of careful focusing and alignment and are unaware of the resulting error. Using a criterion of 95% of replicated readings, it is found that errors of up to 0.50 D occur under the best testing conditions and up to 1.00 D in a clinical situation.

RELATIONSHIP TO CORNEAL APEX

The corneal apex is defined as the point of maximum corneal curvature or shortest radius. If there is no maximum point but rather a central area of constant radius, the apex will be the centroid of that area. The corneal apex is generally located near the geometric center of the cornea but may be decentered a significant distance in any direction. There is no predictable relationship between the apex and the pupillary axis or line of sight and when the videokeratograph is aligned with a cornea its relationship to the apex is unknown.

A misalignment of the videokeratograph with the corneal apex produces asymmetry of the videokeratograph image and may give rise to a false interpretation of the corneal shape. The origin of this artifact can be demonstrated by a model cornea of ellipsoidal shape as shown in Figure 2-5. Figure 2-5A illustrates the ideal but infrequent arrangement in which the videokeratograph is aligned so that its optic axis coincides with the corneal apex. This coincidence would only occur when there is zero angle lambda, so that the CSC falls on the pupillary axis. When angle lambda is any value except zero the CSC is displaced from the pupillary axis so that the videokeratograph is offset laterally from the apex as in Figure 2-5B.

However, at this position the image of the target rings would appear decentered in the monitor, prompting the operator to adjust the alignment to appear as in Figure 2-5C, the most frequent alignment relationship in which the videokeratograph optic axis is normal to the cornea but not directed at the corneal apex. If the corneal apex were located on the pupillary axis, this misalignment of the videokeratograph from the corneal apex would be due to angle lambda. However, since the apex may be located some distance from the pupillary axis, the videokeratograph misalignment is simply due to the apex decentration.

In some normal corneas there is a rather large decentration of the corneal apex from the pupillary axis, which results in a videokeratograph map which has considerable asymmetry. If corneal astigmatism is present, as illustrated in Figure 2-6, the astigmatism will appear to be asymmetric in type and produce the characteristic irregular bowtie pattern in the

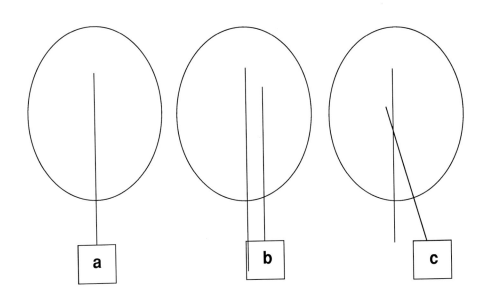

Figure 2-5A,B,C. A misalignment of the videokeratograph with the cornea apex produces asymmetry of the videokeratograph image and may give rise to a false interpretation of the corneal shape.

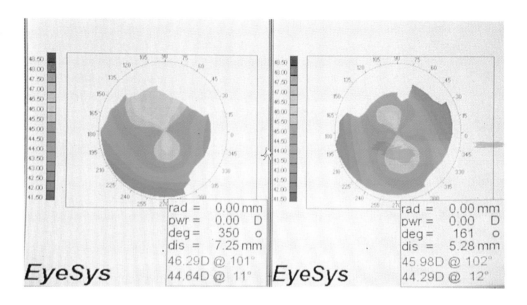

Figure 2-6. Apparent asymmetric astigmatism with regular videokeratograph alignment (left) can usually be transformed to a fairly regular astigmatism by changing fixation (right), which shows that the asymmetric astigmatism is simply the result of an eye in which the regular alignment of the videokeratograph is oblique to the corneal axis of symmetry.

corneal map (Figure 2-6, left). Unfortunately, with a regular videokeratograph alignment there is no way of determining whether the corneal asymmetry is due to a decentered apex or due to a different rate of corneal flattening in the two hemi-meridians of the major axis.

However, the etiology of the asymmetric astigmatism in the corneal map may be clarified if the eye fixation is shifted so that the corneal apex is aligned with the optic axis of the videokeratograph, as shown in Figure 2-6, right. The apparent asymmetric astigmatism has now been transformed to a fairly regular astigmatism, which shows that the asymmetric astigmatism is simply the result of an eye in which the alignment of the videokeratograph is oblique to the corneal axis of symmetry. Hence, an apparent asymmetric astigmatism as judged from the corneal map may occur for either of two reasons:

1. There is an inherent asymmetry of the corneal topography in which there are different rates of corneal flattening in the two hemi-meridians of the major axis.
2. There is an apparent asymmetry of the corneal topography due to a decentration of the optic axis of the videokeratograph from the corneal apex during regular alignment.

RELATION TO REFRACTIVE SURGERY

Of current interest is how the location of the corneal optical zone position in refractive surgery or RK relates to the entrance pupil position in videokeratography.[1,2] In refractive surgery, as in videokeratography, it is the line of sight that should be used as a reference axis for centering the corneal optical zone[8] and not the visual axis, as has been sometimes recommended.[9]

The line of sight corresponds to the center of the bundle of light from an object point in real space that passes into the

eye and forms the retinal image, as was shown in Figure 2-1. This bundle of light in three-dimensional space forms a cone if the pupil is round. If the pupil is oval or has any other shape, the bundle of light will have the same cross-sectional shape as the pupil. It is this bundle of light that is of concern in RK or refractive surgery since its intersection with the cornea defines the corneal area which is involved in forming the retinal image. This corneal area must be avoided in RK and must be included as a minimum in photorefractive surgery.

The alignment system for photorefractive surgery differs from videokeratography in that ideally the patient's fixation point is on the optic axis of one monocular of the microscope which is coaxial with the laser, and it in turn is aligned with the center of the patient's entrance pupil. There is coincidence of the optic axis of the monocular and the patient's line of sight, but the microscope's monocular optic axis is usually not normal to the corneal surface. There is no displacement of the entrance pupil due to alignment. Similarly, when the entrance pupil of a patient is observed directly by the examiner's naked eye, his own line of sight is coincident with the line of sight of the patient but not necessarily normal to the corneal surface. It is only the alignment of the videokeratograph in a normal relationship to the corneal surface that creates the apparent displacement of the entrance pupil.

Because of the arrangement of the videokeratograph alignment system, an ablation area which is centered on the line of sight would appear to be shifted away from the videokeratograph optic axis by the same amount as the center of the entrance pupil. The decentration of the ablation area from the line of sight can be found from the difference in the distances of the ablation area and the entrance pupil center from the videokeratograph optic axis.[10]

In many instances the displacement of the entrance pupil in videokeratography has no practical consequences other than its decentered appearance in the videokeratograph monitor. An understanding of the reason for the entrance pupil displacement should allay the practitioner's fears of a possible misalignment of the system.

REFERENCES

1. Uozato H, Guyton DL. Centering corneal surgical procedures. *Am J Ophthalmol.* 1987;103:264-275.
2. Maloney RK. Corneal topography and optical zone location in photorefractive keratectomy. *J Refract Cor Surgery.* 1190;6:363-371.
3. Mandell RB. The enigma of the corneal contour. *CLAO J.* 1992;18:267-273.
4. Wilson MA, Campbell MCW. Change of pupil centration with change of illumination and pupil size. *Optom & Vis Science.* 1992;69(2):129-136.
5. Charlier JR, Behague M, Buquet C. Shift of the pupil center with pupil constriction. *ARVO Abstracts Invest Ophthalmol Vis Science.* 1994;35(4):1278.
6. Morico A, Carones F, Brancato R, et al. Is there any offset of the center of pupillary entrance after pharmacological induced myosis? *ARVO Abstracts Invest Ophthalmol Vis Science.* 1994;35(4):2018.
7. Fry GA. *Geometrical Optics*, Philadelphia, PA: Chilton; 1969:110.
8. Mandell RB. Apparent pupil displacement in videokeratography. *CLAO J.* 1994;20(2):123-127.
9. Pande M, Hillman JS. Optical zone centration in keratorefractive surgery. *Ophthalmology.* 1993;100:1230-1237.
10. Moreno ML, et al. Effect of decentration of the ablation on contrast sensitivity after excimer photorefractive keratectomy for mild to moderate myopia. *ARVO Abstracts Invest Ophthalmol Vis Science.* 1994;35(4):2141.

CHARACTERIZING ASTIGMATISM: KERATOMETRIC MEASUREMENTS DO NOT ALWAYS ACCURATELY REFLECT CORNEAL TOPOGRAPHY

CHAPTER

3

Donald R. Sanders, MD, PhD
James P. Gills, MD
Robert G. Martin, MD

Until now, corneal astigmatism has routinely been measured by keratometry. Keratometry uses only four data points, each approximately 1.5 mm from the center of the cornea, two on the apparently steepest axis and two on the axis 90° away. Astigmatism is defined as the difference in the two axes in diopters. In many cases, this measurement is adequate.

However, this definition of astigmatism depends on the implicit assumption that the cornea is symmetrical, although not spherical. Unfortunately, many corneas are asymmetrical, and the greater the asymmetry, the greater the potential for keratometric error.

Corneal topography maps the entire surface of the cornea and thus provides an extremely detailed picture of the shape of the cornea. This visual image of the cornea can provide more data than keratometry, and often reveals that keratometry can be misleading.

SYMMETRICAL ASTIGMATISM

Of course, conventional keratometry often describes the shape of the cornea quite accurately. For example, the corneal topography image in Figure 3-1 shows symmetrical, with-the-rule astigmatism in the typical bowtie pattern. Keratometry indicates 2.5 D of astigmatism at axis 90, which is consistent with this image. In another case, keratometry was 1.5 D at axis 180, indicating against-the-rule astigmatism. The topographical image, Figure 3-2, indeed shows against-the-rule astigmatism of the classic bowtie pattern. Another, less typical, pattern of against-the-rule astigmatism is shown in Figure 3-3. Notice that the steepest areas are wedge-shaped. Figure 3-4 shows the topographical images of the right and left eyes of another patient. Note the common finding of nonsuperimposable mirror symmetry (enantiomorphism). In all of the preceding examples of symmetrical astigmatism, keratometry provided an adequate, if not always complete, description of the astigmatism present.

ASYMMETRICAL ASTIGMATISM

However, in cases of asymmetrical astigmatism, corneal topography often yields data that are not apparent from keratometry, even when the keratometry provides a reasonable estimate of the degree of astigmatism. For example,

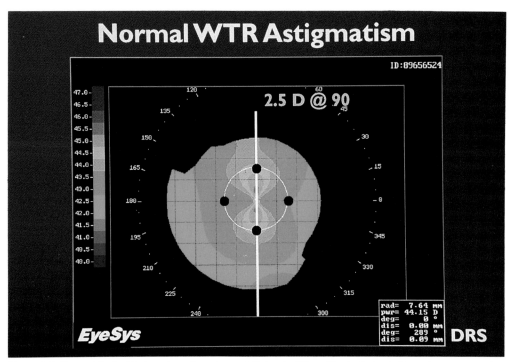

Figure 3-1. Symmetrical with-the-rule astigmatism at 90° (vertical line). Black circles indicate keratometric data points.

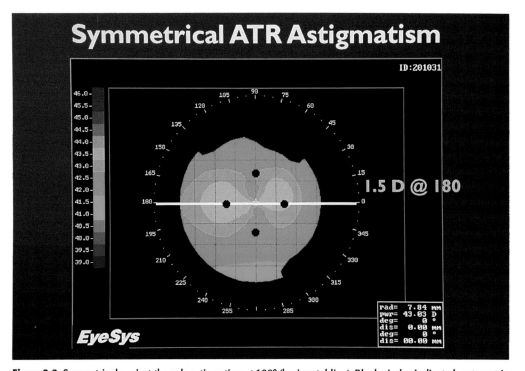

Figure 3-2. Symmetrical against-the-rule astigmatism at 180° (horizontal line). Black circles indicate keratometric data points.

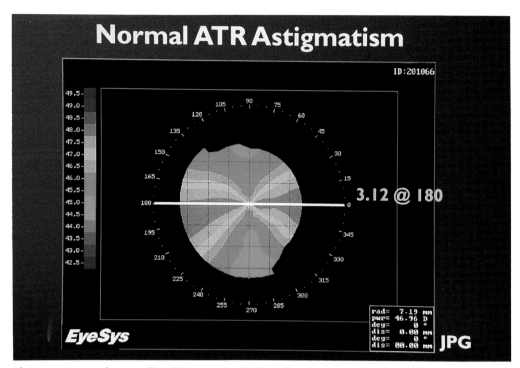

Figure 3-3. Unusual against-the-rule astigmatism with wedge-shaped steep areas. Horizontal line indicates keratometric axis measured at 180.°

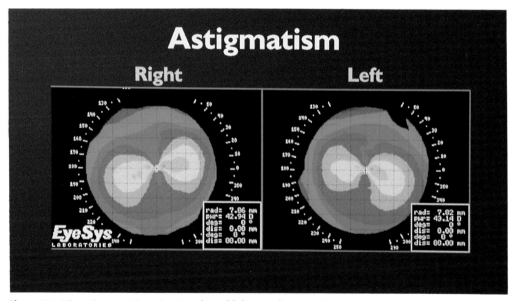

Figure 3-4. Mirror-image astigmatism in right and left eyes of same patient.

Figure 3-5 shows another case of with-the-rule astigmatism. Keratometry indicates 3.5 D of astigmatism at axis 108, but the topographic image reveals more information than just the magnitude and direction of the astigmatism, namely that this cornea is steeper superiorly than inferiorly.

Figure 3-6 demonstrates the same case with some other display options. In the upper left is the color-coded contour map with simulated keratometry values overlaid showing some asymmetrical astigmatism, with greater astigmatism superiorly. In the upper right is the threshold map, demonstrating the astigmatic pattern. The bottom left shows a corneal profile map with the corneal astigmatism asymmetry mapped out. Lower left provides simulated keratometry values at the 3-, 5-, and 7-mm optical zones.

Figure 3-7 demonstrates another asymmetrical cornea. The steep areas are very discrepant in size. For the patient in Figure 3-8, the keratometry reading is 1.62 D at axis 180, but the corneal topography image clearly shows asymmetrical astigmatism with the steepest area at the 340° axis.

MISLEADING KERATOMETRY

Figures 3-9 and 3-10 show corneas in which no true astigmatism can be identified on the topographic images, yet both have non-trivial keratometric astigmatism. Figure 3-9 has keratometric astigmatism of 0.87 D at axis 18. However,

the topographic image clearly shows that the cornea is steep superiorly, with a gradient of 2 D from the top to the bottom of the cornea. Figure 3-10 has keratometric astigmatism of 1.37 D at axis 179. The cornea is in fact steep inferotemporally and flat superonasally, with a gradient of 2.5 D. Clearly the keratometry measurements do not reflect the corneal surface characteristics.

Figure 3-11 illustrates the value of corneal topography in avoiding possibly inappropriate surgery. The keratometric measurements demonstrated 1.5 D of astigmatism at axis 170. Corneal topography reveals a very unusual pattern of superior steepness and inferior flatness. The gradient of 4 D lies approximately 90° away from the keratometric axis. If a surgeon attempted to correct the keratometric astigmatism with relaxing incisions at the 170° axis, which is where the keratometer indicated the astigmatism to be, it would probably prove to be ineffective with this strange astigmatism pattern. In this case, a single or two T-cuts superiorly with none inferiorly has the greatest probability of improving the astigmatism. Incisional refractive surgery should be approached with caution in such a case, however, as this might be an unusual variant of keratoconus. Corneal topography is the only clinically available tool that could have detected this problem.

Figure 3-12 is a preoperative image that was unavailable

Figure 3-5. Asymmetrical with-the-rule astigmatism, steeper superiorly. Line indicates keratometric axis measured at 108.°

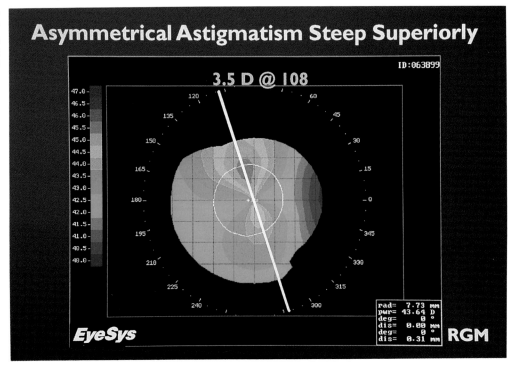

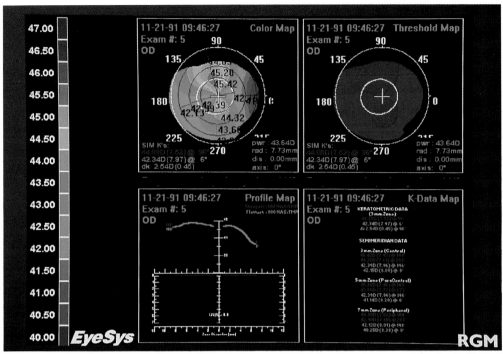

Figure 3-6. Other display options for case shown in Figure 3-5. Top left, contour map; top right, threshold map; bottom left, corneal profile map; bottom right, keratometry at 3-, 5-, and 7-mm optical zones.

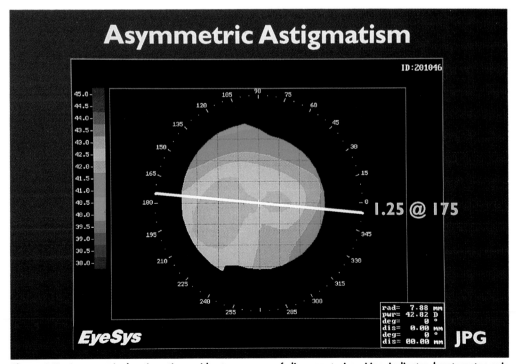

Figure 3-7. Asymmetrical astigmatism with steep areas of discrepant size. Line indicates keratometry axis measured at 175.°

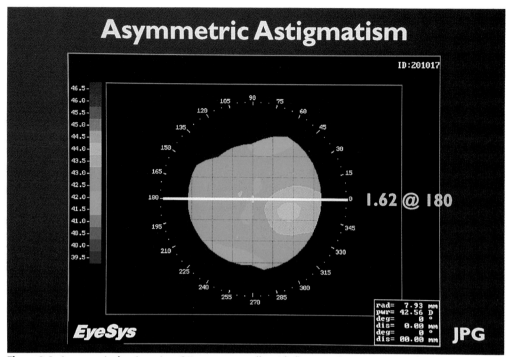

Figure 3-8. Asymmetrical astigmatism OD, steeper nasally with flat central cornea. Line indicates keratometric axis measured at 180.°

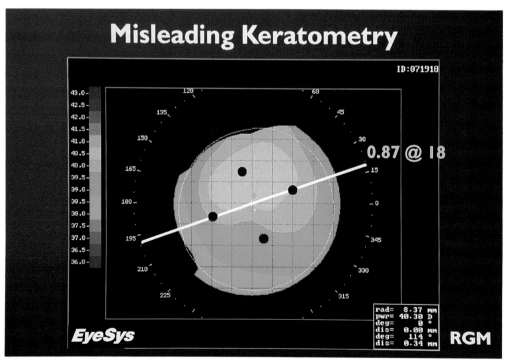

Figure 3-9. Misleading keratometry. The cornea is steep superiorly, with a 2 D gradient from top to bottom. Keratometry indicated astigmatism of 0.87 D at axis 18 (line). Black circles indicate keratometric data points.

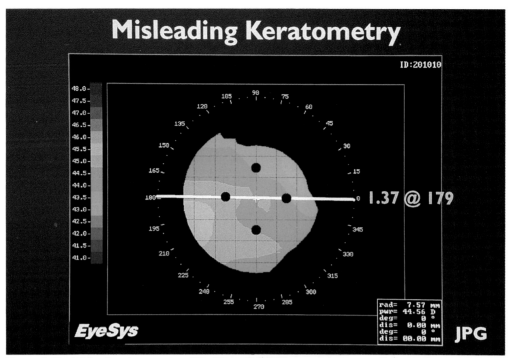

Figure 3-10. Misleading keratometry OD. The cornea is steep inferotemporally and flat superonasally. Keratometry indicates astigmatism of 1.37 D at axis 179 (line). Black circles indicate keratometric data points.

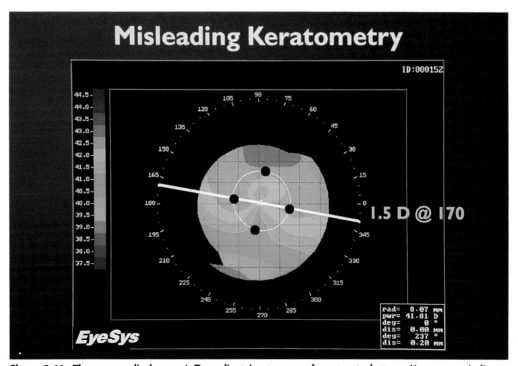

Figure 3-11. The cornea displays a 4 D gradient in steepness from top to bottom. Keratometry indicates astigmatism of 1.5 D at axis 170 (line), 90° away from the steepest gradient on the topographic image. Black circles indicate keratometric data points.

to the surgeon, who placed corneal relaxing incisions at 70,° where keratometry indicated the astigmatic axis to be. Unfortunately, this patient probably had an asymptomatic keratoconus without mires distortion, and corneal relaxing surgery resulted in further corneal distortion and an increase in the keratometric cylinder.

Figure 3-13 demonstrates a cornea in which the astigmatism axes are not orthogonal, a relatively common occurrence post penetrating keratoplasty. Any astigmatism reduction plan would have to be based on corneal topography, as keratometry is incapable of accurately identifying the location of the steep and flat areas.

Figure 3-12. Possible asymptomatic keratoconus in patient who had no mires distortion. Line indicates keratometric axis measured at 70.°

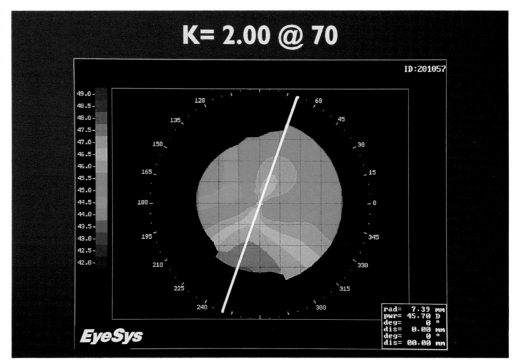

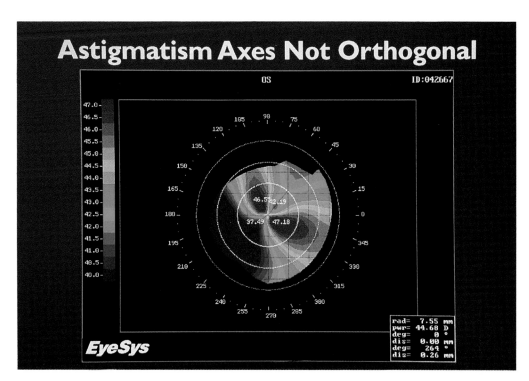

Figure 3-13. A cornea in which the astigmatism axes are not orthogonal. Since keratometry assumes symmetrical astigmatism, it could not characterize the true shape of this cornea. Any astigmatism reduction plan would have to rely on corneal topography to identify the locations of the corneal distortion.

CONCLUSION

The examples presented in this chapter demonstrate the value of corneal topography to the clinician. Many corneas cannot be adequately described by keratometry because of their deviation from symmetry, underscoring the critical importance of topographic data in planning corneal relaxing surgery. These examples may explain much of the variability, and in some cases the ineffectuality or harmful results, of some incisional refractive procedures. The avoidance of ineffective or inappropriate surgery is a major contribution of corneal topography, but certainly not the only one. Research is now underway to explore the potential contribution of corneal topography to the predictability of refractive surgical procedures. In addition, corneal topography can be used to follow the postoperative course of surgery. In some cases, corneal topography may be used to explain apparent discrepancies between keratometric measurements of surgically modified astigmatism and postoperative visual acuity.

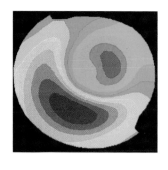 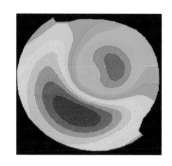 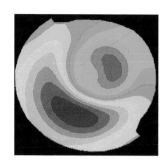 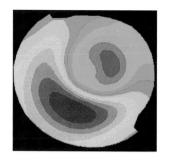

SECTION II

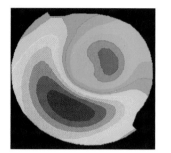 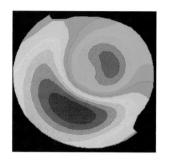

CURRENT TECHNOLOGY

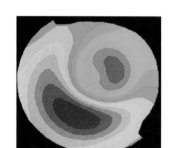 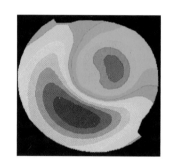

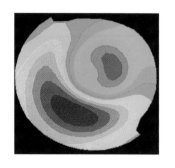 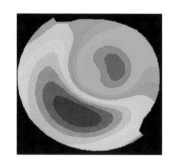 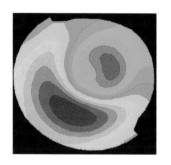 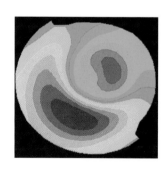

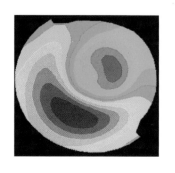 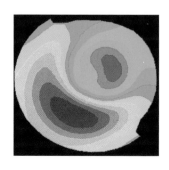 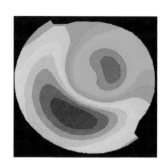 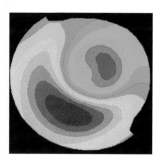

CORNEAL TOPOGRAPHY AS MEASURED BY THE EYEMAP EH-270

Sami G. El Hage, OD, PhD, DSc
James J. Salz, MD
Michael W. Belin, MD
John A. Costin, MD
Michael G. Gressel, MD

The EyeMap EH-270 computerized corneal mapping (Alcon Labs) is an on-line, near real-time corneal topography analyzer. It projects 23 rings onto the cornea. The inner ring has a diameter on the cornea of 0.31 mm and the outer ring has a diameter > 10 mm depending on the shape of the cornea. It is important to note that the number of rings by itself has no real value. What is important is how many of the projected rings are really imaged, and even more importantly, with what accuracy these images are measured (Figure 4-1). Typical measurements are performed on 36° semi-meridians, but up to 360° semi-meridians can be calculated; both options are available. Up to 8280 points are calculated (Figure 4-2) and used to describe the three-dimensional configuration of the cornea. Tabulation formats (Figure 4-3) can be displayed, printed, or stored in memory. An auto-positioning system is incorporated in the corneal topographer to improve repeatability of corneal measurements. The software consists of: a system control program, topographic analysis display system, topographical data, archival and retrieval system, a sophisticated user menu interface, an operating system, an image digitizer, a graphic controller, a pointing device, and diagnostics. Once obtained, the data are fit to a high-order polynomial for each meridian. Then each datum is integrated to determine the three-dimensional configuration of the cornea along each meridian. If desired, this configuration can be compared to a sphere for demonstration purposes. The time of analysis is 2 seconds.

Assessing and describing the accuracy of this corneal topographer presents a set of problems not previously encountered in keratometry. An important one is that the surfaces of the calibrating balls usually used for calibration duty may be manufactured and measured by means less precise than the topographer. Often they are assumed to be as described by their makers.

In the past, irregularities of these surfaces have not been a problem because the instruments that they were intended to calibrate lacked the sensitivity to detect many irregularities or alert the user to inaccuracies. Where the concern was for an approximate average, as is the case in keratometry, relatively small irregularities of the calibrating balls were of little importance. Clinicians tend to compare a new instrument to an old one with which they are familiar, but in the case of this corneal topographer such a comparison might be similar to checking the measurements of a micrometer with a wooden yardstick.

In calibrating the corneal topographer, precision steel and graphite balls are used. Table 4-1 presents three consecutive measurements of a surface specified as 40.50 D, or 8.33 mm of radius. To aid practitioners who are used to thinking of corneal curvature in terms of diopters, the computer scales the measurements to 0.12 D, the value claimed as the accuracy of the instruments. The validity of this claim is only as good as the balls upon which the calibrations were established. Considering the care with which the balls were selected, the claim should be valid. Both diopter and radius scales are presented in most of the graphic displays.

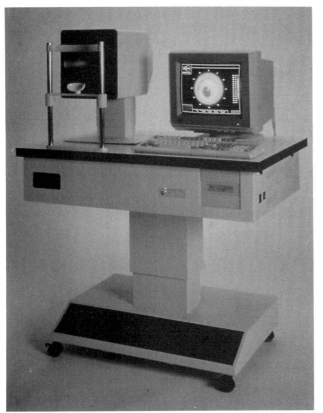

Figure 4-1. The Alcon EyeMap™ EH-270 computerized corneal topographer.

VIDEO DISPLAYS

Several displays are available in the main menu. All displays are color-coded to aid in their interpretation. The color code adopted in this instrument is red for steep curvature and blue for flat curvature. However, the software has the capability to change the color scheme to any desired configuration.

Dioptric Plot

The dioptric plot of the cornea may be obtained from the main menu. The location of the cursor, in terms of distance from the center as well as azimuthal angle, is presented in a box at the bottom of the graph along with the difference the cornea makes with the oscillatory circle at any given location. The color code of the plot can, at a glance, show the practitioner where the steep and flat areas are located on the cornea. For example, in a normal cornea the central portion will be red, the intermediate yellow/green, and the periphery blue (Figure 4-4).

A unique feature of the dioptric plot is the ability to display both the sagittal and tangential radii of curvature. The tangential measurements are more sensitive to change in the shape of the cornea and hence can show better the "elbow" in post-refractive surgery (Figure 4-5).

Figure 4-2. A digitized video-keratograph. Up to 8280 points are calculated on the cornea.

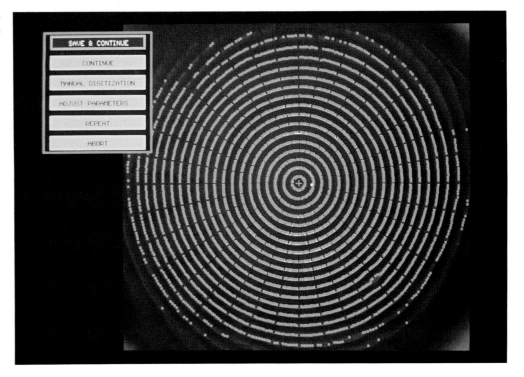

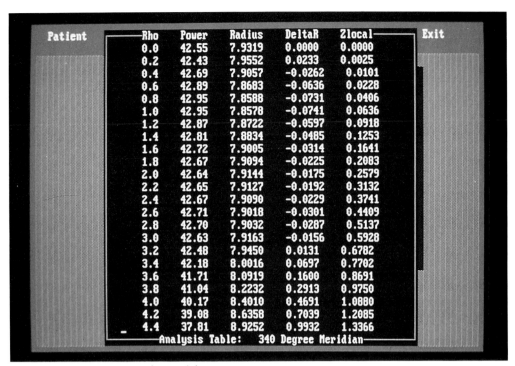

Rho	Power	Radius	DeltaR	Zlocal
0.0	42.55	7.9319	0.0000	0.0000
0.2	42.43	7.9552	0.0233	0.0025
0.4	42.69	7.9057	-0.0262	0.0101
0.6	42.89	7.8683	-0.0636	0.0228
0.8	42.95	7.8588	-0.0731	0.0406
1.0	42.95	7.8578	-0.0741	0.0636
1.2	42.87	7.8722	-0.0597	0.0918
1.4	42.81	7.8834	-0.0485	0.1253
1.6	42.72	7.9005	-0.0314	0.1641
1.8	42.67	7.9094	-0.0225	0.2083
2.0	42.64	7.9144	-0.0175	0.2579
2.2	42.65	7.9127	-0.0192	0.3132
2.4	42.67	7.9090	-0.0229	0.3741
2.6	42.71	7.9018	-0.0301	0.4409
2.8	42.70	7.9032	-0.0287	0.5137
3.0	42.63	7.9163	-0.0156	0.5928
3.2	42.48	7.9450	0.0131	0.6782
3.4	42.18	8.0016	0.0697	0.7702
3.6	41.71	8.0919	0.1600	0.8691
3.8	41.04	8.2232	0.2913	0.9750
4.0	40.17	8.4010	0.4691	1.0880
4.2	39.08	8.6358	0.7039	1.2085
4.4	37.81	8.9252	0.9932	1.3366

Analysis Table: 340 Degree Meridian

Figure 4-3. Tabulation format of corneal data.

Avg.   Radius: 8.338   Power: 40.48   Sigma: 0.034

Axis	Radius	Power	Delta	Axis	Radius	Power	Delta
0	8.33	40.51	0.03	180	8.32	40.58	0.03
10	8.33	40.50	0.04	190	8.31	40.63	0.03
20	8.34	40.48	0.04	200	8.31	40.60	0.03
30	8.35	40.44	0.03	210	8.31	40.59	0.03
40	8.36	40.39	0.04	220	8.32	40.57	0.03
50	8.36	40.35	0.04	230	8.32	40.56	0.02
60	8.37	40.34	0.04	240	8.33	40.54	0.02
70	8.36	40.35	0.03	250	8.34	40.49	0.03
80	8.36	40.37	0.03	260	8.35	40.44	0.03
90	8.35	40.43	0.03	270	8.35	40.44	0.04
100	8.35	40.44	0.03	280	8.35	40.41	0.04
110	8.34	40.47	0.03	290	8.35	40.41	0.03
120	8.34	40.49	0.03	300	8.35	40.41	0.03
130	8.33	40.51	0.03	310	8.35	40.42	0.03
140	8.33	40.51	0.03	320	8.35	40.43	0.03
150	8.33	40.52	0.04	330	8.34	40.47	0.05
160	8.32	40.56	0.04	340	8.34	40.48	0.04
170	8.32	40.57	0.03	350	8.33	40.50	0.04

Table 4-1. Measurements of spherical surface of 8.3 mm in radius.

Figure 4-4. Dioptric plot of a normal cornea.

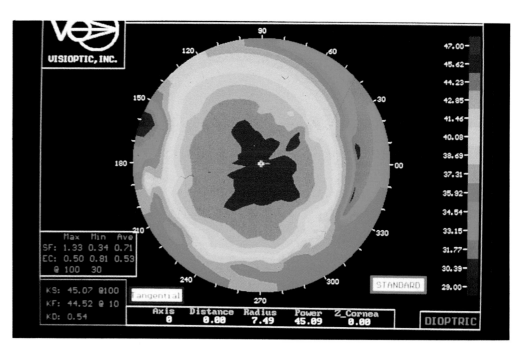

Dioptric Plot with Side-by-Side Image Plot

In this plot, the image and the diopter plot of the cornea are displayed side by side. This feature allows the practitioner to visualize the relationship between the image and the dioptric plot by identifying, for instance, corneal incisions with the color display (Figure 4-6). In this example, the post-radial keratotomy (RK) incisions are visible on the image (eight cuts) and the corresponding color display on the dioptric plot. Perhaps it could also validate the extent of the relationship between the subclinical keratoconus observation on the dioptric plot and the rings' regularity on the image.

Three-Dimensional Display

This plot is specific to the EH-270, because the system of analysis provides the z values. The three-dimensional wire graph of the cornea is displayed for an overview. This graph

Figure 4-5. Dioptric plot of a post-PRK patient. Tangential measurement.

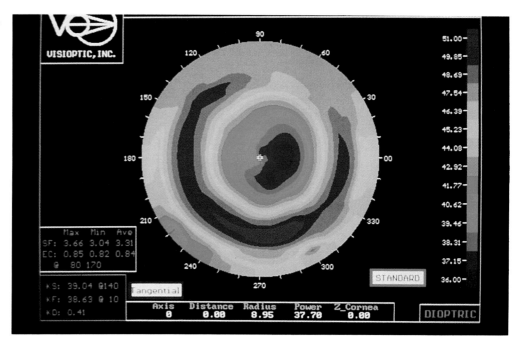

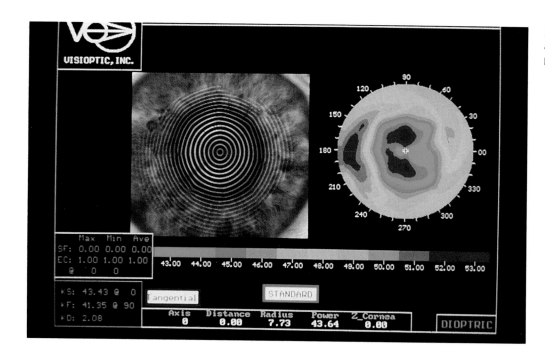

Figure 4-6. Side-by-side image and dioptric plot of a post-RK patient.

can be rotated on the x and y axis in 10° steps, providing a view of the cornea from different angles. Figures 4-7 through 4-9 show the three-dimensional display of a normal cornea, a post-photorefractive keratectomy (PRK) cornea, and a lattice degenerative cornea, respectively.

Contact Lens Fitting Display

This view is one of the first interactive contact lens fitting displays that provided practitioners with reduced diagnostic fitting of rigid gas-permeable contact lenses. No trial set is needed, and the parameters of the contact lens are displayed: base curve, optical zone, power, peripheral curves, and diameter. The displays show, side by side, the dioptric plot on the left and the fluorescein pattern on the right (Figure 4-10). The color-coded scale is shown on the left side and the tear thickness scale on the right side. With a simple keystroke, the user can change any of the contact lens parameters and instantaneously see the changes of the fluorescein pattern and the thickness of the tear film underneath the contact lens, eliminating the trial and error in office sessions. The simulation of the fluorescein pattern is presented on the screen, and, if desired, the three-dimensional fitting of the contact lens can also be displayed on the screen (Figure 4-11).

Comparative Dioptric Plot

Two different comparative dioptric plots are available. The first compares the left and right cornea of the same patient, or a given cornea pre- and postoperatively, or the difference between sagittal and tangential maps in the same cornea (Figure 4-12). The second compares four different

corneas. The comparison could be for a given cornea at four different follow-up visits, or both of the patient's corneas before and after a specific procedure. Moreover, the practitioner can obtain the difference between any given pair of corneas by moving the cursor to a given location on the dioptric plot (Figure 4-13).

Difference Plot

The difference plot is of particular interest. It allows the practitioner to examine the effect of a given procedure on the corneal shape and provides a better understanding of the results of certain refractive surgical procedures. The difference plot displays the difference between a pre- and postoperative procedure of a given cornea. The practitioner can see the difference in the dioptric value and assess the result of the procedure. Again, the unique feature of this topographer can be used in the display, that is, the sagittal versus tangential values (Figure 4-14).

Meridional Contour

This display is a cross-section of the cornea on a particular meridian chosen by the practitioner (Figure 4-15). In this example, the meridian is the axis 0° to 180°. This display provides a profile view of the cornea. The bottom box shows the axis on which the cursor is located, the distance from the center, the radius of curvature in millimeters, the power of the cornea, and the z of the cornea. Also, the difference between the oscillatory circle, the radius of curvature, the power, and the z of the cornea can be shown.

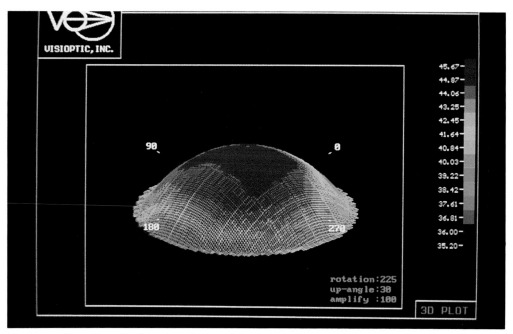

Figure 4-7. Three-dimensional configuration of a normal cornea.

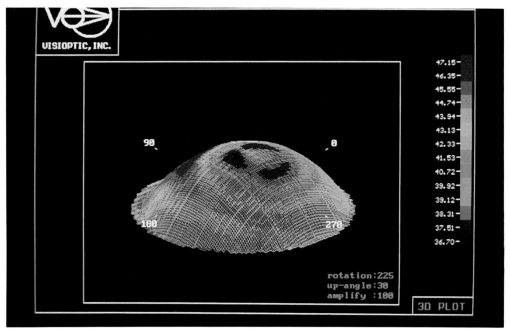

Figure 4-8. Three-dimensional configuration of a post-PRK cornea.

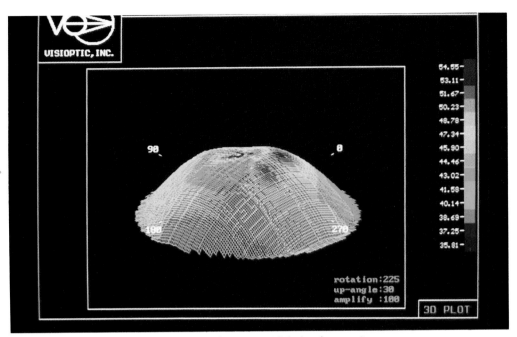

Figure 4-9. Three-dimensional configuration of a cornea with lattice degeneration.

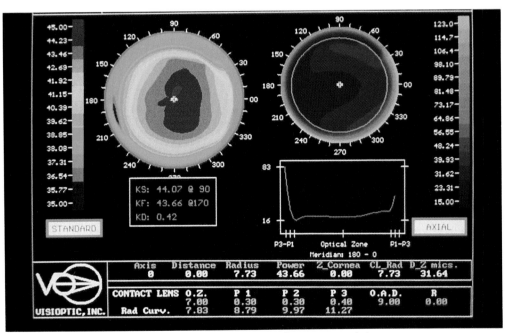

Figure 4-10. Side-by-side dioptric plot and contact lens fitting fluorescein simulation.

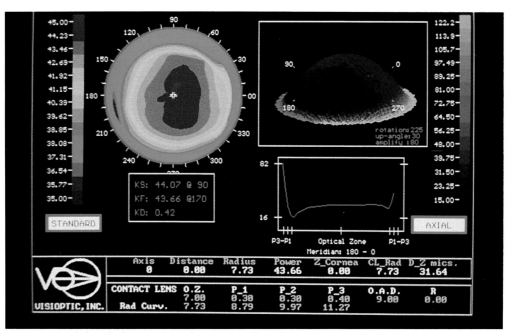

Figure 4-11. Side-by-side dioptric plot and contact lens three-dimensional fitting fluorescein simulation.

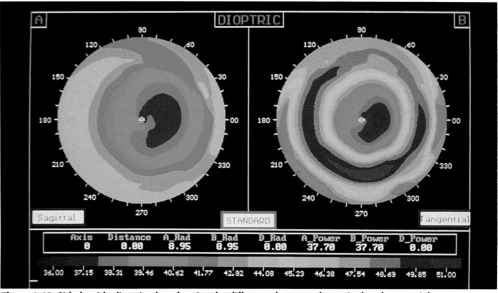

Figure 4-12. Side-by-side dioptric plots showing the difference between the sagittal and tangential measurements for the same cornea.

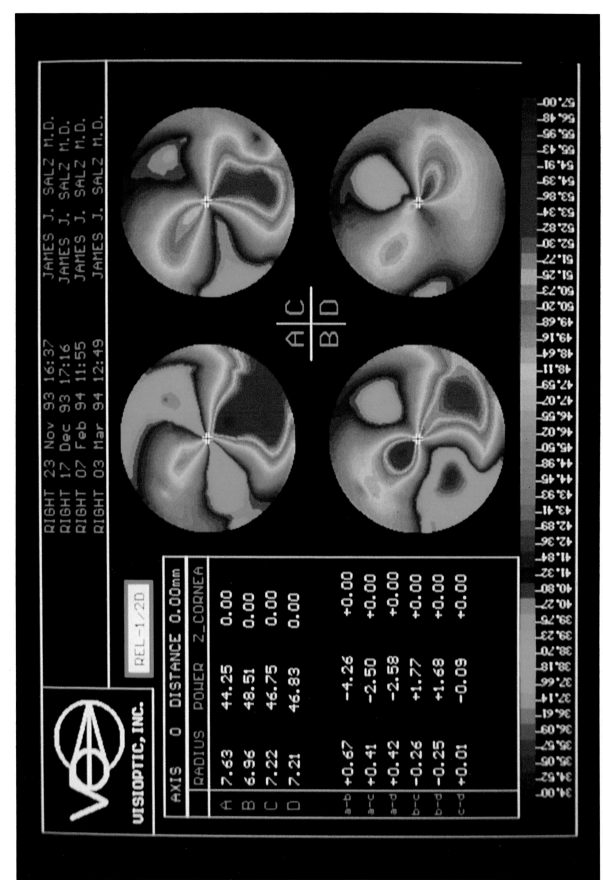

Figure 4-13. Quadruple dioptric plot comparing four different dioptric plots.

CLINICAL APPLICATIONS

Many clinical uses for the EH-270 corneal topographer are suggested by its design and the increase in information it offers over previous devices for measuring the corneal surface. The following list delineates some of the applications now in consideration:

1. Use as a principal guide in a laser technology in refractive surgery
2. Provide the necessary pre- and postoperative corneal measurements needed to improve current refractive and cataract surgery techniques
3. Provide the measurements to guide postoperative manipulation of the cornea to reduce astigmatism
4. Refine IOL calculations to improve accuracy, especially for new multifocal types
5. Provide the information for rapid, accurate, and sophisticated fitting of contact lenses, especially aspheric designs
6. Use as a powerful graphic case presentation to patients.

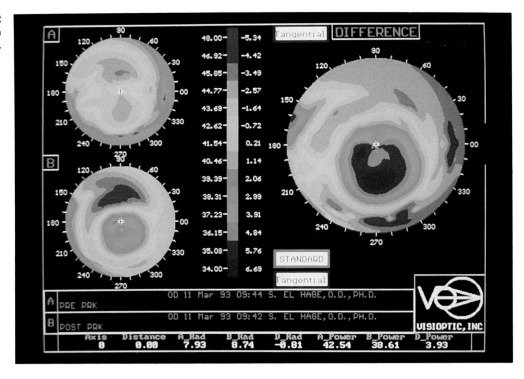

Figure 4-14. Difference plot showing the difference between pre- and postoperative PRK.

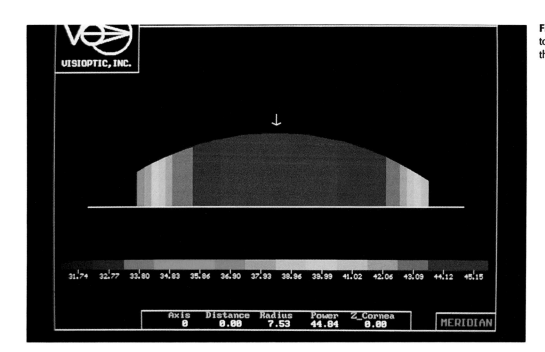

Figure 4-15. Meridional contour showing a cross-section of the cornea at a given meridian.

Case Examples

Figures 4-16 through 4-22 demonstrate corneal topography of corneal pathology, refractive surgery, and excimer laser surgery cases.

MEASUREMENT

Any measurement of corneal topography needs to fulfill the following requirements:

1. No assumption on the shape of the cornea
2. An accurate measurement at the corneal periphery
3. An instantaneous measurement of the total surface of the cornea
4. An image free of most geometrical aberrations
5. An autopositioning for measurement repeatability.

Telecentric Method of Corneal Topography

The important factor in videokeratoscopy resides in the quality of the captured images, the method of analysis of the images, and the required accuracy on the corneal topography. In order to assure an acceptable level of accuracy for the measured cornea, the methods of analyses are designed on a relation between the projected object used and that of the surface of the cornea.[1]

If one uses a series of rings as an object, the radius of curvature of the cornea is calculated from the arrangement and dimensions of the rings and their images. In an optical image, all the rays emitted from a point of the object converge to a conjugated image point.

As the object (optical head), the aspheric conical ring design was selected because it corresponds best to the experimental conditions, and it is easy to empirically verify that this shape can reduce most of the aberrations: spherical aberrations, coma, astigmatism, field curvature, and distortion.

The EH-270 Method of Analysis

In the EH-270 method of corneal analysis, the shape of the surface is dependent on the analysis of several points in a given region of the cornea. The position of these points is determined in reference to a plane tangent to the cornea and perpendicular to the optic axis of the reflected image. That is, any given point is located on this plane by its distance from the optic axis. This point is designated coordinate y in the calculations. The mathematical analysis seeks to determine the distance from the point on this plane to the reflective surface, designated coordinate x. It is the collective values of x along a given meridian of interest that describe the shape of the reflective surface of the cornea. The apex of the cornea is

Figure 4-16. A typical inferior corneal steepening ("form fruste" keratoconus).

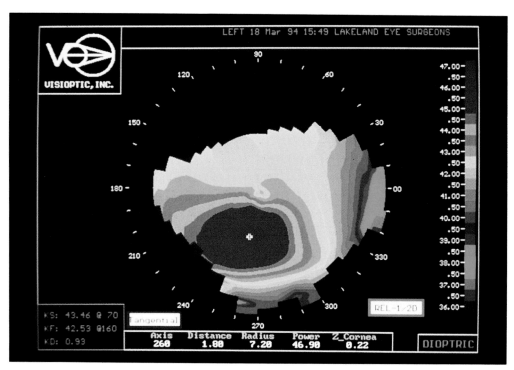

located at x = 0 and y = 0. To compute corneal topography, it is essential to know the exact location of the set of object rings in space. This location is defined for each ring by its distance from the optical axis (called b) and the distance from the ring to a plane perpendicular to the optic axis through the apex (called a).

The points in object space from which the reflective image originates are formed on a cone-shaped target held before the cornea. Precisely placed on this cone are 23 transilluminated rings. The light from each of these rings is diffused in character so that some part of the emitted light will reach the area of interest on the cornea, normal to that point. The distance from these originating points to point 0,0 (value a) is determined by new proprietary sensing devices within the instrument and the computer. The cone is moved by commands from the computer by means of a precision stepping motor, which, through a mechanical arrangement, moves the entire object cone, thus changing the distance between the cone and the eye to a preselected value for a. Also, the cone containing the object point must be centered on the optic axis of the cornea. This position is also monitored by sensing devices within the instrument. The entire optical head of the instrument is mounted on an x,y table driven by a precision stepping motor responding to the commands generated by the computer. When the cone is in

the proper position to satisfy the requirements of value a and is centered on the optic axis, the data are secured, or "grabbed," in a few milliseconds. For this positioning operation to be successful, the computer and mechanical combination must be remarkably fast. The instrument is designed to be insensitive to normal saccadic movements of the eye but can be frustrated by nystagmus. In the event that these automatic systems are ineffective for any reason, an override manual "firing" sequence is provided.

One of the unique optical elements of this instrument is the placement of the aperture. The stop of the objective is not near the principal plane as is usually done, but rather in the back focal plane. The entrance pupil is therefore at infinity, and the chief rays reflected from the cornea are parallel to the optical axis. As it pertains to measurements of the corneal curvature, this arrangement was first presented by El Hage in 1967.

This arrangement has an important consequence. Normally, the aperture stop is placed at the objective, so that the height (y) is not recorded directly, and the angle that the chief ray forms with the optical axis is a factor in the analysis. In this instrument, y is obtained directly on the array of receptors (CCD). One advantage is that a slight error of focus will have a negligible effect on the captured image height.

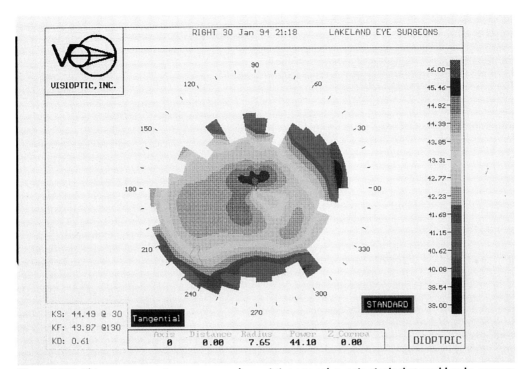

Figure 4-17A. This case represents a very unusual preexisting corneal myopic nipple that would make accurate prediction of postoperative refraction following cataract surgery virtually impossible without corneal topography. Left eye.

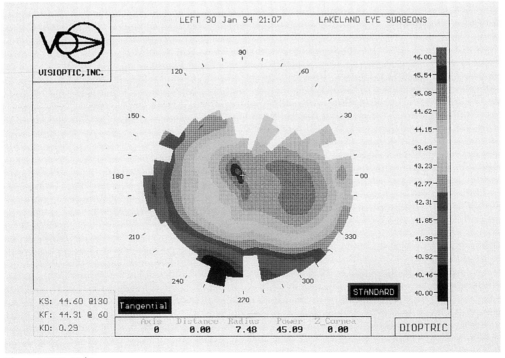

Figure 4-17B. Right eye.

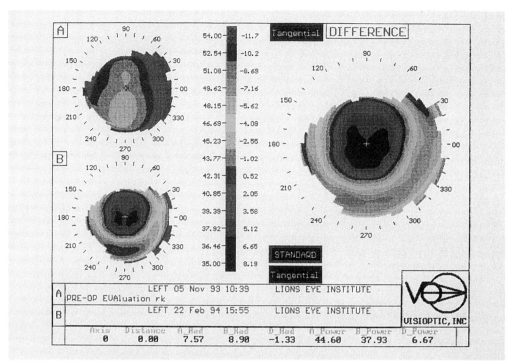

Figure 4-18. Pre- and postoperative RK, suggesting shallow superior incision.

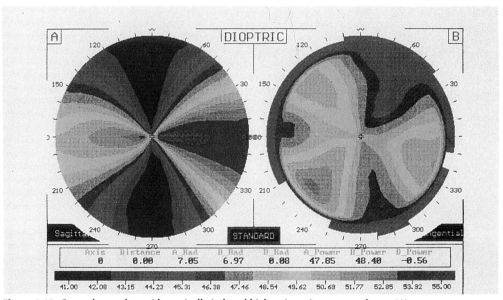

Figure 4-19. Corneal transplant with surgically induced high astigmatism, pre- and post-AK.

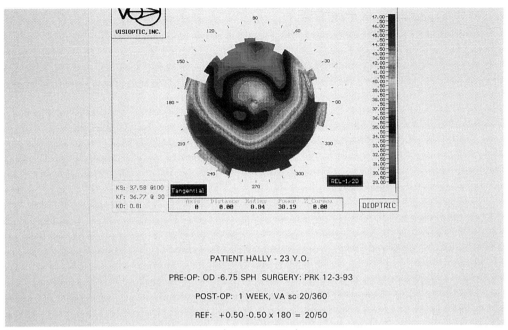

PATIENT HALLY - 23 Y.O.

PRE-OP: OD -6.75 SPH SURGERY: PRK 12-3-93

POST-OP: 1 WEEK, VA sc 20/360

REF: +0.50 -0.50 x 180 = 20/50

Figure 4-20. PRK with central steepening, 5 weeks postoperatively.

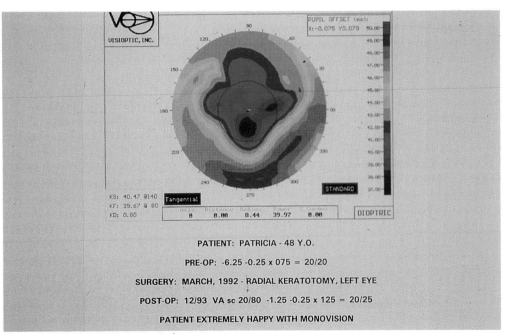

PATIENT: PATRICIA - 48 Y.O.

PRE-OP: -6.25 -0.25 x 075 = 20/20

SURGERY: MARCH, 1992 - RADIAL KERATOTOMY, LEFT EYE

POST-OP: 12/93 VA sc 20/80 -1.25 -0.25 x 125 = 20/25

PATIENT EXTREMELY HAPPY WITH MONOVISION

Figure 4-21. RK 2 years postoperatively.

Figure 4-22. Subclinical kerato-conus, side-by-side dioptric plot with image.

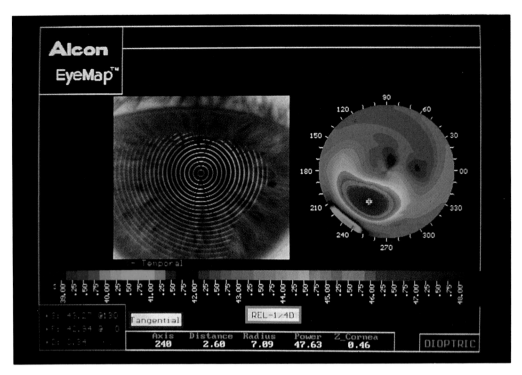

CONCLUSION

The purpose of this corneal topographer is to improve the accuracy and repeatability of corneal surface measurements over a large area of the cornea. With the advancement of computer technology and the use of a computerized, near real-time system, practitioners are able to make more detailed, accurate, comprehensive, and rapid analysis of corneal topography for use in diagnosis, refractive surgery, contact lens fitting, and other procedures.

REFERENCE

1. El Hage S. Recherche de l'équation mathématique de la cornée à partir d'une méthode photokératoscopique. En conférence faite au premier Congrès National d'Optique de Contact, Tours 1968. *Opt Lun.* 1969;192.

THE EYESYS 2000 CORNEAL ANALYSIS SYSTEM

Spencer P. Thornton, MD, FACS
Joseph Wakil, MD, MEE

A s the company with the world's largest installed base of corneal topography systems, as well as the only major company totally dedicated to corneal topography, EyeSys Technologies provides systems that deliver accurate, reproducible results; practical, high-performance features; simplicity and ease of use; and affordability. The EyeSys 2000 Corneal Analysis System—EyeSys' state-of-the-art fourth generation product—combines the proven technology of previous EyeSys products with innovative improvements.

THE EYESYS 2000 CORNEAL ANALYSIS SYSTEM OVERVIEW

The EyeSys System 2000 utilizes a three-camera design to provide automatic focusing and in-office calibration to enhance accuracy and reproducibility (Figure 5-1). The Microsoft Windows-based software system was specifically designed for simplicity and ease of use and allows the operator to create personalized examination paths or protocols to streamline operation. The operator can create custom displays and reports such as the Holladay Diagnostic Summary and the Standard Topographical Analysis for Refractive Surgery (STARS®) Display. In addition, the system will plug into the parallel printer port of IBM compatible personal computers (PCs), allowing clinicians to purchase their own PC hardware ("plug and play" capability).

HIGH PERFORMANCE HARDWARE

Three-Camera Technology with Profile View

A microminiaturized three-camera imaging system design (Figure 5-2A) provides two simultaneous views of the patient's cornea—a frontal view and a temporal view. These multiple views enable the system to precisely locate the patient's cornea in three dimensions, automatically focus the videokeratoscopic image, and then automatically correct the image processing for any images that were not at the point of optimal image focus.

In the three camera design, the front camera is aligned with the center of the acquired ring image to provide the traditional ring mire image for the patient's cornea. The two remaining cameras are positioned on either side of the videokeratoscope to provide a simultaneous side view profile of the patient's cornea. The optical axes of the three cameras intersect at 90° at the point where optimal focus for the system is achieved (Figure 5-2B). In addition to automatic focus and correction capabilities, the side view profile image will allow true corneal profile measurement for the 90° meridian and sagittal height measurement from the corneal apex to limbus.

Optimal Corneal Coverage

Video cameras use grids of discrete sensors called pixels to sense the light reflecting off of objects. The finite number of available pixels in these cameras (512 x 512 pixels) creates a challenge for companies designing corneal topography systems. Ring mires that are too small in diameter are difficult to detect due to the limited pixel resolution. Ring mires that are too closely spaced tend to blur together when reflected off distortions present with keratoconus or post-surgical corneas.

Given these video camera limitations, this system is designed with an optimal corneal coverage and ring mire spacing (Figure 5-3). For normal corneas (42.5 D) the ring mires begin at the 0.5-mm zone (0.25 mm from center) and extend to the 9.6-mm zone (4.8 mm from center). Within this range the system is able to precisely locate 360 data points on each of the 18 ring edges (6480 data points) for accuracy over a wide range of corneal curvatures and pathologies.

Figure 5-1. The EyeSys 2000 Corneal Analysis System combines high performance with ease of use and affordability.

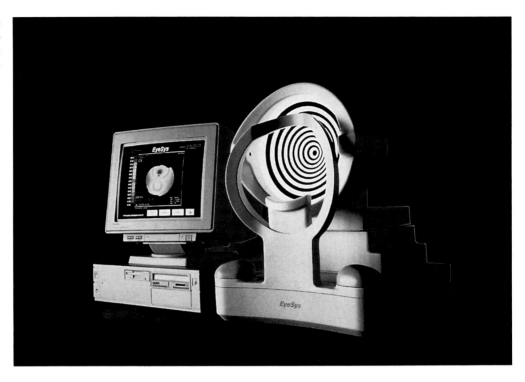

HIGH PERFORMANCE SOFTWARE

Overwhelmed by the wealth of corneal topographic data presentations, clinicians have been asking for a standard means to diagnose corneal pathologies and evaluate postsurgical results. The System 2000 provides a series of comprehensive diagnostic and surgical analysis displays: the Holladay Diagnostic Summary and the STARS display designed by Dr. Daniel Durrie. In addition to standard topographic data report formats, the System 2000 software provides displays such as the Tangential, High Resolution Absolute, Adjustable Normalized, and Difference Map displays. For added flexibility, displays and reports can be customized.

Holladay Diagnostic Summary

Because the cornea provides more than 75% of the eye's refraction, it is critical that clinicians have an accurate description of the cornea's refractive power, shape, and optical quality. Designed in conjunction with Jack T. Holladay, MD, the Holladay Diagnostic Summary is meant to provide a view of these aspects of the cornea (Figure 5-4). Clinical applications of the Holladay Diagnostic Summary are described in Chapter 19.

STARS Display

The STARS display was specifically designed for the refractive surgeon to provide a retrospective view of the cornea to help analyze surgical results and the healing pattern caused by refractive surgery. The STARS display is a five-map display containing a preoperative examination and two postoperative examinations on the top row, and two difference maps on the bottom. The operator selects the preoperative, postoperative, and follow-up examinations and the STARS display calculates the surgical and healing changes, that is, the corneal changes induced by surgery (preoperative to first postoperative) and the changes occurring between the postoperative exams (Figure 5-5).

Preoperative and Postoperative Examinations

A single standard scale used for the preoperative and the two postoperative examinations provides an easy-to-read serial view of the patient's corneal changes.

Surgical Change and Healing Change Maps

The corneal changes from the preoperative examination to the first postoperative examination (surgical change) and from the first postoperative to the second postoperative examination (healing changes) are calculated and displayed as two subtracted difference maps. The scales from the difference maps are centered on the mean difference in central keratometry values for each pair of exams, providing maximum resolution for analyzing the changes. As in all EyeSys displays, a synchronous mouse cursor provides precise point-to-point comparisons of corneal power and curvature.

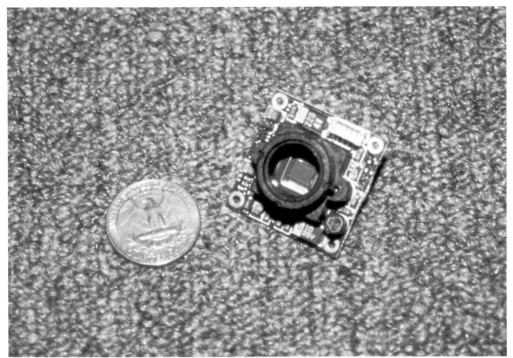

Figure 5-2A. Microminiaturized three-camera imaging system. Each CCD camera is approximately the size of a quarter.

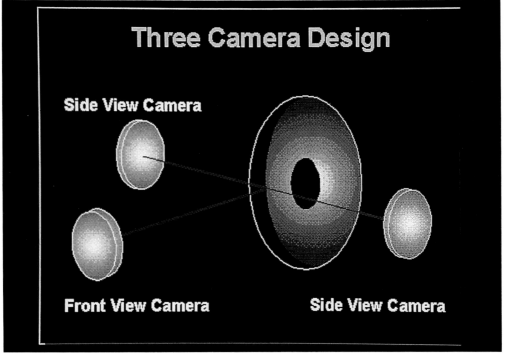

Figure 5-2B. The optical axes of the three cameras intersect at 90° at the point of optimal focus to properly align the imaging system.

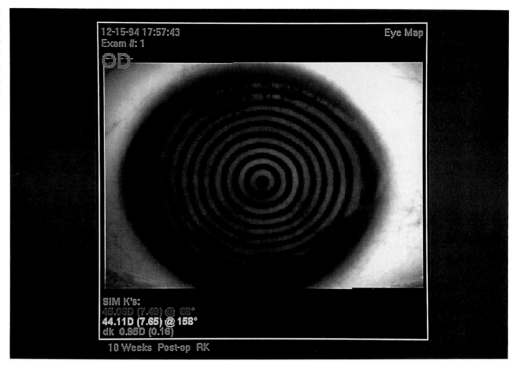

High Resolution Absolute Scale

Since technicians most often perform the patient's topographic examination, clinicians rely on the printed data report in the patient's chart to analyze the topographic changes between examinations. The High Resolution Absolute Scale provides a consistent means for analyzing data across numerous corneas. This scale combines colors and patterns to form a standard color scale ranging from 35 to 52 D in clinically significant 0.5 D increments (Figure 5-6). Using the High Resolution Absolute Scale, the clinician can quickly perform true color-coded diagnoses and comparisons between corneal topography maps.

Adjustable Normalized Scale

Sometimes additional resolution is needed for analyzing topographic data maps of keratoconus or post-surgical patients. EyeSys provides adjustable Normalized Scales for more precise data analysis of the cornea. The Normalized Scale automatically adjusts for each cornea under examination by centering the scale on the mean corneal curvature and adjusting the increments to include the entire range of corneal curvature (Figure 5-7). The Normalized Scale defaults to 0.5, 1.0, or 2.0 D steps depending on the cornea's curvature range. The step size and center value can be easily modified, enabling the user to zoom in on a particular area of curvature for a more precise analysis.

Tangential Color Map

The software provides two measures of the cornea's radius of curvature to allow clinicians to choose the most appropriate color map for the cornea being analyzed. The radius of curvature most often used for representing corneal topography is called the axial or sagittal radius of curvature. This measurement is used for generating the Normalized and High Resolution Absolute Scale color maps. The alternative measurement, the tangential radius of curvature, is depicted in the Tangential Color Map (Figure 5-8).

The axial radius may be thought of as the steel ball equivalent radius because the radius at any corneal point would be equal to that of an equivalent steel ball whose center lies on the videokeratograph axis. Since the equivalent steel ball must always be centered on the axis of the videokeratograph, the axial radius of curvature is axis dependent. The axial radius of curvature works well for the central cornea but an alternative method, the tangential radius of curvature, is required for evaluating the peripheral zone of irregular corneas.

The tangential radius of curvature is not axis dependent since it reads directly as though the videokeratograph was realigned for every point on the cornea, allowing the Tangential Color Map to provide more detail about the true peripheral corneal shape. Using the Tangential Color Map to obtain more detailed information regarding true corneal

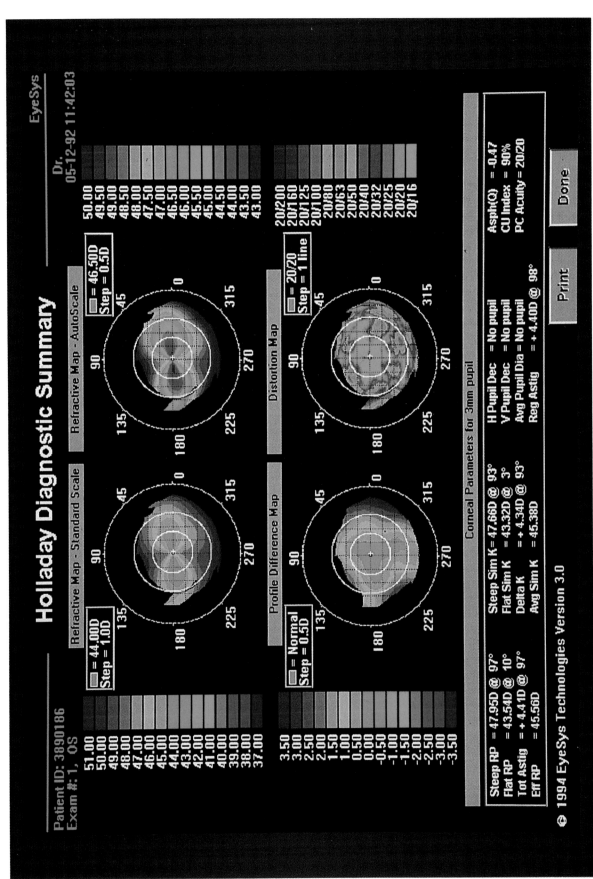

Figure 5-4. RK case displayed using the Holladay Diagnostic Summary.

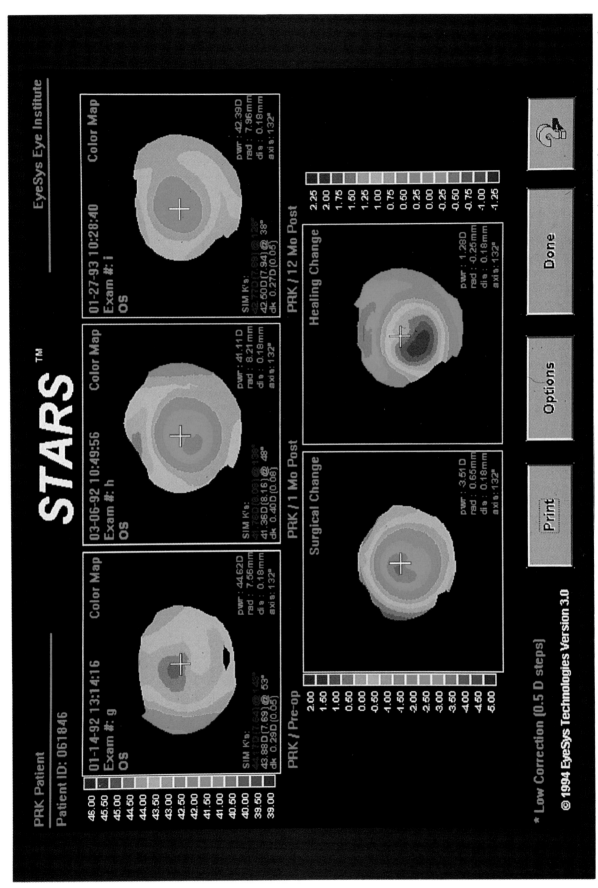

Figure 5-5. STARS display of a PRK case. Top left shows preoperative corneal topography, top middle shows 1-month postoperative appearance, and top right shows 12-month postoperative appearance. The first change map (lower left) demonstrates the surgically induced corneal changes, while the second change map (lower right) demonstrates the corneal changes between the two postoperative exams, in this case indicating regression of surgical effect.

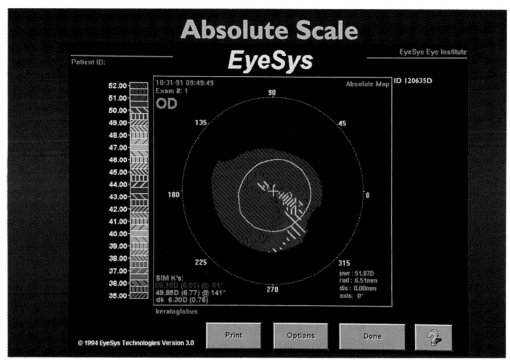

Figure 5-6. The High Resolution Absolute Scale provides simple color-coded diagnosis by employing colors and patterns to form a scale with a clinically significant 0.5 D step size and a 35 to 52 D range. Pathologic corneas, such as this case of keratoglobus, are easily identified. This cornea is entirely outside the normal power range of the scale.

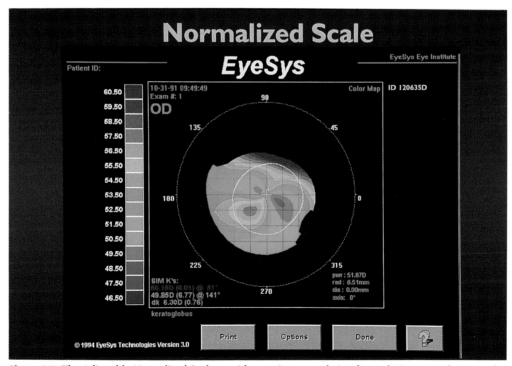

Figure 5-7. The Adjustable Normalized Scale provides maximum resolution for analyzing corneal topography. The center of the scale is set to the mean curvature value of the cornea being analyzed while the step size is automatically adjusted to ensure the entire range of corneal curvature is displayed. Compare this figure with Figure 5-6, which shows the same case in the absolute scale.

Figure 5-8. The Tangential Color Map Display analyzes the cornea using a tangential radius of curvature measurement to provide the more accurate description of corneal shape for irregular or distorted corneas such as this keratoconus patient.

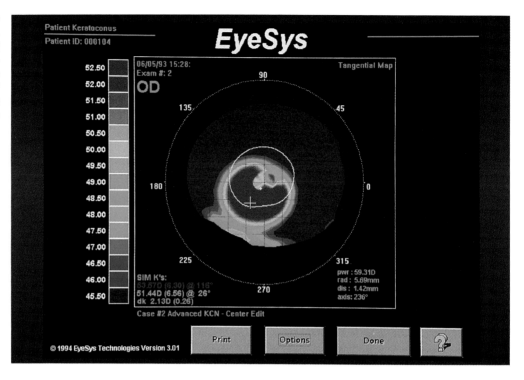

shape is particularly useful when analyzing keratoconus or post-surgical cases (Figures 5-9A and B).

Difference Maps

Clinicians require a means to effectively track changes in corneal topography over time. Single and dual difference maps provide this capability by displaying the serial examinations and a subtracted change map. In this way, changes in pathology and post-surgical cases can be easily documented (Figure 5-10).

Customizable Displays and Reports

Data display screens can be modified while viewing a patient's examination without requiring the operator to memorize keyboard function keys. To modify the screen, the operator selects the display options button from the bottom of the display screen. From the display options screen the operator can easily change the map type, the selected examination, the map layers, or the color scale parameters (Figures 5-11 and 5-12). Customizable displays and reports in conjunction with the personalized examination protocols help to ensure that the clinician receives the desired patient data from each examination.

Multi-Map Comparison Tools

EyeSys allows the operator to perform point-to-point comparisons of corneal topography between serial color maps and difference maps by including a cursor box in the bottom right corner of each map (Figure 5-13). The cursor box contains details about the precise curvature, power, and location of the cursor for each map on the screen.

ACCURACY AND REPRODUCIBILITY

Focus Verification

Focusing and positioning errors are the leading causes of inaccurate corneal topographic data. Previous Corneal Analysis Systems saved an image of optical crosshairs with each eye image. The EyeSys System 2000 allows for permanent focus and corneal apex position verification by saving the side view profile image (Figure 5-14). Because the operator easily verifies and permanently documents the quality of each examination, the quality of a topographic examination is assured.

Precise Ring Edge Detection

Since a single pixel change in ring mire location can equate to a significant change in calculated corneal power, sub-pixel accuracy is critical when locating ring mires. The EyeSys System 2000 utilizes ring edge detection when processing corneal topographic data because the sharp contrast (black/white) of the ring's edge can be located much more precisely than the ring's center. The precision of edge detection ensures greater accuracy when measuring corneal shape (Figure 5-15).

Artifact Detection and Correction

Since computer processing in topography systems is not infallible, EyeSys provides the operator with the capability to edit the processed eye image if necessary (Figure 5-16). In this way, the operator can detect and remove artifacts caused by eyelash shadows or corneal scars to prevent erroneous data from appearing in the corneal power maps. This capability helps to ensure artifact-free corneal topographic data.

Automatic System Calibration

Since in-office calibration is critical to any diagnostic instrument, the system can be calibrated using a set of laboratory manufactured and tested objects ranging in curvature from 37 to 55 D to ensure accuracy over a wide range of patient corneas. A push of a single button will automatically focus, capture, and process several images for each calibration surface while in perfect focus, as well as while too far in and too far out of focus. Using the calibration data obtained from this automatic procedure, sophisticated algorithms compensate image processing for poorly focused patient examinations.

SIMPLICITY AND EASE OF USE

Auto-Focus and Auto-Correction

The system uses the side view image to precisely locate the patient's cornea in three-dimensional space. The operator can easily determine from the display whether the image is too far in or too far out of focus. When satisfied with the image alignment, the operator presses the joystick acquisition button. Within a fraction of a second, the system automatically moves the videokeratoscope into optimal focus and captures the image.

The optimal focus and position may not always be achievable due to involuntary eye movement or severely distorted corneas. For these cases, the automatic correction feature ensures accurate and reproducible data. Using the side view profile image to determine the precise location of the patient's cornea at the instant of image acquisition, the image processing algorithms compensate for focusing errors.

Side-By-Side Patient/Operator Position

Technicians prefer the side-by-side patient operator position to the traditional confrontational configuration because it provides convenient access to their patients as necessary for lifting obscuring eyelids or verifying patient head positioning. In addition to this benefit, the side-by-side configuration allows the system to be placed against a wall, thus occupying a smaller amount of office space and allowing the patient to easily view their topographic color map on the system monitor (Figure 5-17).

Exam Protocols with Auto Save and Print

Clinicians require that patient examinations and the training of new operators be completed as quickly and easily as possible. In response to these needs, the software includes an examination protocol setup feature (Figure 5-18). Each examination protocol can be personalized for the practice, patient pathology, or specific doctor's needs. Once configured, the examination protocol provides a guided tour through the desired sequence of events for a successful exam. Examination tasks such as acquiring the patient's photograph, viewing a specific data display, printing, and saving the examination data can be performed automatically by selecting the desired protocol button.

Patient Identification Photo

Because accuracy is a critical characteristic for medical record databases, the patient identification photograph is an integral part of every patient record. The patient photograph is obtained by inserting a small patient photo adapter into the center of the Placido. This feature helps to ensure that the proper patient record is selected when reviewing and saving topographic examination data.

Microsoft Windows-Based Software

The EyeSys System 2000 software capitalizes on the ease of use of Microsoft Windows while increasing the simplicity of the processes by utilizing examination protocols and large intuitive buttons to reduce required training. The worldwide acceptance of Microsoft Windows ensures compatibility with a variety of computer hardware and software applications.

AFFORDABILITY AND UPGRADABILITY

Peripheral Corneal Topographer Technology

With the EyeSys System 2000, all proprietary image processing and multi-media electronics are located within the Image Acquisition Unit rather than in the computer. The system attaches via the parallel port to any qualified IBM-compatible computer running the software. Clinicians can choose computing power, data storage, and printing options based on the specific needs of their practice. Upgrades and network adaptability are more easily attained since there are no longer any proprietary electronic cards in the computer.

Patient Database Software

A full-featured patient database contains records for all patients examined with the system. To simplify access to the patient data files, the database includes a complete listing of the data storage location of all examinations, including data stored off-line.

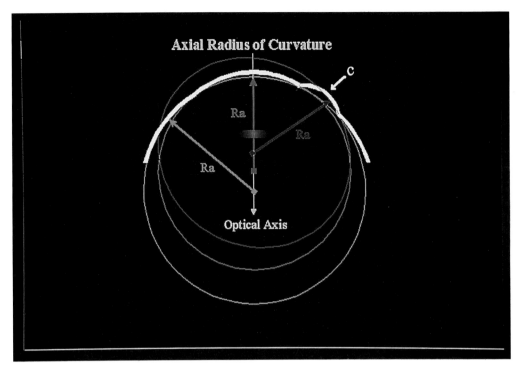

Figure 5-9A. The difference between tangential and axial radius of curvature can be more easily demonstrated in cases of asymmetric steepening such as keratoconus.

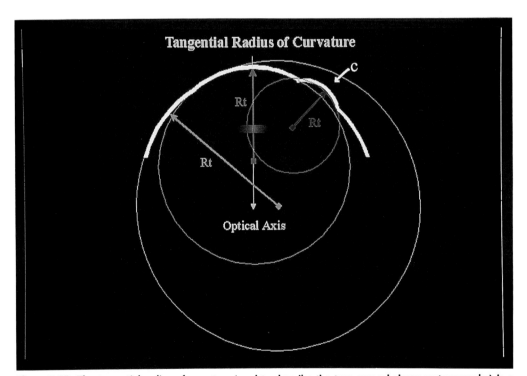

Figure 5-9B. The tangential radius of curvature (used to describe the true corneal shape or topography) is a measurement of the radius of curvature (Rt) of any point on the cornea with respect to that point, which is graphically represented by fitting the cornea with a series of best fit spheres to local shape characteristics without restricting their center locations as shown in this simulated keratoconic cornea (cone = c).

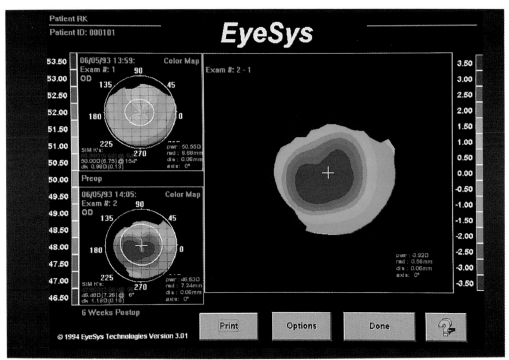

Figure 5-10. Difference maps enable clinicians to easily evaluate changes induced with corneal surgery. This display shows the pre- and postoperative RK surgery examinations for a patient demonstrating 4 D of flattening at 6 weeks.

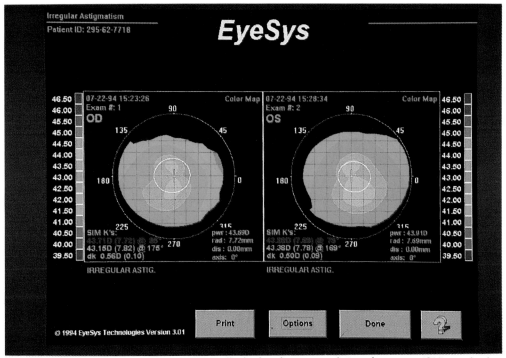

Figure 5-11. The Two Map Display is automatically displayed upon completion of a two eye (OU) examination.

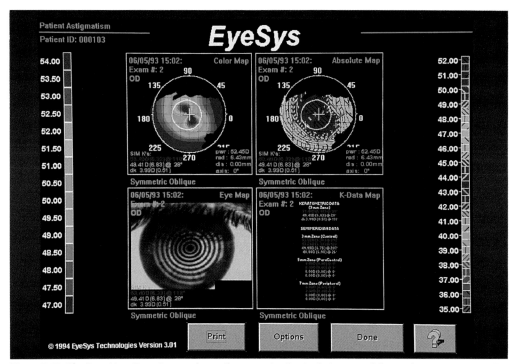

Figure 5-12. The Four Map Overview can be easily customized to include many different data report types. This overview includes a normalized color map, an absolute scale map, an eye image, and semi-meridian keratometric data for a cornea with symmetric oblique astigmatism.

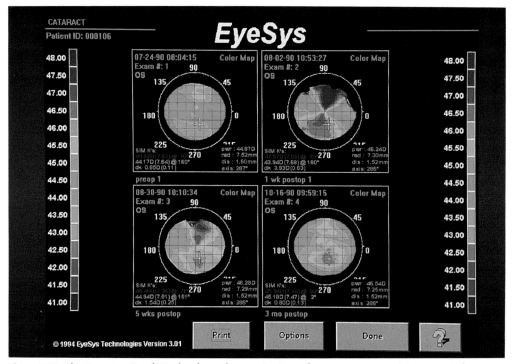

Figure 5-13. This Four Map Trend Display shows the examinations of a cataract case receiving one-stitch surgery. A too-tight suture caused corneal steepening, resulting in some postoperative asymmetric astigmatism, which can be documented by reading the multi-map cursor values.

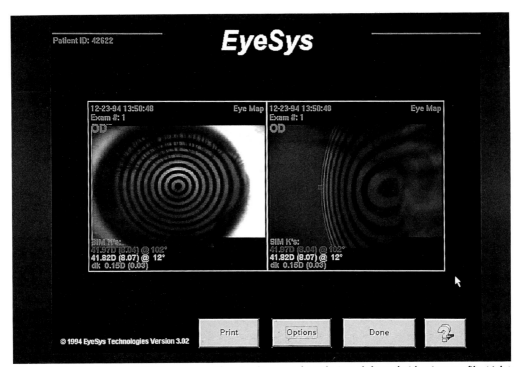

Figure 5-14. The EyeSys 2000 System provides simultaneous frontal view (left) and side view profile (right) images. The red dot on the profile image marks the location of the corneal apex. The Side View Profile Image provides clinicians with a permanent record of image alignment and focus, as well as valuable information about the corneal apex and 90° meridian.

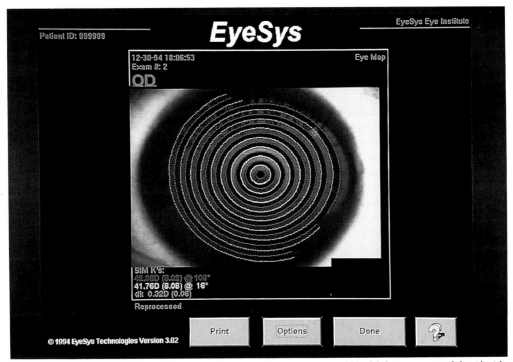

Figure 5-15. The EyeSys System 2000 precisely locates the sharp edges of black/white contrast of the Placido mires reflected off the cornea.

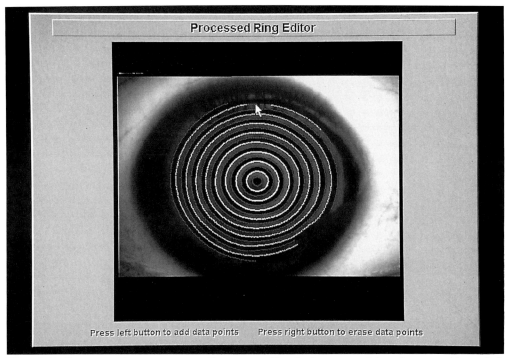

Figure 5-16. If necessary, the operator can easily remove artifacts in the processed ring edges caused by eyelash shadows or corneal scars. Arrow points to area where data points were added.

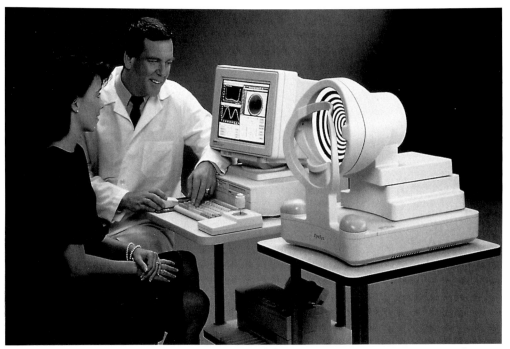

Figure 5-17. The convenient side-by-side configuration of the EyeSys System 2000 improves patient/operator interaction.

Patient Selection

A complete database of patient corneal topographic data is only useful if it can be easily accessed. A "zoom" function aids the user in finding individual patient data. As the operator enters the patient's name or ID, the software instantly displays the closest match in the database.

Patient Photo Identification

To ensure that the selected patient file belongs to the desired patient, the software displays the patient identification photograph in the upper right corner of the patient locator screen (Figure 5-19).

Database Backup

Because physical degradation of internal storage devices can occur, a quick and effective method for backing up the patient database index files for each patient in the database is included, enabling a quick recovery of the index information if damage should ever occur to the internal hard drive.

Export/Import Conversion Capabilities

With the changing health care environment, managed care and co-management of patients is becoming more frequent today. A convenient import and export capability for patient data files provide a means for EyeSys users to share patient records with other offices or surgical centers.

CONTACT LENS FITTING SOFTWARE

In addition to providing valuable clinical information for diagnoses, surgical planning, and documentation, topography systems can be a valuable tool for designing contact lenses because of the precise detail with which they can describe corneal shape.

The System 2000 has a comprehensive contact lens fitting and analysis program. Soft lenses and soft torics can be selected and RGP lenses can be quickly designed specifically for the patient's cornea. The EyeSys Corneal Analysis System software's interactive fluorescein simulation depicts how the RGP lens design will fit on the patient's cornea. Contact lenses can then be selected and ordered utilizing a comprehensive Tyler's Quarterly database.

Fitting Protocols

Since contact lens fitting is not an exact science, the software allows fitters to develop their own individual fitting preferences and lens type screening criterion (Figures 5-20 and 5-21). The clinician can establish customized fitting preferences such as plus or minus cylinder notation, cylinder limits for soft and RGP torics, and sagittal tear film thickness for desired RGP apical clearance. A simulated fluorescein

pattern depicts how the custom RGP lens will appear on a typical patient cornea.

Lens Categories

The software provides both soft and RGP lens fitting. Based on the cylinder limits established in the personalized fitting protocols, the patient's refraction, and the patient's corneal topography, the Contact Lens Fitting Software will recommend either soft, soft toric, RGP, or RGP toric lenses.

Simulated Fluorescein

Complete simulated fluorescein analysis can be performed for RGP and RGP toric lenses. The software also provides an interactive analysis with both automatic or manual lens tilt and manual lens positioning (Figure 5-22). The design parameters of the suggested contact lens can be easily modified while viewing the changes induced in the simulated fluorescein display.

Trial Lens Fitting

Trial lens fitting results can easily be entered to further refine the suggested lens design. These parameters include overrefraction and lens specifications. Trial fitting evaluation of soft torics can be performed using the manufacturer's trial lens set or after the actual lens has been dispensed to the patient. If using the manufacturer's trial lens set, the amount of lens rotation and orientation of the lens scribe mark can be entered to further refine the calculated cylinder axis (Figure 5-23).

Complete Tyler's Quarterly Database

To simplify the ordering process, the entire Tyler's Quarterly database is integrated into the software (Figure 5-24). Lenses can be selected by lens brand name or manufacturer. The contact lens fitter can select the base curve, lens diameter, and lens color from a list of available lenses. In addition to extensive information on manufacturer and lens brand, a manufacturer's fitting guide is also included.

Ordering

The software will automatically include the manufacturer's name and phone number in the order form if the fitter so desires. The contact lens fitter can customize the order form by simply entering the phone and fax numbers for a specific contact lens lab or distributor. The form can then be printed or faxed directly to the manufacturer, distributor, or lab for processing (Figure 5-25).

REFRACTIVE NOMOGRAM SOFTWARE

The EyeSys RK Planner Series is a set of advanced computer programs which automate the process of planning

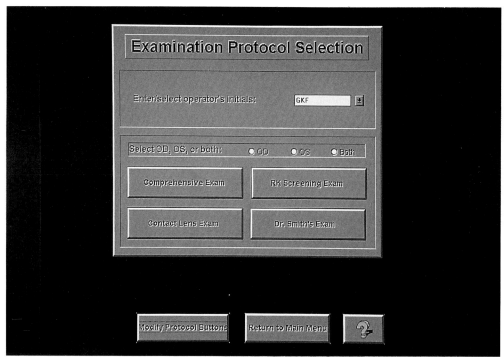

Figure 5-18. Customizable examination protocols ensure that the desired reports are created for each patient.

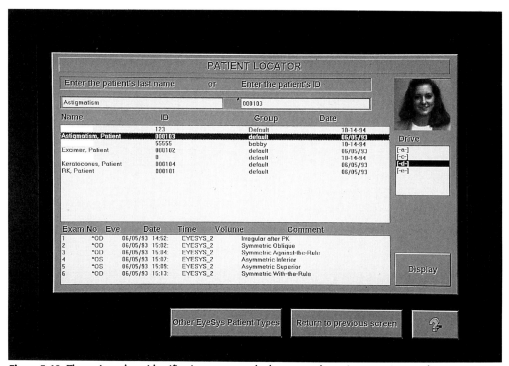

Figure 5-19. The patient photo identification permanently documents the patient examination data.

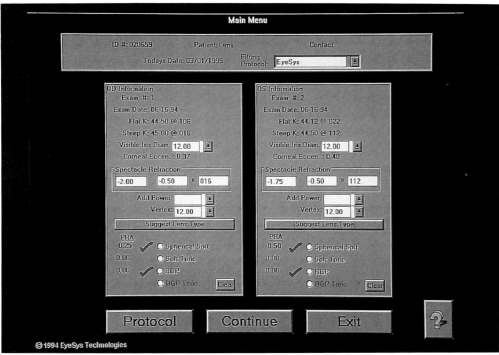

Figure 5-20. Contact lens fitting main menu.

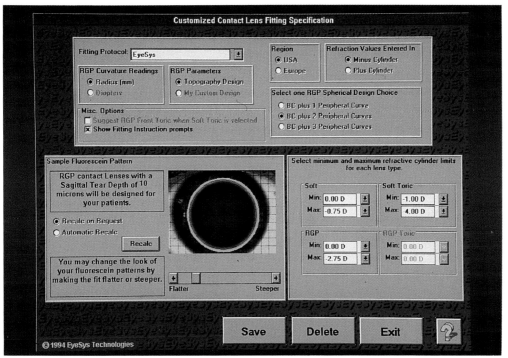

Figure 5-21. Contact lens fitting protocol screen.

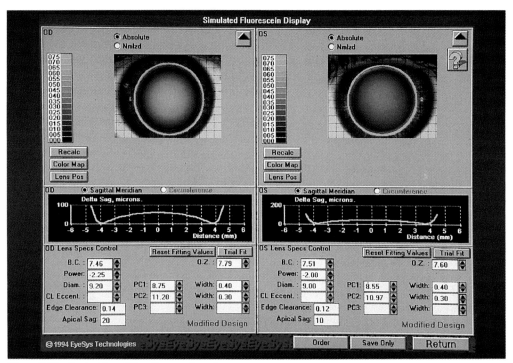

Figure 5-22. Contact lens fitting fluorescein pattern screen.

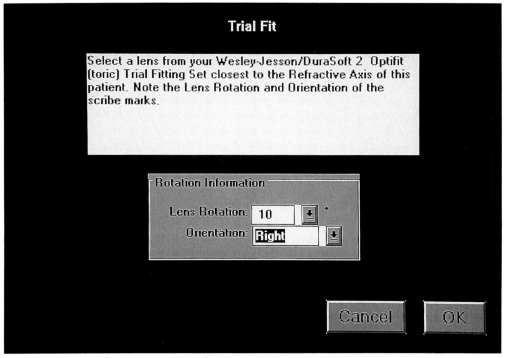

Figure 5-23. Trial lens fitting parameter entry form.

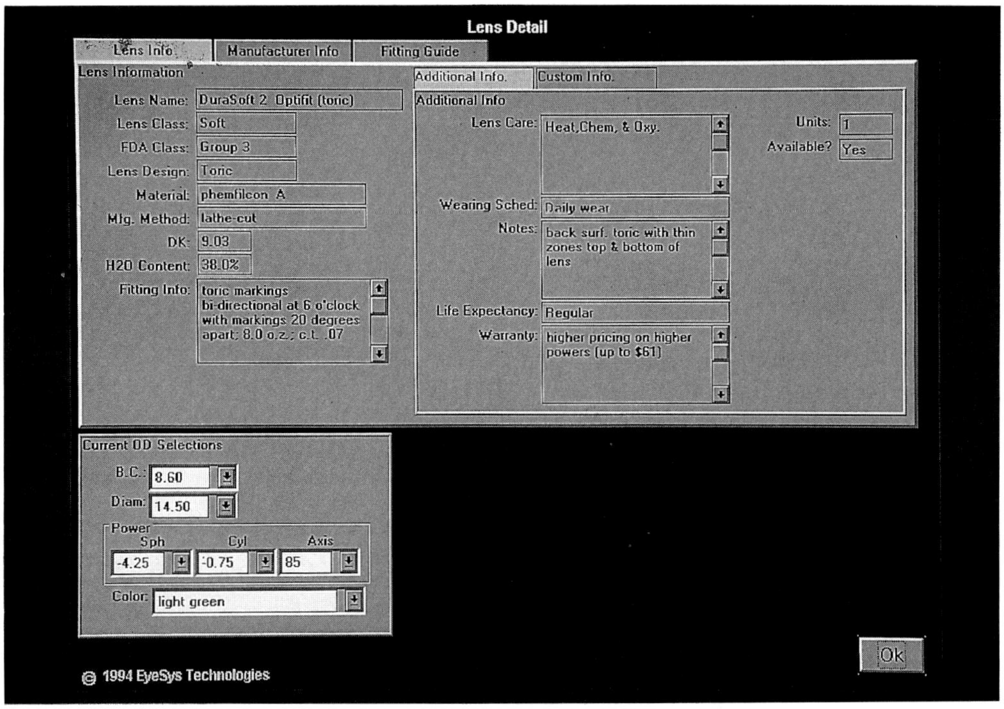

Figure 5-24. Contact lens fitting screen showing Tyler's Quarterly database information.

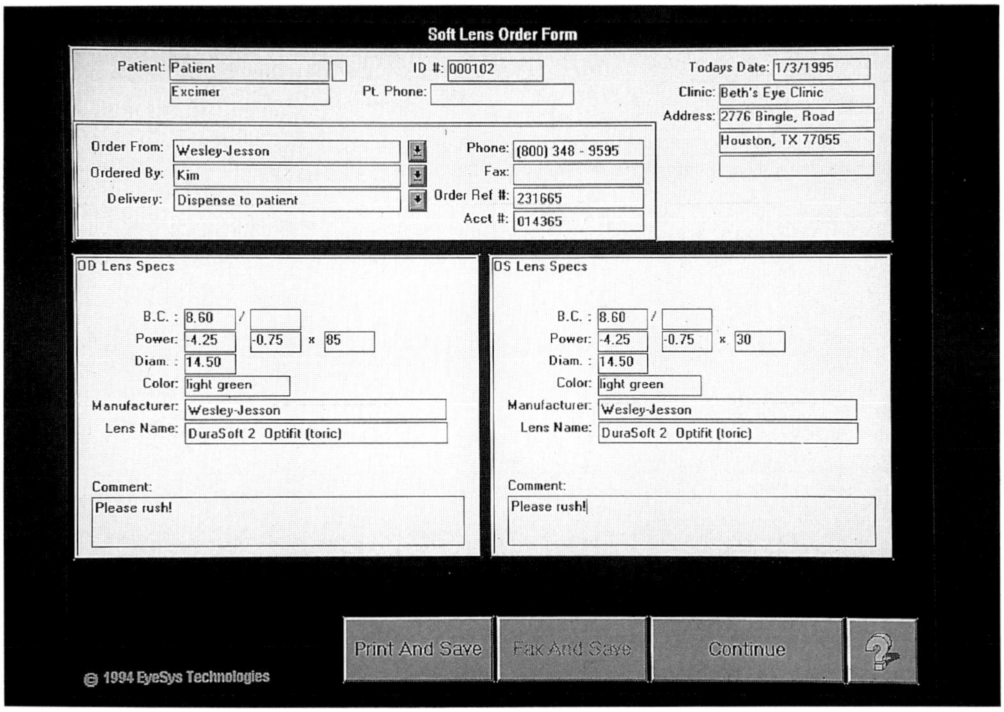

Figure 5-25. Contact lens fitting order form.

Figure 5-26. RK Planner patient data entry screen.

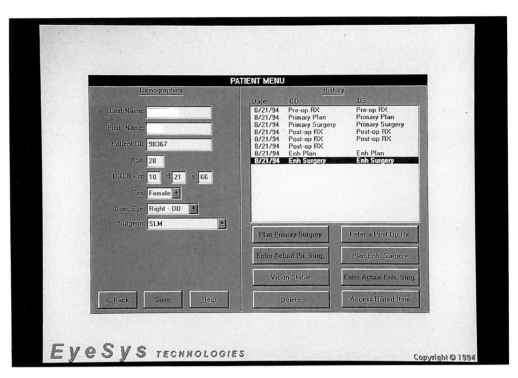

and documenting refractive surgery procedures. The series includes RK and AK nomograms from leading refractive surgeons: Kerry Assil, MD; J. Charles Casebeer, MD; Lee Nordan, MD; and Spencer Thornton, MD.

The EyeSys RK Planners allow surgeons to generate a refractive surgery plan for use during surgery while permanently documenting the patient's surgical history (Figure 5-26). The surgical planning worksheet provides optical zone, cut direction, and incisional patterns presented in a clear graphical format. The desired refractive surgery plan can be selected from the available plan options. At any point in the program, the operator can view a comprehensive interactive help system for additional detail on pachymetry, blade settings, nomogram modifiers, and program operation (Figure 5-27).

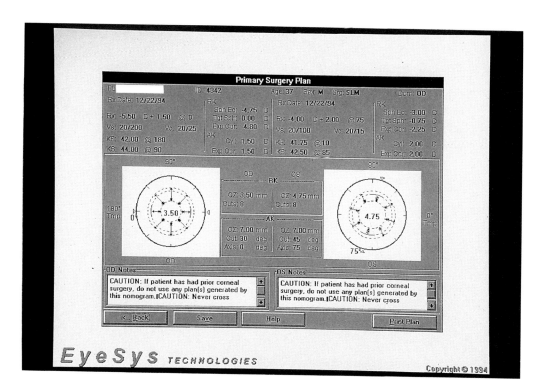

Figure 5-27. RK Planner surgical plan.

CONCLUSION

In recent years, corneal topography has proven to be a powerful tool for the advanced eyecare practitioner by providing indispensable information for refractive and corneal surgical applications, the diagnosis and treatment of corneal pathologies, and the fitting of contact lenses. EyeSys has improved both software and hardware in their latest offering to make the system easier to use, provide new displays and new information to clinicians, and enhance accuracy.

MasterVue Topography Systems

Glenda G. Anderson

The MasterVue Premier Dual Camera System (Humphrey Instruments), operating under the Microsoft Windows environment, is designed to be easy to use while advancing the technology of corneal topography (Figures 6-1 and 6-2). Winner of the 1994 Photonics Circle of Excellence Award for "excellence, innovation, and achievement in a sector of photonics technology," the MasterVue system represents the state-of-the-art in Placido disk-based systems.

The Dual Camera System featured in the MasterVue improves the accuracy in the central region of the cornea by combining the higher effective resolution of a four-power magnified camera image with the extra-wide angle provided by a full-view camera. This patent-pending design is capable of detecting central corneal islands as small as 1.0 mm in diameter with as little as 0.5 D change from the underlying sphere.[1]

The software-enhanced Autofocus is a second patent-pending feature of the MasterVue system. This design uses a protruding "cone-of-focus" and the principle of parallax to calculate the actual working distance of the device from the two-dimensional captured image. This dynamic working distance provides exceptional repeatability across the entire 1.0 mm depth of focus of the instrument.[2] If the image is in sufficient focus that the rings can be detected, the resulting topography will be accurate to within 0.25 D.

IMAGING WITH THE MASTERVUE SYSTEM

Figure 6-3 illustrates the MasterVue imaging system. A 20-ring Placido image is projected onto the cornea and reflected back to the CCD camera. A beam splitter directs the light into two different optical paths. One path is sent through a 4x magnifying lens before being imaged by the central corneal camera. The other path is directed to the full-view

CCD camera. These two camera images are combined to generate a corneal power map.

Focusing

The software-enhanced Autofocus feature ensures an accurate map even when the image is slightly out of focus. The 10th ring, the cone-of-focus, protrudes outward from the Placido disk. With the principle of parallax, the software calculates the position of the 10th ring relative to the 9th and 11th rings. As the cone is brought closer to the cornea, the 10th ring appears closer to the 9th ring, and as the cone is brought further from the cornea, it appears closer to the 11th ring. This relationship is used in a backward propagation of the conversion algorithm to calculate the actual working distance of the system for that individual image. The topography algorithm can then produce an accurate image as long as the operator is within ± .5 mm of focus, thus providing the operator with up to 1.0 mm permissible variation in focus.

Alignment

The software-enhanced Autoalignment feature simplifies the image capturing process. The operator simply positions the device while viewing the image of the eye in the monitor. When the center of the crosshair falls anywhere within the smallest ring and the rings appear visually in focus, the operator captures an image. The software then locks onto the center. This process typically provides the user with a 0.6 mm permissible variation in horizontal and vertical positioning. If the quality of the focus or centering is found by the software to unacceptably affect the accuracy of the resulting topographic map, the system will warn the operator and attach a LOW or MED confidence label on the data displays.

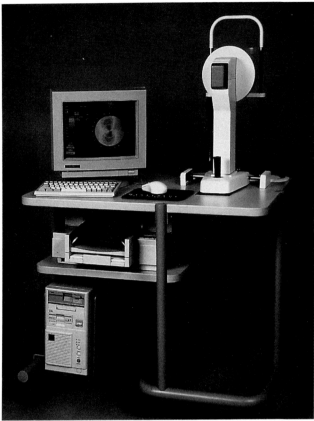

Figure 6-1. MasterVue Premier Dual Camera System.

Data Conversion

The MasterVue image processing locates the leading and trailing edge of each of the 20 rings imaged in the low magnification camera and the central five rings in the high magnification camera at every 2° interval. More than 8000 points are measured and calculated in this process. This edge location information is then used to calculate the center of mass of intensity for each ring. The low and high magnification data are then combined into a single table.

The data conversion algorithm translates the ring location data table to a table describing the three-dimensional shape of the cornea. This algorithm has been proven to provide a more robust three-dimensional solution to the highly complex problem of the irregular or surgically altered cornea.[3]

COLLECTING EXAMS

QuickVue

For routine screening, or high-volume operation, the QuickVue option allows the user to capture and view a single exam in less than 20 seconds. After viewing the topography map, the user has the option of printing the exam without saving or saving the exam to the patient database.

Full Exam

The full exam option automatically saves the exam, as the patient and exam information must be entered before the image is captured. Up to four images can be obtained and reviewed for clarity and focus before selecting one image to process into a corneal power map. In this way, images that are poorly focused, have artifacts from shadows, or have significant missing ring data can be eliminated, thereby yielding the most accurate and precise map.

VIEWING EXAMS

Corneal Power Maps

Like other topography systems, MasterVue displays the topographical data as a color-coded corneal map with "hot colors" (yellow, orange, and red) representing steeper areas, green representing intermediate areas, and "cool colors" (light and dark blue) representing flatter areas (Figure 6-4). The standard scale ranges from 38.5 to 50.0 D in 0.50 D increments, using 24 solid colors for display. This scale is of sufficient range and detail to characterize most corneas.

Corneas with pathology or that have had refractive surgery may fall outside the range of the standard scale. The AutoSize option automatically scales the image to the entire range of data from its minimum to maximum values in increments as small as 0.25 D (Figure 6-5). The user can also create a custom scale, using any dioptric interval or maximum and minimum values. Information at any point on the cornea is available by placing the mouse cursor at that point. This information consists of the dioptric power, radius of curvature in millimeters, distance from the vertex (center of map), location of the semi-meridian, and distance from the center of the pupil (see Figure 6-5).

Numerical View

The Numerical View presents the same information as the corneal power map but displays the data in numerical dioptric power values. These numerical values are also color-coded to correspond to the steepness and flatness of the cornea.

Keratometric View

The Keratometric View displays information similar to that provided by a keratometer. The system averages points along all semi-meridians in the 0 mm to 3 mm, 3 mm to 5 mm, and 5 mm to 7 mm optical zones in order to find the steepest and flattest semi-meridians. The data are then displayed graphically, with the steepest semi-meridian indicated in red and the flattest in blue. A simulated keratometer reading is also displayed.

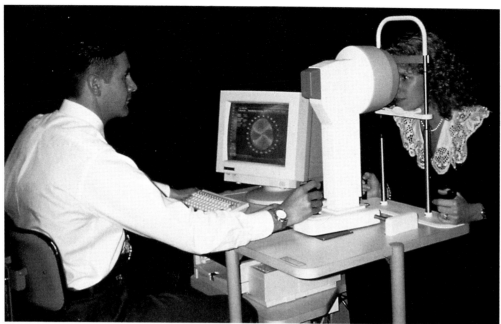

Figure 6-2. Obtaining an exam with the MasterVue system.

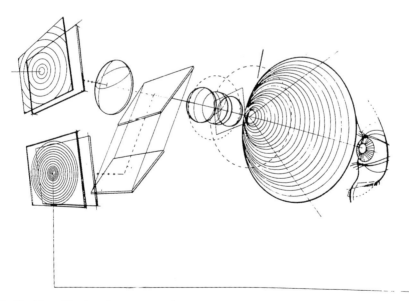

Figure 6-3. The MasterVue imaging system. A beam splitter directs the light from the Placido image to two different paths. On one path the light is sent through a 4x magnifying lens before being imaged by the central corneal camera and the other path is directed to the full view CCD camera. These two camera images are combined to generate a corneal power map.

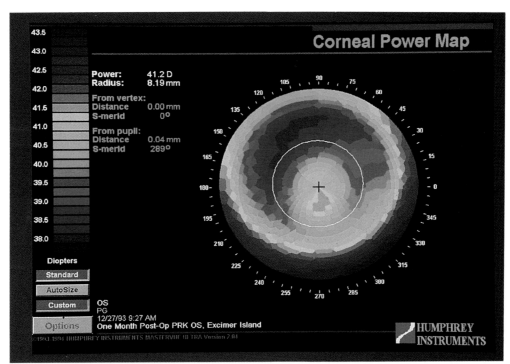

Figure 6-4. A color-coded corneal map in the MasterVue system. This corneal map represents a post-PRK eye with a "central island." The blue areas indicate flattening caused by the PRK, while the central yellow area is a steeper region. The numbers in the upper left show the power and radius of the cornea at the mouse cursor and the location of the cursor. The mouse cursor can be placed at any spot on the map.

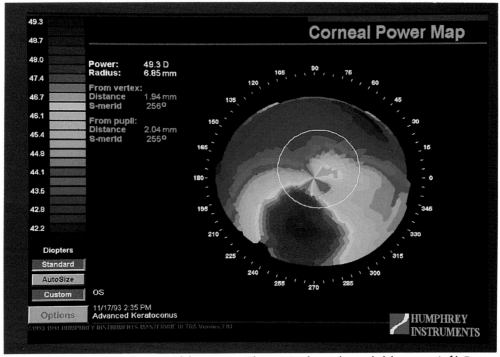

Figure 6-5. A corneal map of an eye with keratoconus. The autosize feature has scaled the cornea in $\frac{1}{3}$ D steps to show the detail in the cone.

Photokeratoscope View

The Photokeratoscope View represents the actual captured image of the cornea in a black and white display. The reflection of the 20 rings and cone-of-focus is visible in this view.

Profile View

The Profile View displays the dioptric power or radius of curvature changes over the corneal surface, using a line graph to show the axis and optical zones for the flattest and steepest corneal meridians.

MultiVue Displays

Most patients will have more than one exam. Patients with corneal pathology are generally followed through the course of their treatment, and patients receiving surgery will be evaluated preoperatively and through successive postoperative visits. Up to four exams will automatically be displayed together in the Trend with Time display. This display allows the physician to easily evaluate changes to the cornea over a period of time (Figure 6-6).

The Difference display allows the physician to evaluate changes to the cornea from any two exams. The earlier exam is subtracted point for point from the later exam and the result displayed along with the two exams. The difference map can be displayed in a standard scale range of ±2.0 D in increments of 0.5 D, or an auxiliary diopter scale adjusted to accommodate the widest range of the two exams. The Difference display is particularly useful for evaluating surgically induced changes (Figure 6-7), regression of surgical effect, progression of pathology, or contact lens-induced warpage.

The OD/OS compare display shows both eyes of a patient side by side. This view displays the currently active exam and the most recent exam of the fellow eye (Figure 6-8). This option is particularly useful for evaluating symmetry between the eyes, and for detecting corneal pathology that is often bilateral, such as keratoconus.

The Exam Overview display combines the corneal power map, numerical view, keratometric view, and the photokeratoscope view as a single display (Figure 6-9). The user can also produce a custom display using up to four views in any combination.

MANAGING EXAMS

A database containing information about the location of every patient exam is stored on the hard drive. The 420MB hard drive itself can store over 2000 exams. Inactive exams can be archived to floppy or a high capacity removable storage system. The diskette label is then automatically stored in the database, making later retrieval of archived exams easy. Exams can be archived individually, or sent in a group according to user-defined criteria. Additional data management features include a tape back-up system for backing up the hard drive, an export/import function for sending exams from one MasterVue unit to another without removing them from the hard disk, and a data maintenance utility for editing or deleting patient information.

OUTPUT

A Hewlett-Packard DeskJet 560C color printer is included in the system for creating high quality color printouts. In addition, there is an option for sending the output to a bitmap file, which can then be sent to a slide bureau for filming. Output can also be sent to a tiff file for import into nearly any graphics package. This option is useful for those developing various patient marketing tools, such as radial keratotomy (RK) brochures.

NETWORKING

A built-in modem enables communication between two MasterVue topography units. With this feature, two physicians in different offices can confer on a patient, with the topography available to both. The modem can also link satellite offices together, aiding transfer of topography information between sites.

The modem can also be used to call the company for technical support. With a direct link into the computer system, technical support personnel can better identify any problems and find solutions faster. In most instances, problems can be resolved within minutes without the need for a service representative to visit the office.

Other Humphrey instruments will soon be able to communicate with the MasterVue. For example, refraction data from the Humphrey auto-refractor can now be electronically transferred and stored with the patient's exam data on the MasterVue.

OPTIONAL MODULES

Contact Lens Fitting Module

The optional contact lens fitting module uses the topography data in its algorithm for improved fitting. Three fittings are available: topographic fitting using proprietary nomograms, keratometric fitting using manufacturers' nomograms, and custom fitting allowing a user-defined nomogram to be input for fitting based on the user's preferences.

Traditionally, contact lenses have been fit using keratometric data. However, since keratometry provides very limited data (only four points in the 3-mm zone) about the

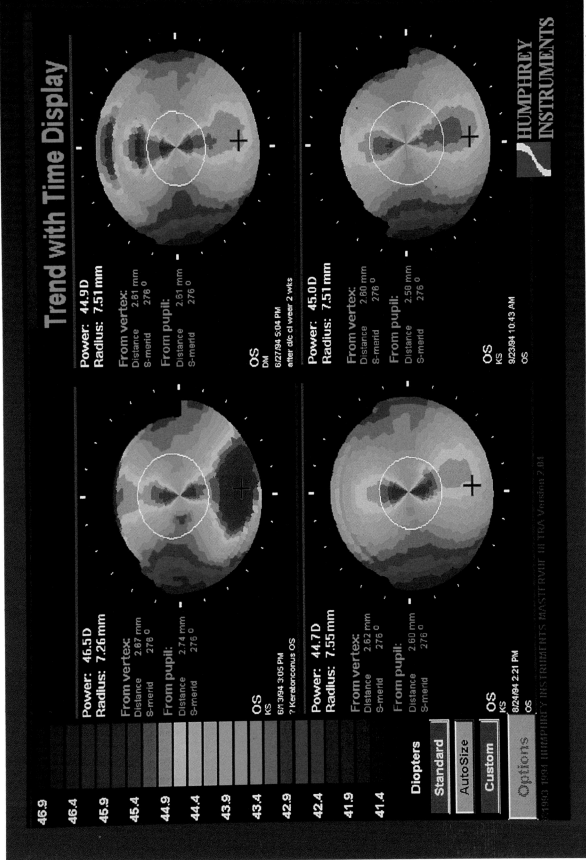

Figure 6-6. A keratoconus case displayed in the Trend with Time View. Upper left shows keratoconus before treatment with contact lens. Upper right shows appearance after 2 weeks of contact lens wear. Lower left and lower right show corneal topography after 2 months and 3 months, respectively, of contact lens wear.

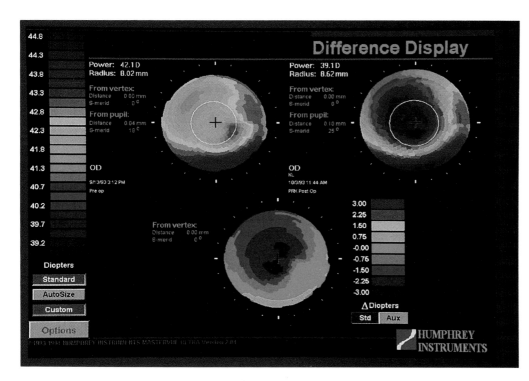

Figure 6-7. A PRK case displayed with the Difference view. Upper left shows preoperative corneal appearance, upper right shows 3-week postoperative appearance, and bottom shows difference map illustrating induced corneal changes. Blue on the change map indicates induced flattening.

contour of the cornea, it lacks accuracy in asymmetric corneas. MasterVue's innovative topographic fitting uses the patient topography data, thus taking into account the entire contour of the cornea (0.3 to 8.3 mm). This method offers improved results, particularly on corneas that have been surgically altered (Figure 6-10).

The fluorescein view displays a simulated fluorescein pattern using the fitting data. The clearance plot also shown in this view indicates the microns of clearance between the anterior surface of the cornea and the posterior surface of the contact lens across any meridian. Figure 6-11 displays the fluorescein view of the same case in Figure 6-10. The dark green on the simulated fluorescein pattern indicates minimal clearance, signifying a good fit. This pattern corresponds to less than 20 μm of clearance at any point on the 0° to 180° meridian, shown on the clearance plot. Any meridian can be chosen for display in the clearance plot by dragging the red ball around the fluorescein pattern with the mouse.

RK Nomogram Module

The optional RK nomogram module includes custom programmed software for virtually all of the principal RK nomograms taught today. The user interface has been made consistent across all the nomograms, making each easy to learn and operate. Having several nomograms installed in one system facilitates comparison among the different programs.

Nomograms from other sources can also be custom installed. Thus, a physician who uses his own nomogram can add it to the package to ease surgical planning.

Clinical Outcomes Module

The optional clinical outcomes module currently under development will provide practitioners with a tool to analyze patient outcomes across the breadth of their practice. Using the powerful database management capabilities of the MasterVue, the physician can analyze changes in topography, astigmatism, corneal regularity, as well as refraction and visual acuity across groups of patients and through periods of time. These variables can be presented as individual trend lines for outcomes reporting or analyzed for correlations using more sophisticated statistical tools.

FUTURE DEVELOPMENTS

"Islands of automation" is the term that best describes the instrumentation found in most medical practices today. Highly automated diagnostic instruments perform complex measurements operating in isolation from one another, the common first stage of automation recognized in industries as seemingly unrelated as automobile assembly, microprocessor fabrication, advertising agencies, and discount retailing. This stage is typically followed by the "Piece-wise Communication" stage in which individual automated instruments are

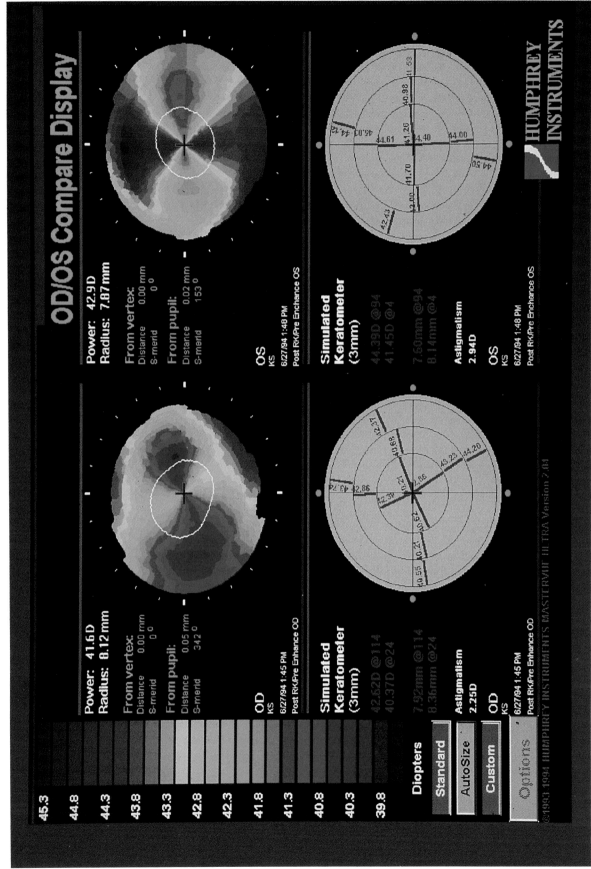

Figure 6-8. The OD/OS Compare display. This patient has had RK in both eyes, accounting for the lack of symmetry between eyes.

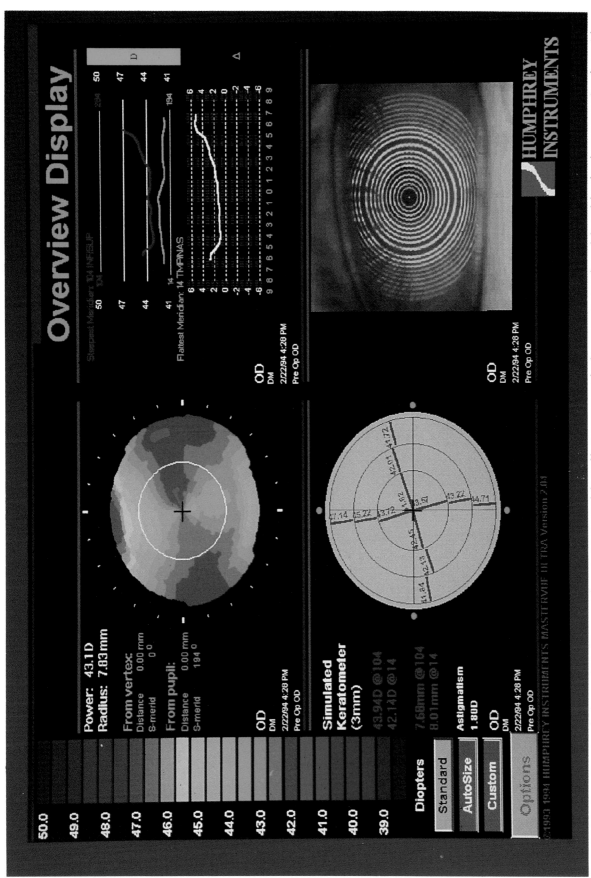

Figure 6-9. The Exam Overview display combining the corneal power map (upper left), profile view (upper right), keratometric view (lower left), and the photokeratoscope view (lower right).

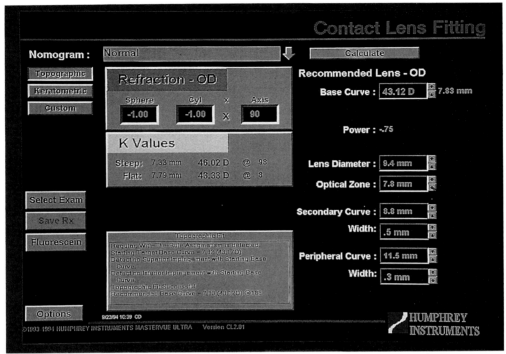

Figure 6-10. Contact lens fitting data using a topographic fit.

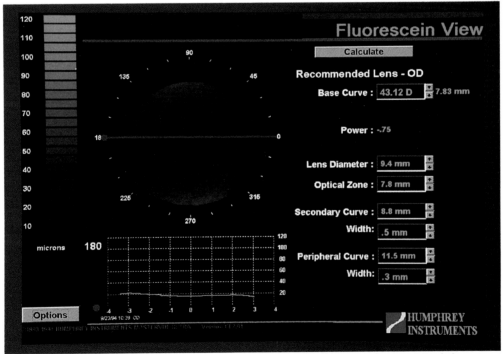

Figure 6-11. Simulated fluorescein view of same case in Figure 6-10. Solid green indicates minimal clearance signifying a good fit.

other medical specialties in the adoption of this piece-wise communication and electronic handling of patient medical files. As successful practices open satellite offices to meet the needs of a more mobile patient population, the need to access current patient history files at multiple locations drives a growing interest in electronic medical files. As referral networks play an integral role in eye care, the efficient transmission of patient history and exam data will become a vital element of effective patient management.

The MasterVue Smart Topography system can play a central role in the management of electronic exam files, satellite offices, and an active referral business. When electronically linked to the other diagnostic instruments in the exam room, the system provides an eye care practice with the powerful database management, image capture, and communication capabilities that make electronic exam management possible.

SUMMARY

Humphrey Instruments, a division of Carl Zeiss, Inc., is committed to providing the worldwide eyecare profession with instruments and software that enhance the practice of medicine and improve patient care.

The MasterVue Smart Topography system advances the state-of-the-art in corneal topography. Features such as the dual camera system and software driven Autofocus assure the practitioner of exams with improved accuracy and repeatability. Additional hardware and software features such as the included modem, data management functions, and optional modules enhance the ease of use and extend the value of the system to the clinical physician.

REFERENCES

1. Kaatmann S. *Comparison of videokeratoscope accuracy using spheres, torics and bicurved surfaces.* Published White Paper Optical Radiation Corp; 1993.
2. Belin MW, Hannush SB, Maloney RK, Riveroll L. *Evaluation of computerized videokeratoscopy decentering and defocusing error.* Presented at Castroviejo Corneal Society; October 1994.
3. Van Saarloos PP, Constable IJ. Improved method for calculation of corneal topography for any photokeratoscope geometry. *Optometry and Vision Science.* 1991;68(12):960-965.

PACHYMETRY AND TRUE TOPOGRAPHY USING THE ORBSCAN SYSTEM

Richard K. Snook

A better understanding of the optical and mechanical properties of the cornea is essential to the advancement of surgical processes now being developed. The ORBSCAN (Orbtek, Inc.) technique for pictorial representation of corneal topography in true as opposed to derivative terms will provide some of these needed data.

The reflective systems embodied in most of the topographic mapping devices of recent years do not produce true surface maps. Consider a topographic map of a mountain. The shape of the terrain is implicit in the contour lines which are parallel slices of the shapes to be depicted. A set of parallel slices of a toric section such as a spectacle lens should be a set of nested ellipses and not a set of bowties. The bowtie representation of the shape in derivative form is implicit to the technique of display used by most current topographic instruments. The accurate representation of corneal shape by the ORBSCAN system provides the parallel slice map form which can convey a better understanding of corneal optical properties. In addition, the ORBSCAN system can provide full surface pachymetry to assist the setting of depth of cut in radial keratotomy (RK) as well as identification of keratoconus which is not well defined by reflective keratometers.

A normal emmetropic cornea mapped by subtraction from a perfectly spherical surface is shown in Figure 7-1. The display of the corneal topography in Z, or sagittal depth terms, as opposed to the more common derivative maps of the Placido-based devices, is not readily apparent. Some realignment of our mental picture is required here to better see the differences and to appreciate the advantage of true topographical, rather than derivative, display of the corneal shape. In use, the figure may be turned in three-space to better visualize the pathology.

Figure 7-2 shows a cornea with irregular astigmatism. The oblique view of Figure 7-2 (showing the same measurement as Figure 7-1) illustrates one of the capacities of this system for rendering visible irregularities of the cornea. The divergence from true spherical form is small relative to the total sagittal depth and so is quite subtle in this direct view. In consequence, a "best fit" sphere at the 3-mm diameter zone is constructed in software and subtracted from the Z axis, or sagittal depth map first shown. This difference mapping is one of several choices open to the user which can serve to illustrate the power of Z axis mapping as is produced by the ORBSCAN technique.

The next four figures are comparison with the sphere format. The central 3-mm zone of Figure 7-3 differs from the perfect sphere by less than 10 μm and the small island at 8:00 is not only minor in magnitude but also outside of the image forming area of the cornea. This is clearly a normal eye where the correction, if any, is simple plus or minus with no astigmatic component.

The second illustration (Figure 7-4) shows an astigmatic cornea with the "cylinder" axis horizontal. The third illustration (Figure 7-5) shows astigmatism of similar magnitude but in the vertical meridian. In the first case, the best line through the areas which depart from spherical is a curve from 197°, passing below the center of vision and extending to 337°. A keratometer reading would not show that the astigmatic shape is not coincident with the axis of vision and could give misleading data when surgery is being planned.

A more complex surface shape change induced by contact lens wear is illustrated in Figure 7-6. The zone at about 4 mm below center is depressed from the desired spherical form by about 100 μm. If converted into radius of axial curvature terms or dioptric value this would represent about eight tenths of a diopter or a change of radius to about

Figure 7-1. Sagittal depth map of normal emmetropic cornea.

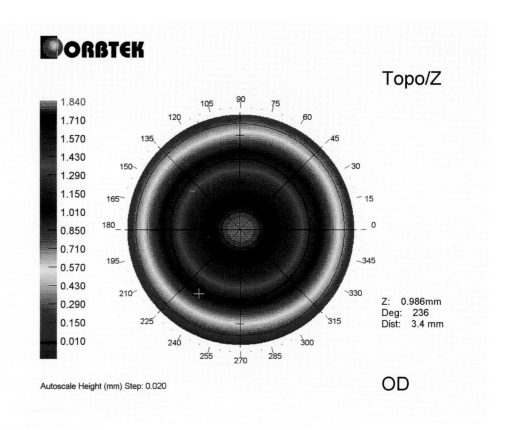

7.29 mm. This amount probably is not significant in terms of focusing power but is quite significant in terms of probable tissue thinning in the depressed area. Is this a cone? Without the corneal thickness attendant to the anterior surface change, the issue is in doubt. The ORBSCAN system will provide the local pachymetric data upon which the determination can be made, which represents a substantial enhancement of the data available to the surgeon for better planning the course of treatment to be employed.

HISTORY OF CORNEAL TOPOGRAPHY ENGINEERING

The general method now used for corneal topography is an extension of the work of Gullstrand in the latter part of the last century. Gullstrand defined the use of photographic measurements for keratometry in 1893.[1] He stated that "The method should, therefore, consist of photographing the corneal reflected images of several objects situated at known distances and, subsequently, measuring the photographic plate."

While he understood the need for long eye to lens distance for best accuracy (the calculations are based on an assumed infinite object distance), he was limited by the available materials. The level of illumination required with the photographic emulsions of the time, as well as the quality

of camera lenses, determined the design of his apparatus more than the "best" configuration as defined by his mathematical analysis.

Gullstrand placed several fixation targets on the surface of the Placido, which was illuminated from the front as opposed to the transillumination scheme currently used. When a glass lens of known shape was measured by his technique, the several images could be fitted into a single smooth surface. When human eyes were photographed, the surface defined was not smooth but was segmented. He stated: "If one disregards the unevenness it is immediately evident that the central part characteristically shows proportionally less variation of curvature, while in the peripheral part a rapidly increasing rate of flattening occurs, so that we can speak of a central optical zone and a peripheral zone of the cornea."

A careful look at the curves demonstrates the effect of several fixation points. Because the fixation axis is displaced from the center of curvature, and because a non-spherical surface is defined as spherical equivalents, the individual parts of the segmented curve are distorted and do not fit into a single smooth curve. This aberration of the reflected target measurement system accounts for a substantial part of the "nasal flattening" shown in keratometric surface reconstructions.

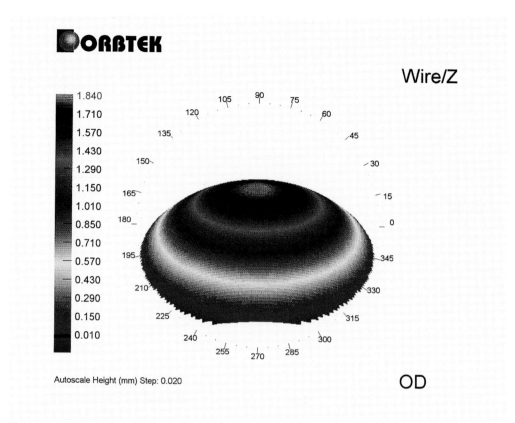

Figure 7-2. Oblique view of cornea with irregular astigmatism.

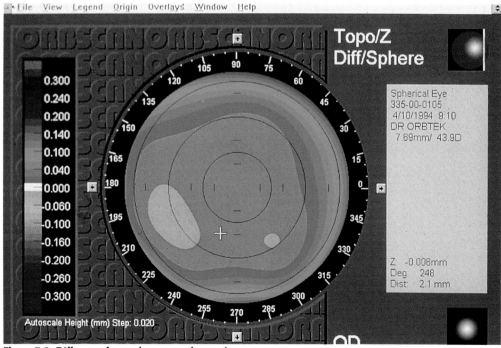

Figure 7-3. Difference from sphere map of normal cornea.

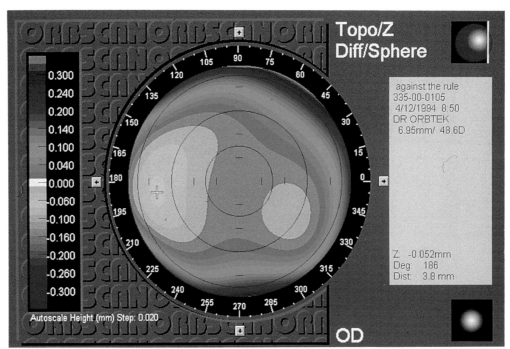

Figure 7-4. Difference from sphere map of cornea with against-the-rule astigmatism.

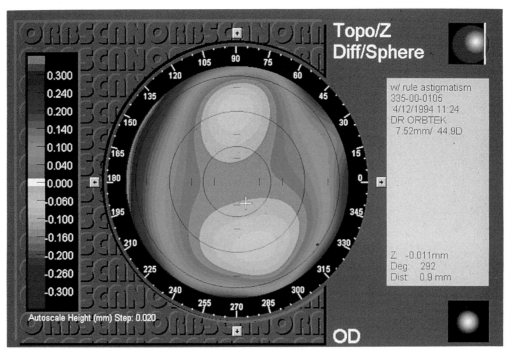

Figure 7-5. Difference from sphere map of cornea with with-the-rule astigmatism.

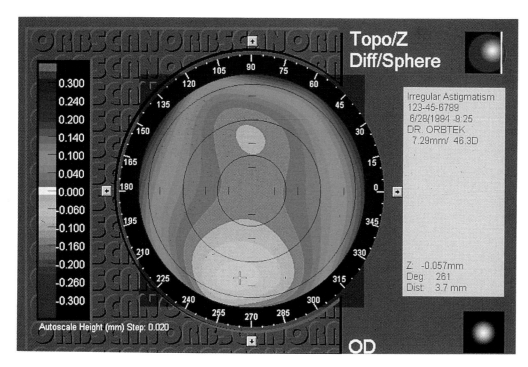

Figure 7-6. Difference from sphere map of cornea with contact lens-induced corneal warpage.

Figure 7-7 shows the basis for the reflective keratometer measurements. An object, F, is placed at a known distance from the corneal surface. The object F is any point on the ring of a Placido or the target in an ophthalmometer. A camera lens located at A views the reflection of the object point F. The ray from F must be reflected from a point C on a surface normal N2 so that the angles FCE and ACE are equal. If the point F is at an infinite distance, the ray FC would cross the optical centerline at a point midway between the points C and D where D is the center of curvature for the surface at point C. At some surface slope, there is no ray which can enter the camera lens (dashed path) for an object of large size. This imposes one limit on peripheral measurements made with "Placido's method."

A second limit is imposed by the geometry of the reflected ray from the center. At the surface normal N2, which is on the optical axis, the entrance and exit angles are smaller than can be defined with the limited resolution of the camera. The variation in axial distance caused by corneal shape causes defocusing and unknown baseline errors for areas remote from center which are not compensated by the mathematical system used to define the surface shape. Attempts to obtain better image quality by changing the target surface shape into conical, hemispherical, or cylindrical form inject other uncompensated errors which are dependent upon the operator error as well as the basic geometry.

Other limitations of Placido's method are well known. The desired topographical map of the cornea should be in

such form as to provide accurate definition of the focusing power so that the data can be used for surgical planning irrespective of the shape of the surface.

Placido-based instruments use an arbitrary value of index of refraction (1.3375) for the reflecting surface. This value yields a fair approximation of single surface focusing power for normal corneal surfaces at points near the 3-mm zone if the instrument is carefully focused and centered.

However, this technique has limitations which are becoming more apparent as they are used more frequently in clinical practice. The distance to the image (reflection of the target disc) is not constant since the surface of the cornea is not spherical as the simplistic analysis assumes. In long baseline systems, the error induced by image plane displacement from the theoretical plane is small, but in short baseline systems it cannot be neglected. This factor imposes a limit on the precision of axial location of the instrument relative to the eye for good accuracy. The camera lens must have large depth of focus so that the several rings are all rendered sharply in the camera. This causes difficulty in assessing the "focus" in the clinical setting even though absolute positional accuracy is imperative for good measurements. The image must be exactly centered or angular position-induced errors of measurement result.

The several "focus aid" systems in use are not effective in practice. Examine the published photographs in brochures and articles and you will find decentering of the eye image is common.

Figure 7-7. Placido's method. A ray from the placido at F enters the camera lens at A, and the relative image size in the camera determines radial curvature at point C. The angles ACE and FCE are equal, and EF, the normal, is perpendicular to the surface tangent N₁. Some rays near tangent N₂ produce such small images in the camera that accurate measurement is not possible. Some rays, such as from X, are near or beyond tangent N₃, do not reach the camera, and no measurement is possible.

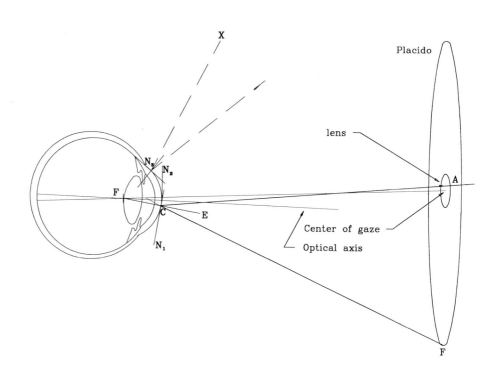

Much of the "nasal flattening" described by Gullstrand and later investigators using similar apparatus may well be an inherent error of the technique. Because the axis of fixation does not coincide with the axis of symmetry, the shape as defined by the reflected target method will be distorted if the corneal surface is non-spherical. To quote Gullstrand, "The cornea in general is not symmetric to the line of sight, in the horizontal or vertical meridians, and that no axis of symmetry of the cornea is evinced," and "I had to be content with calculating the influence of oblique incidence and I was only able to add that the eccentric position of the corneal vertex causes an enlargement of those values which express the degree of asymmetry."

Gullstrand's comment on resolution of measurement is significant in the context of small diameter reflections near the image center: "However, if one is attempting to employ it [ophthalmometry] to measure the radius of different small corneal areas lying next to one another in the same meridian, then the observation errors certainly play an important role. If the individual ophthalmometer finding suffers from errors of observation, then how much more so must this be in the case where it is important to indicate a small difference between two such values. If, for example, the possible error of observation amounts to 1% and the difference to be measured is about 5% of the measured values, it can easily result that

the larger value is 1% too large and the smaller value is 1% too small, so that it is apparent that the difference to be measured can be found two fifths or 40% too large."

In Gullstrand's paper he also said, "During an ophthalmometric measurement the true radius is never found at any point of the cornea." Similarly, the description of the surface in radius of curvature terms as defined by manufacturers of Placido-based keratometers is based on spherical object equivalents with the axis of measurement coincident with the apex of the surface. Displacement of the line of fixation from the axis of symmetry is physiologically normal while assumed centers of curvatures are located on the visual axis line which is seldom, if ever, the locus of the true center.

Measurements of reflection size are made from a solid-state television camera image. These measured points are inherently a series of discrete amplitude analog points arranged in parallel lines called a "raster." When the measurement of the reflex diameter includes the center of a circle the resolution is greatest and is reduced as the line of measurement deviates from the center.

Rowsey et al used a system of rotation of the photographic image of the reflections to overcome the loss of resolution in other meridians, but this method is not possible in direct videokeratometers which employ Placido reflections. As the raster line of measurement gets near the tangent condition at the top and bottom of each circle, the ability to locate accurately the reflection point diminishes. The limitation is even greater as the image size decreases near center so that the uncertainty of measurement is considerable within the central portion of the optical zone. The topographic data are displayed in a derivative format where the implied surface shape is grossly distorted. A series of parallel plane slices through a toric section will result in a family of ellipses, not the bowtie which is shown by most keratometric topographical measurements of today's practice.

The various reflective keratometers now being used in clinical practice do not provide accurate sagittal curvature maps, let alone dioptric maps. The picture is further distorted when the derived axial curvature data are presented in dioptric form. Description of the corneal shape in dioptric terms is not supported by the physics of any keratometer.

The diopter is, at best, a "rubber ruler" since the size of a diopter is a function of the surface in a nonlinear way. One fourth diopter for a 1 D lens is 250 mm but for a 40 D lens it is 0.2 mm. What is one fourth of a diopter? The surface shape must be known in real terms before any such measurement could have validity. Then the change in dioptric terms for a given shape change still would not be reflected by the change of plane of focus caused by the induced shape change.

Keratometer dioptric conversion assumes that the surface is centered and spherical and that a constant can be employed for the index of refraction-derived conversion formula. The assumed value which has different values in some instruments works reasonably well for "normal" corneas at the so-called 3-mm zone but often fails badly when these conditions are not met. The true dioptric values for human corneas can not be measured by the Placido-based techniques used by most instruments because of the inherent errors of the technique.

The optical system of the eye involves several elements, and the shapes and spacings all contribute to the total focusing power of the eye. In the case of RK, the central flattening is not confined to the anterior surface and so the anterior chamber depth changes. The anterior chamber may be thought of as the distance, d, between the lens and the effective lens formed by the cornea. The total focusing power is then derived by:

$$bfl = [f1 (d-f2)]/[d-(f1+f2)]$$

where f1 is the corneal focal length, f2 is the lens focal length, and d is the anterior chamber depth. When the refractive change is small the effect can probably be ignored, but clearly there is some error inherent in the assumption. The nonuniform stress distribution in the cornea is also changed when incisions are made which can also result in unpredicted focusing power results from surgery.

ORBSCAN SYSTEM OF CORNEAL TOPOGRAPHY

To express the focusing power for any corneal shape and relative axis of measurement, the Placido system must be abandoned and a better system employed. The ORBSCAN technique is designed to reduce the errors which are a part of the reflective method of topographical mapping of the cornea. The X, Y, Z maps in true cartesian coordinate terms are a better representation of the surface and focusing power of the cornea as well as providing corneal thickness data for substantially all of the cornea to the limbus.

A beam of sunlight entering a darkened room through a hole in a curtain or shining through a hole in a cloud forms a visible path due to Rayleigh scattering (Figure 7-8). The same principle is used in slit lamp examination of the eye where the scattering of light in nearly transparent tissues renders visible structures that cannot otherwise be seen (Figure 7-9). In the ORBSCAN instrument, modified conventional köhler projectors provide the focal illumination.

The object at the focal plane is one or more optical slits that may be moved by an associated computer-controlled mechanism in a Scheimpflug-corrected path to provide critical focus for all portions of the cornea (Figure 7-10). The image of each slit is made confocal with a television camera which forms a part of the keratometer/pachymeter so that the instrument may examine various areas without repositioning.

The projection lens focal length is as long as possible to reduce the convergence or divergence of the beams over small axial distances. Projection lens focal ratio is calculated by a well-known technique for producing optimal brightness and sharpness of the illuminated area. The diameter of the exit pupil is kept small to diminish the effect of aperture versus focal distance which requires that the lamp brightness be high to provide adequate illumination of the slit image. The total energy at the cornea is quite small and does not approach the threshold of phototoxicity to the eye.

The projector and camera are mounted on a common optical bench to allow the projected thin sheets of light to enter the eye at an angle to the camera axis. The bench assembly is, in turn, mounted on an X, Y, Z mechanism to permit horizontal, vertical, and axial alignment with the eye. The beams of light produce diffuse reflection from each successive portion of the anterior part of the eye through which they pass. The projection systems produce tyndall parallelapiped cross-sections of the cornea as luminous bands against a dark pupil. As the focused beam passes through the cornea, stroma act as scattering centers for the incident light. The index of refraction of these molecules is greater than the saline in which they are immersed and these optical interfaces at a molecular level produce the diffuse light reflex observed.

Much as smoke, water vapor, and dust in the atmosphere act as scattering centers to make the sky blue, these scattered rays are brighter at the shorter wavelengths.

Rayleigh scattering increases inversely as the fourth power of wavelength. At normal incidence, the reflection of light at a boundary between media of differing index of refraction is calculated as follows:

$$R = (n2\text{-}n1)^2/(n2+n1)^2$$

where R is the reflected percentage of the incident beam, and n1 and n2 are the indices of refraction of the two media, respectively. From this relationship it follows that the air to cornea and cornea to aqueous interfaces will reflect a definable portion of the slit beam specularly as well as the amount scattered as previously noted. This effect produces the reflex used in reflective system instruments. The tyndall image is the result of diffuse reflection at the optical discontinuities in the slit beam path, each of which reflect a portion of the incident light. Because the locus of origin and angular relationship of the slit beam relative to the optical axis of the camera is known, the shape of the tyndall image describes the shape of a cross-section of the cornea.

The exit pupil of the fixation target and the slit projectors produces Purkinje images at the surfaces of the cornea and lens (Figure 7-11). The geometry of the system is such that with a normal eye properly aligned for measurement, these Purkinje images will lie in a line coincident with the horizontal centerline of the eye being measured.

The shape of both anterior and posterior surfaces and therefore thickness of the cornea of the human eye can be mapped by means of slit projection. The line of gaze fixation is made coincident with the optical axis of the camera by a target viewed by the subject via a beam splitter. The beam splitter and fixation target are so positioned as to cause the desired alignment of the eye and camera, and thus, the slit beam. The coaxial location of the fixation target insures that the visual axis of the eye being examined is coincident with the optical axis of the television camera. Beams of light formed by projection of an optical slit or slits are focused at or slightly behind the corneal surface. The beams are projected from known points located on a line at a fixed angle, 45°, at the center of motion from the optical axis of a camera, and in the same plane. The optical slits are translated in the object plane by incremental motors under computer control.

Consider a point on the tyndall image as seen by the television camera. The bright line of the tyndall image is displaced laterally by an amount which is a direct function of the sagittal depth of the cornea at the point selected (Figure 7-12). The instantaneous position of the single slit in each captured image is known. The included angle relative to the camera optical axis is then used to calculate the Z, or sagittal depth, from the horizontal and vertical position data for each pixel which defines the edge of the tyndall image, corresponding to the leading edge of the slit.

The optical axes of the camera and the two projectors converge in a single point. A plane containing that point is erected, in fact, in instrument calibration during assembly at the factory. This Z0 plane is perpendicular to the optical axis of the camera. A series of measurements of the slit images in this plane and other parallel planes together with the exact focal distance and camera image magnification data provides the foundation for surface determination.

Figure 7-8. The tyndall image is produced by Rayleigh scattering of the light from a projected slit image.

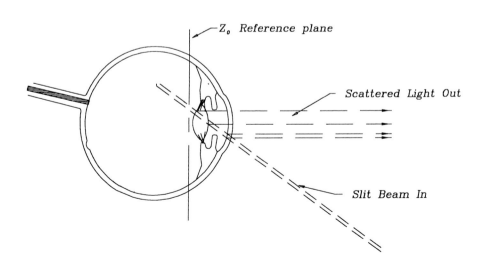

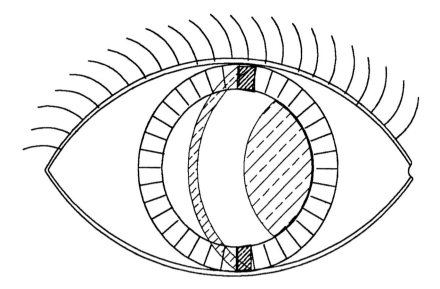

Figure 7-9. The cross-section of the cornea and lens is seen as a hazy area against the overall eye image.

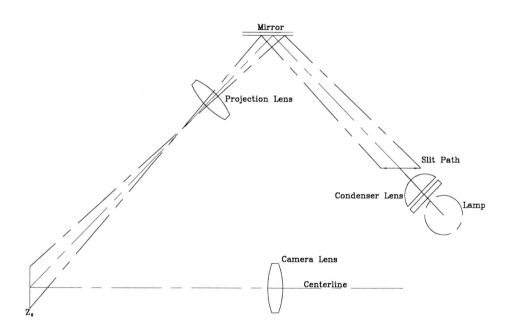

Figure 7-10. The projected slit image is corrected for depth of focus by scheimpflug rule motion of the slit in the object plane of the projectors. The slit path is not perpendicular to the axis of projection but is inclined by an amount calculated to produce the best image quality at the eye.

If the slit beam strikes a surface closer to the camera than the Z0 reference plane, the image will be displaced laterally by an amount directly related to the axial distance. This distance in corneal measurements is the sagittal depth of the cornea at each point plus a constant offset which can be subtracted to derive true X, Y, Z data for each image point in each tyndall image of the sequence of 20 exposures. Ten exposures are made from each side for the complete measurement series for a corneal shape and thickness determination. By measuring a large number of points with each of a sequence of slit positions, 10 from each side, the X, Y, Z locus of thousands of points on the surface of the cornea are determined and stored for mapping the surface.

Alignment

As a part of the design of the instrument, two additional half-height slits are positionable in the projector focal planes. These are used for alignment of the instrument by the operator. The position of each is set by the computer so that when the two are brought into vertical alignment at the center of the corneal image by positioning of the instrument, the axial distance to the corneal surface is known and the depth of focus of the camera is great enough to render sharply the tyndall image, irrespective of the sagittal depth of the cornea being measured. In addition, fiducial markings in the image of the eye on the computer monitor provide centering information to the operator. This system for establishing instrument position is much more accurate than the focus aids of the reflective systems even though the ORBSCAN technique is much less sensitive to instrument alignment for accurate rendition of the topography of the cornea.

The Purkinje image of the fixation target is made coincident with the merged, half-height slit tyndall images and the limbus of the eye is thereby also centered in the display at the time of measurement. This method assures the measurement will be within the optical and mathematical range required for accuracy.

The eye will move slightly over the time required for the capture of the several images. By a proprietary computer technique the sequence of images captured by the system is aligned mathematically to compensate for the microsaccadic motion. If the movement is greater than the system can compensate for, the operator is advised to repeat the measurement.

Topographic and Pachymetric Maps

The location of selected portions of the limbus and other reference points is used for this proprietary determination and the fitting of the data into a single three-dimensional surface. This surface, which is a true topographical map of the cornea,

is displayed and also serves as the foundation for thickness calculation for the pachymetric data. The surface shape information is also made available in the less accurate radius of curvature form for comparison with data from other instruments by selection from a menu of displays.

The creation of a surface by ORBSCAN topographic measurement provides the basis for the derivation of pachymetric and radius of curvature maps. To derive the radius of curvature in the form provided by Placido-based instruments, the exact surface data provide the needed data for the less accurate form of data display. The data are first converted from cartesian to polar form with the corneal apex as the center. Alternatively, the centroid of the limbus may serve as the central point of the data set. Along each selected hemi-meridian, the X, Y, Z data points are selected from storage for display. The number of hemi-meridians used may be varied depending on the desired resolution weighed against time to calculate and display. Where the computed surface from the derived Z axis data are smoothed by cubic splines the tangents are implicit for providing surface normal tangent angles. Where the data are in simple cartesian form, the tangent angles are computed for points at selected intervals along the hemi-meridian line (Figures 7-13 and 7-14). The following calculations will provide radius of axial curvature for the selected points:

$$R = (r^2 + 4h^2)/8h$$

where h is the sagittal difference from the apex and r is the half chord of a corneal point, both related to the radius of axial surface curvature R. Clearly, the radius of curvature need not be mapped since only the surface normal angle is required for thickness calculation. The radial distance, r, and the radius of curvature, R, are the short side and hypotenuse of a right triangle. The supplement of the angle formed by the half chord and the resultant R is the complement of the angle between the normal and a line parallel to the axis. This angle is added to the projection angle to form the true angle of incidence of the slit beam ray. The calculations to derive corneal thickness involve simple trigonometry and the application of Snell's law of refraction.

The angular relationship of the trailing edge of the tyndall image to the surface defined in the keratometric measurements provides the entrance angle for ray tracing the illumination path in the cornea and, hence, thickness at each point. Differentiation of the smooth curve defined by the Z measurements on any hemi-meridian is the foundation for the surface normal derivation needed to calculate the ray entrance angle for the trailing edge of the slit. Substituting the hypotenuse of a defined triangle from adjacent Z values along the line from center does introduce a small error in the normal

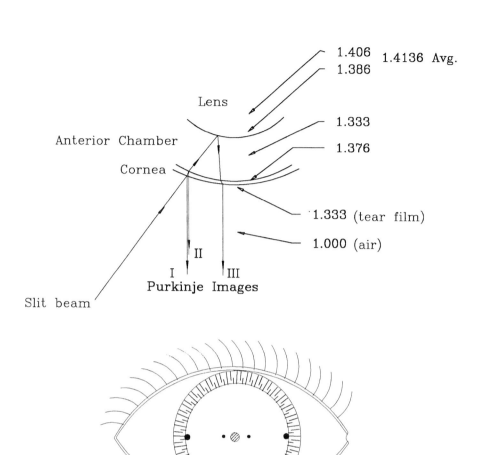

Figure 7-11. Purkinje images are formed at each optical surface by reflection of the illuminating source. In the ORBSCAN system, the two slit projectors yield pairs of reflections which are indicative of the geometry of the eye.

as defined from the true surface tangent, but the magnitude of the error is within the error budget defined by clinical requirements. For research use the data can be calculated to a more exact value, but the time of calculation is much greater and is not required for the usual clinical application of the pachymetric data.

The axial radius of curvature determination sequence is as follows: after conversion from cartesian to polar form, the selected hemi-meridian is broken into segments based on central angle. At each of a number of points on the hemi-meridian the X, Y, Z locus is derived and stored. A cylinder of revolution centered at the corneal apex with a 5-mm radius is superimposed on the defined surface. The intersection of the cylinder and the surface defines the Z0 reference for each measurement. This location for the Z

reference was chosen as least likely to change between measurements even after surgery. Because of the location chosen, the Z values outside the 10-mm diameter zone have negative values. The Z values are scaled to the reference plane from the original Z0 plane of measurement. The sagittal depth, d, at each point on each selected half chord is calculated by subtraction from the new Z reference. Z differences for any selected resolution desired are selected and the resultant angles calculated for the topographical map. If the value of d is small (near center), the surface reference is mathematically rotated relative to the zero plane by some arbitrary angle before calculation of the surface angle.

The previously given formula, $R = (r^2 + 4h^2)/8h$, is applicable for central areas only since it assumes that the sine of the angle and the angle are approximately equal for the

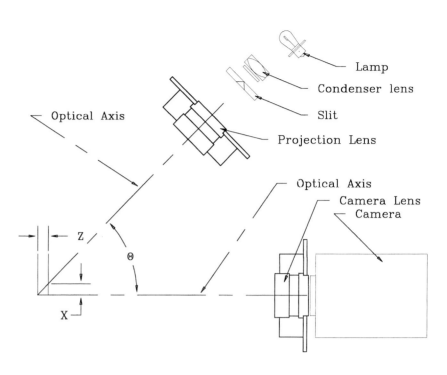

Figure 7-12. A schematic illustration of one of the slit projectors. The camera image of the tyndall image is displaced laterally (X), by an amount (Z) which is a function of sagittal depth at the point of intersection of the slit beam and the cornea.

application of Snell's law and that the source is at a large distance. Both of these are untrue in the real world. A better approximation is derived by:

$$f' = z + x \times \cot(\theta i - \theta t)$$

where θi is the incident angle and θt is the transmitted ray angle. The coordinate system is Z axis from the apex at 0,0. The R value for each point selected on the several hemi-meridians are then stored for map generation. In general, the surface curve from the Z values can be fitted to a conic section. The formula describes a conic surface with the vertex at 0,0 and the center at (R0/(1-e^2),0). The value of eccentricity, e, has been given the range of 0.25 to 0.7 in various sources. The assumption that the entire surface can or should be represented by a single surface of rotation is questionable except for gross approximations since there could not be any corneal astigmatism for this to be close to reality. A best fit spherical surface with user chosen characteristics can be subtracted from the modeled surface to emphasize deviations such as are present in astigmatic corneas. Keratoconus is also emphasized by the subtraction and is confirmed, if present, by the pachymetric map of the same area.

In calculating the posterior surface, the displacement of the projected ray by the refraction of the cornea is computed. The virtual image of the slit at the posterior corneal surface is laterally displaced by an amount which is related to the angle

of incidence and the local tissue thickness. The rear surface distance D' is derived from the incident ray angle i.

The Purkinje images (Figure 7-15), formed at the tear film and the anterior surface of the lens together with limbus location relative to fixation target reflex, serve as landmarks for sequence fitting with the understanding that the second Purkinje image will merge with the first and that the locus of the third and higher images will be determined by the plane of focus of the eye. The anterior surface of the lens will be displaced axially by the accommodation of focus. Anterior chamber depth is also altered by the effect of surgical alteration of the surface curvature. The exact sequence fitting scheme is proprietary.

To provide infinity plane fixation, a target illuminated by the LED is imaged with a single lens so that the target is seen by the subject at infinity plus or minus the spectacle correction. The correction can be made by axial displacement of the lens via a calibrated control knob adjusted by the operator. Thus, the image can be at optical infinity so that the subject will not be accommodating. The operator would have to adjust the fixation image plane to compensate for the refractive error of the subject. The Purkinje images are a guide for X,Y motion when compared with the limbus centroid but they can produce misleading fit for some patients. The proprietary algorithm provides for the solution

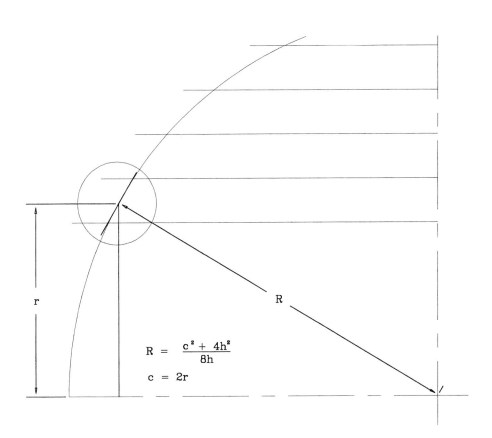

Figure 7-13. The sagittal depth, h, of a point defined by a half chord r is used to derive the axial radius of curvature. The tangent slope is derived from these data to find the relative angle of incidence of the slit beam.

$$R = \frac{c^2 + 4h^2}{8h}$$

$$c = 2r$$

of sequence fitting by weighting and analysis of motion in pixel terms for each measurement series.

OTHER NON-PLACIDO TOPOGRAPHY

The construction of true topographical surfaces is also possible by the PAR system of pattern projection. The PAR device employs fluorescein dye in the tear film rather than slit projection. Projection systems, unlike reflective systems using Placidos, are quite tolerant of positioning errors since the measurements are substantially independent of relative position of the instrument. The term positioning is used in place of the more common focusing, since the focus is determined by the system design and not instrument location as is the case in reflective systems. The ability to provide true surface topography coupled with the ease of use of these instruments is the most important advance over the common Placido-based technology.

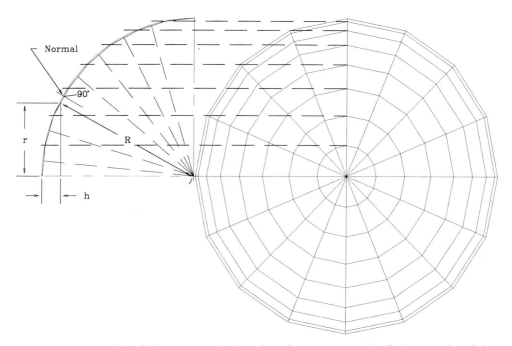

Figure 7-14. The normal is by definition perpendicular to the surface tangent. A series of points are selected along each of a set of hemi-meridians, and the sagittal depth together with the radius of axial curvature are calculated for each selected point. The number of points calculated can be chosen for speed or resolution depending on the user's needs.

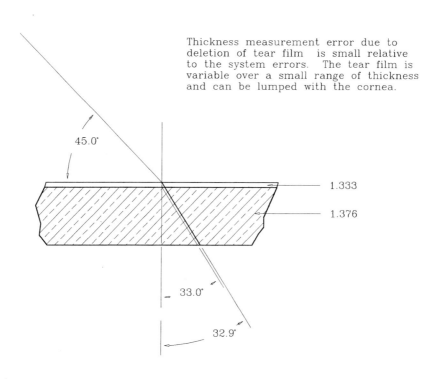

Figure 7-15. Thickness measurement error due to deletion of tear film is small relative to the system errors. The tear film is variable over a small range of thickness and can be lumped with the cornea.

ENDNOTE

In 1896, Gullstrand published an article entitled "Photographic-Ophthalmometric and Clinical Investigations of Corneal Refraction." This paper describes what is currently called "Placido's method of photo keratometry." The quotations given are from the 1964 translation by William M. Ludlam. The Gullstrand paper is the foundation for all keratometric systems which use a reflected target for surface measurements.

BIBLIOGRAPHY

Belin W, Zloty P. Accuracy of the PAR corneal topography system with spatial misalignment. *CLAO.* 1993;19(1):64-68.

Belin W, et al. The PAR technology corneal topography system. *Refr & Corneal Surg.* 1992;8:88-96.

Douthwaite WA. A new keratometer. *Am Jn of Optom & Physiological Optics.* 1987;64(9):223-230.

Emsley HH. Visual optics. *Butterworths.* 5th ed. 1979;1:336-364.

Hecht E. Optics. *Schaum's Outline Series.* McGraw-Hill;1975.

Maguire LJ, et al. Graphic presentation of computer analyzed keratoscope photographs. *Tech Ophthalmol.* 1987;105:711-715.

McKay T. Selecting and using a videokeratoscope for mapping of corneal topography. *Jn of Ophthalmic Nursing & Technol.* 13(1):23-30.

Roberts C. Characterization of the inherent error in a spherically-based corneal topography system in mapping a radially aspheric surface. *Jn of Refr & Corneal Surg.* 1994;10:103-116.

Snook RK. *Video Keratometer.* US Patent No. 5,110,200 (assigned to EyeSys, Inc).

Tate GW, et al. Accuracy and reproducibility of keratometer reading. *CLAO.* 1987;13(1).

PAR CORNEAL TOPOGRAPHY SYSTEM

Michael W. Belin, MD
James L. Cambier, PhD
John R. Nabors, MS

The PAR Corneal Topography System (PAR Vision Systems Corporation, New Hartford, NY) uses close-range photogrammetry and digital image processing to measure and produce a topographic elevation map of the entire corneal surface.[1-4] Traditional Placido ring-based systems measure the *angle* of the corneal surface using a reflected light image and use the angular measures to compute curvature and reconstruct the surface. In contrast, the PAR system makes direct point-by-point measurements of surface *elevation* using a stereo triangulation technique. A three-dimensional model of the surface results directly from these elevation data and curvature can then be calculated from the model. This particular approach to surface measurement, based on video-format stereo image pairs, has been termed "rasterstereography."

Among the advantages of the PAR system are the generation of true elevation-based topography, virtually instantaneous image acquisition to prevent any artifact due to eye movement, coverage of the entire cornea including the critical central optical zone and extending outward to a diameter of 10 to 12 mm, ability to measure irregular and de-epithelialized corneas, and suitability for intraoperative use.

CTS TECHNOLOGY

Measurement Technique

The CTS uses a form of stereotriangulation, a standard photogrammetric method of extracting three-dimensional object information using two or more overlapping photographs or views of the object taken from different vantage points. Typically some feature of interest is located in each photograph and, using geometric information about the camera position associated with that photograph, a ray is constructed in three-dimensional space which extends from the camera to the feature. Multiple rays from multiple cameras are constructed and their intersection point, which defines the location of the feature, is calculated. The result is an (x,y,z) coordinate for the feature.

Adaptation of the stereotriangulation technique to the cornea requires some special steps. First, the cornea is featureless; there are no landmarks which can be identified and located by multiple cameras and used to perform the ray intersection, so we must create features on the surface by projecting a structured light pattern onto the cornea which will produce unique, identifiable features on the surface. The PAR system uses a grid pattern composed of horizontal and vertical lines spaced about 0.2 mm (200 μm) apart. Each grid intersection comprises a surface feature which can be located in multiple images and used to generate an (x,y,z) coordinate.

In order for the triangulation technique to work, the surface features used must emit light in multiple directions so they can be observed by multiple cameras at once. In most imaging applications the surfaces being measured scatter incident illumination in all directions, and the images can be formed using this scattered light. This mechanism, in fact, is employed in standard photography. But the cornea is not an effective scatterer; it is nearly transparent and the image we see looking into the eye is generated almost entirely by light scattered from the iris. In order to produce light emissions from the surface of the cornea, the PAR system uses a thin film of fluorescein placed on the surface, with the images collected using standard fluorescence-based photography. The secondary fluorescence from the dye is emitted in all

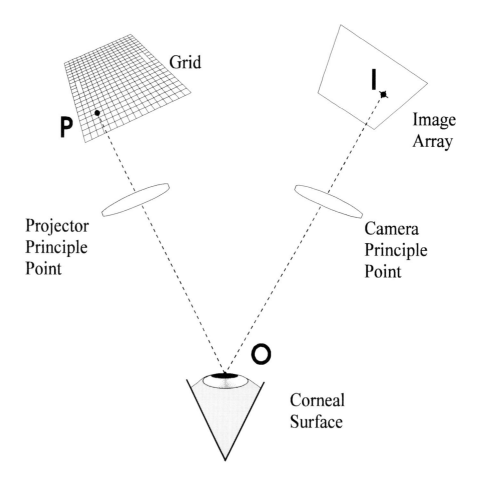

Figure 8-1. CTS triangulation geometry.

directions, just as scattered light would be, so it can be imaged from multiple locations. The grid pattern is projected through a blue excitation filter, and the imaging is performed using a yellow barrier filter so only the secondary fluorescence is observed.

The CTS approach could be implemented by using one optical system to project the grid pattern onto the cornea and create the surface features to be measured, and two or more camera systems to measure the locations of the features. A significant simplification can be achieved by recognizing that the grid projection system is mathematically equivalent to a camera, with the physical grid (a precision silver-chrome pattern deposited on a glass substrate) corresponding to the image. Hence the system can be reduced to two optical systems, one projecting the grid onto the cornea and the other imaging it from another vantage point.

Figure 8-1 illustrates the geometry of this system. Each grid intersection is projected along a ray PO from the grid to the surface of the cornea, and is imaged along a ray OI by the camera. From the known geometry of the projection and imaging systems, the two rays can be intersected in three-dimensional space to compute the (x,y,z) coordinates of the

surface point O. In typical operation, the grid pattern is projected using flash illumination. An image of the projected grid is captured, digitized, and processed using a set of proprietary software algorithms. The processing detects the imaged grid intersections and translates them into a two-dimensional array of elevation values. These raw elevation values, which are referenced to an imaginary plane orthogonal to the optical axis of the eye, represent the true topography of the anterior surface of the cornea.

System Configuration

A typical hardware configuration for the CTS consists of a Windows-based PC with video digitizer and system interface boards, a flash power supply, the CTS optical head which mounts on a slit lamp or operating microscope, and a color printer. Figure 8-2 shows the slit lamp-mounted optical head with computer display and Figure 8-3 shows the complete system configuration. The hardware can be adapted to an existing slit lamp or operating microscope by use of the appropriate mechanical fixtures and optical components to obtain the proper working distance and magnification.

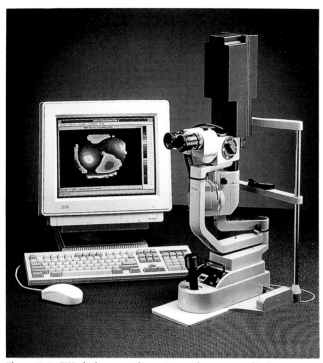

Figure 8-2. CTS slit lamp configuration and computer display.

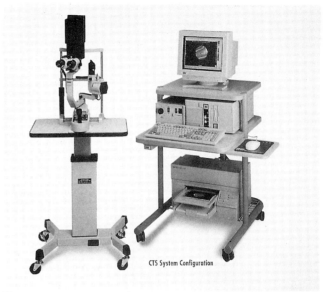

Figure 8-3. CTS system configuration.

Display Methods

As stated above, the topographic model of the cornea produced by the CTS consists of an array of elevation values which define the height of each surface point relative to an imaginary plane located behind the cornea. While this topographic information provides an accurate representation of the corneal shape, it is difficult to display these data in a manner that shows the subtle variations in corneal shape which are clinically significant. Because the cornea is approximately spherical, it proves useful to calculate an average or equivalent sphere for the corneal surface, and display the actual surface with the equivalent sphere as a reference. Elevation deviations, both positive and negative, from this equivalent sphere can then be color coded and displayed. This display shows exactly how the cornea deviates from a perfect sphere, and is extremely useful in evaluating keratoconus, astigmatism, and other anomalies.

Figures 8-4 through 8-8 illustrate typical data from a cornea exhibiting a moderate degree of astigmatism. Figure 8-4 is the fluorescence image showing the grid superimposed on the cornea. The raw elevation data (as measured from the imaginary plane) are shown as a color map in Figure 8-5. Note that because the available color scale must be expanded to accommodate the full range of elevations from the apex to the periphery, it cannot show the subtle variations which are important. Figure 8-6 shows the elevation data displayed with the average sphere as a reference, and we see the

positive and negative deviations from the sphere. If this cornea were perfectly spherical this map would be all one color, but in this case the saddle shape characteristic of astigmatism is readily apparent.

Figure 8-7 is a corneal curvature map based on sagittal curvature, and Figure 8-8 is one based on tangential curvature. The sagittal curvature map is obtained for each point by computing the distance from the surface along the normal to where it intersects the optical axis and using this result as the radius of curvature.

Other authors have pointed out that use of the term "sagittal" to describe this curvature calculation is incorrect,[5] and that Placido ring-based systems have a fundamental inability to correctly measure either sagittal or tangential curvature. But this use of the term has become so widespread in the industry that it has been adopted by PAR as well.

The tangential map is obtained by computing the local or instantaneous radius of curvature along the meridian from the second derivative of the elevation function. Sagittal curvature is used for refractive power calculations in all topography systems, and tangential curvature is also provided in several. Tangential maps are typically more sensitive to local changes in curvature.[6] In the discussions that follow, curvature maps will be referred to as just that, curvature, rather than as refractive power. A number of authors have pointed out that the calculation of refractive power from localized curvature using paraxial models is incorrect and highly inaccurate, particularly in the periphery.[7] It should be understood that the appearance of dioptric values in the following examples is intended as an approximation, provided only for comparison purposes.

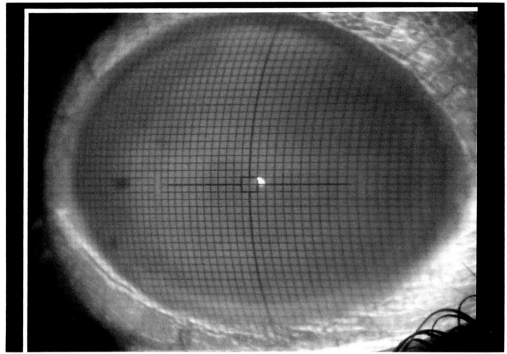

Figure 8-4. Fluorescence image. Note complete coverage of cornea by projected grid.

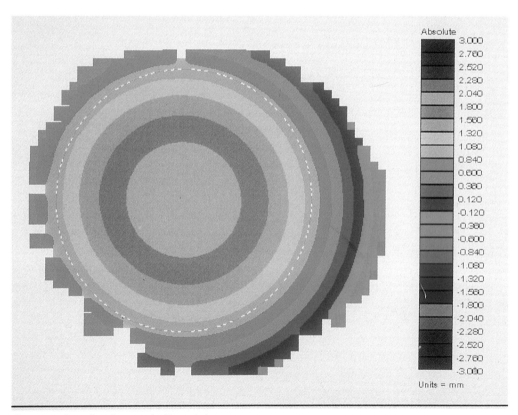

Figure 8-5. Raw elevation map for Figure 8-4.

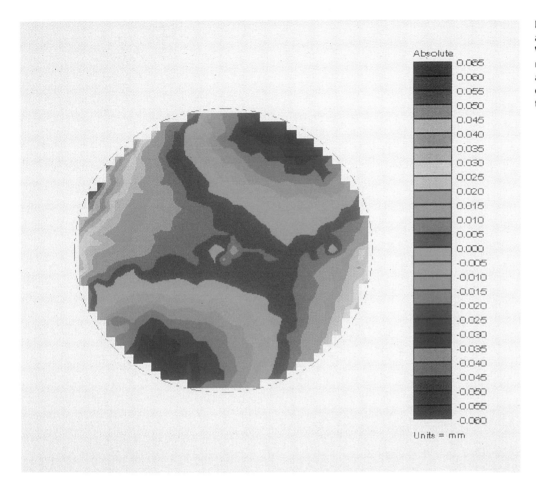

Figure 8-6. Elevation map using average sphere as reference. Warm colors (reds and yellows) represent elevations above the average sphere, and cooler colors (blues and violets) elevations below the average sphere.

The refractive properties of the cornea at a particular point can be accurately described only by determining how an incident ray is bent either toward or away from the normal to the surface, in accordance with Snell's law. The direction of the normal at a point can be determined only from knowledge of the true topography, i.e., elevation data, at that point. The PAR system is able to produce accurate elevation data, and offers a unique potential for generating far more accurate characterizations of corneal refractive properties than those currently available.

The ability of the CTS to generate accurate topographical information is rooted in a rigorous calibration procedure. This procedure enables the system to model the optical system and correct for various optical distortions. The optical design is very flexible and can be configured to operate over a wide range of working distances, permitting its adaptation to a wide variety of slit lamps and operating microscopes.

CTS DESIGN FEATURES

The rasterstereographic approach taken by PAR in the CTS design provides several inherent advantages and improvements over other corneal topography technologies.

Ability to measure true topography. The elevation data provided by the PAR system are unique in that they permit the generation of a precise, accurate, three-dimensional model of the cornea. In addition to the advantages described above relating to refractive power calculations, true topography represents an important tool in photorefractive surgery using excimer lasers. Since laser sculpting ultimately takes place in the elevation domain, the PAR CTS is the natural tool for specifying, predicting, and measuring the effects of laser ablation.

Coverage of the entire corneal surface. The PAR CTS can measure the surface topography of the entire corneal surface from limbus to limbus with uniform accuracy. The area of coverage includes the central optical zone and in some instances portions of the sclera.

Flexible optical configurations. The CTS technology allows for extremely flexible optical design. Because it is not limited by the fundamental geometric constraints imposed by reflectance-based systems, the CTS optical design is very compact and flexible. The system can be configured to match the working distance of a number of different types of slit lamps, or can be constructed with longer working distances

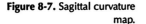

Figure 8-7. Sagittal curvature map.

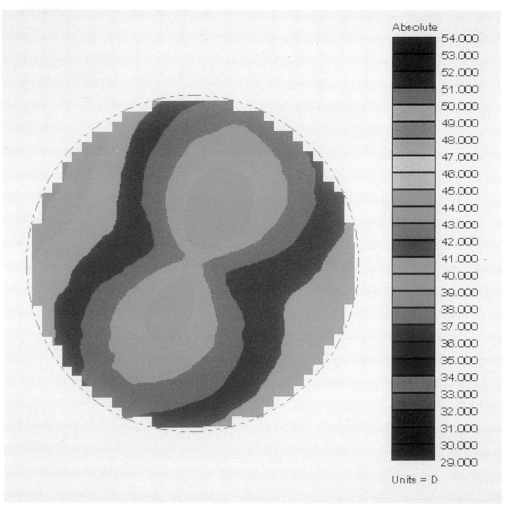

for use on operating microscopes. Both the working distance and the spacing of the projection and imaging systems can be modified for attachment to excimer laser systems, permitting a direct interconnection between the laser and topography system.

Ability to image irregular corneas. The PAR CTS measures surface elevation using a very robust rasterstereographic technique, and can accommodate large surface deviations. It can also be used on corneas which are non-reflective due to scarring, epithelial defects, or irregularities in shape.

Instantaneous image acquisition. The CTS captures all of the required image data from the cornea in approximately one millisecond (0.001 sec), using flash illumination. There is no possibility of significant eye movement during this period of time.

Ease of use. The CTS can measure the surface topography accurately regardless of the cornea's orientation relative to the instrument, as long as the grid is in focus. Visual alignment aids are provided to assure accurate definition of the line of sight and consistent orientation to permit comparison of multiple elevation models from the same cornea.

CLINICAL APPLICATIONS

The CTS is offered in configurations suited to ophthalmic diagnostic use, intraoperative use for either conventional ophthalmic surgery or photoablative procedures, and optometry screening and evaluation. Elevation and curvature maps indicative of a variety of clinical conditions are presented in the following.

Normal Cornea

Figure 8-9 shows an elevation map and sagittal curvature map for a normal cornea. The elevation map displays a band of relatively solid color along the 120° meridian. The astigmatism here is slight as indicated by the shallow drop off

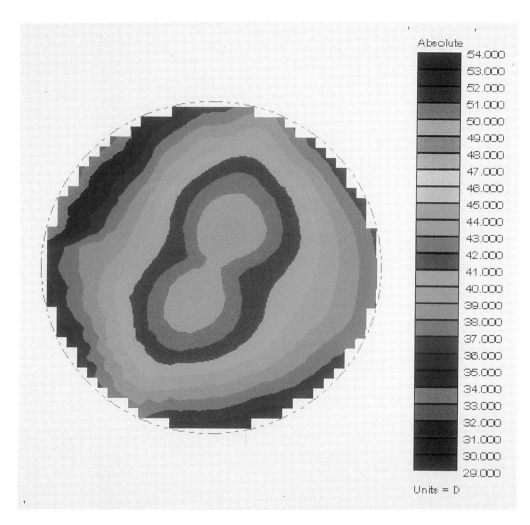

Figure 8-8. Tangential curvature map.

in the 50° meridian. Along this meridian there is only a 14 μm drop in elevation from the line of sight point to the 8 mm circle. The curvature map shows a hint of an astigmatic bowtie along the 50° meridian, and only a small amount (0.6 D) of oblique astigmatism.

Astigmatism

Figure 8-10 shows an elevation map and sagittal curvature map exhibiting about 2 D of astigmatism with the steep axis along the 90° meridian. The elevation map shows a consistent band of green running horizontally. The elevation

profile along the 90° meridian varies from -28 μm (4 mm superior) to +1 μm (line of sight) to -23 μm (4 mm inferior). The greater change in the upper half of the cornea will show as superior steepening. Horizontally, the elevation change is somewhat asymmetric with the nasal portion being somewhat higher and wider than the temporal. The curvature map shows a characteristic with-the-rule bowtie running along the 90° meridian. The superior half of the bowtie is wider and more prominent. Note the 41 D (dark green) area on the nasal side. This area of flatter curvature is caused by the higher elevations seen in this area of the elevation map.

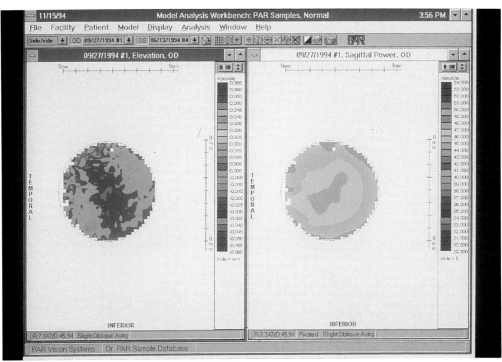

Figure 8-9. Elevation and curvature maps for normal cornea.

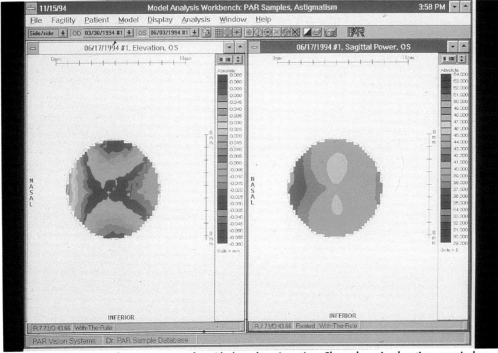

Figure 8-10. Elevation and curvature maps for with-the-rule astigmatism. Sharp drops in elevation superiorly and inferiorly correspond to lobes of highest curvature.

Keratoconus

The elevation map in Figure 8-11 shows a prominent central cone, located just inferotemporally from the line of sight point. The map shows the cone to be circular, and with a diameter of about 3.5 mm. The apex of the cone is about 80 μm above the surrounding cornea, and is about 1.3 mm from the line of sight. The curvature map shows the steepest area of the cornea to fall between the actual apex of the cornea and the line of sight. Another cone, shown in Figure 8-12, is widely spread and located inferotemporally from the line of sight. Also present is some oblique astigmatism indicated by the blue band along the 45° meridian. The cone is 3 mm wide and 5 mm long and also follows the 45° meridian. The apex of the cone is more than 90 μm higher than the surrounding cornea. In the curvature map the location of the cone is misrepresented because of the combined effects of the cone and the oblique astigmatism. The steepest area of the cornea is in the superotemporal quadrant, but the elevation map shows that the cone is actually located in the inferotemporal quadrant. While the steepest area of the cornea is correctly identified in the curvature map, this area does not coincide with the location of the cone.

Post-Radial Keratotomy

Figure 8-13 shows a post-radial keratotomy (RK) fluorescence image. Note how the cuts appear prominently in the image; they do not, however, interfere with the extraction of elevation data. The elevation map (Figure 8-14) shows a characteristic doughnut shape with a prominent gap at 90.° This area of undercorrection is most probably due to incomplete healing of that incision. From the black and white image (see Figure 8-13) you can see that the end of that incision is somewhat spread. Two lobes of higher elevation can be seen horizontally, about 50 μm higher than the central depression. The curvature map shows a with-the-rule astigmatism pattern with areas of flattening corresponding to the horizontal lobes of raised elevation. The steepest area of the cornea corresponds to the depressed area of the doughnut that appears at 90.°

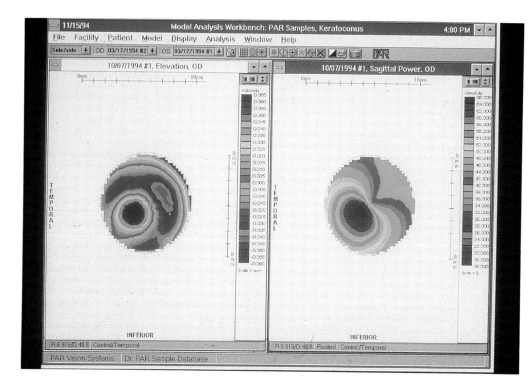

Figure 8-11. Elevation and curvature maps for keratoconus. Diameter and height are readily measurable from the elevation map.

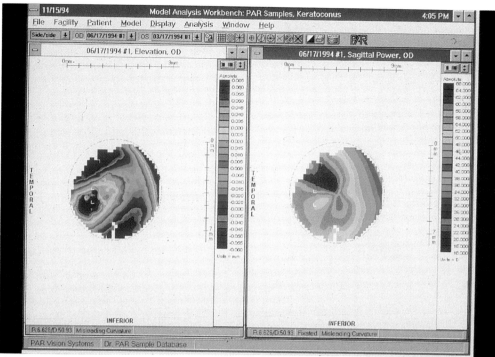

Figure 8-12. Elevation and curvature maps for keratoconus with oblique astigmatism. Note that in the curvature map the location of the cone is not accurately represented because of the presence of the astigmatism.

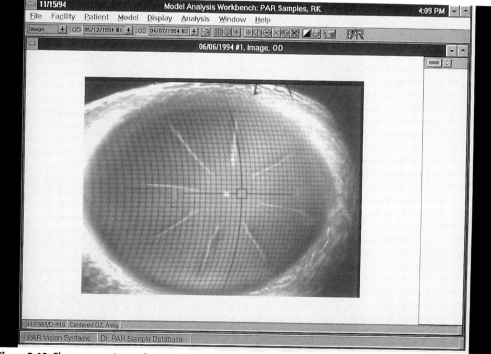

Figure 8-13. Fluorescence image for post-RK. Incisions are readily discernible but do not interfere with extraction of elevation data.

Post-Automated Lamellar Keratoplasty

The elevation map in Figure 8-15 shows the characteristic doughnut shape with a central depression that is well aligned on the line-of-sight point. This central depression results from the removal of corneal tissue by the refractive pass of the keratome. Note the area of higher elevation on the nasal edge of the central depression, corresponding to the hinge of the automated lamellar keratoplasty (ALK) cap. Also note that the area of depression, while well aligned on the line-of-sight point, is not perfectly circular. There is a small degree of vertical elongation of the depression, which will result in some localized against-the-rule astigmatism within the 4 mm circle. Note that this corresponds to the area covered by the central depression. The curvature map shows an area of against-the-rule astigmatism with slight inferior flattening (40.8 D), which shows as a green "bowtie" with a blue inferior lobe. Note that this pattern is fairly limited to the 4 mm circle. Overall, the map shows slight superior and inferior steepening beyond 6 mm.

Intraoperative Topography

Preliminary studies have suggested that CTS topographic measurements obtained immediately following penetrating keratoplasty can be used effectively in suture adjustment to minimize postoperative astigmatism. Other users have demonstrated the measurement of topography immediately after RK, ALK, and astigmatic keratotomy.

Figure 8-16 shows preoperative elevation and sagittal curvature maps for an ALK patient. Note the irregular astigmatism with bowtie pattern extending from 90° to 300°. The elevation and curvature maps in Figure 8-17 were obtained intraoperatively immediately after replacing the flap. Note the prominent central flattening. Figure 8-18 shows the same eye about 1 week postoperative. There is some nasal shift in the flattest part of the cornea but the maximum amount of correction is still about 10 D.

Excimer Photorefractive Keratectomy

A very important application of CTS is measurement of topography of the cornea immediately after photorefractive keratectomy (PRK).[8] The applications of this capability include assessment of the effects of re-epithelialization on corneal topography, and precise measurement of the ablation process by comparison of pre- and post-ablation topography.

Figure 8-19 shows fluorescence images before and after PRK, with the post-PRK image clearly showing the edge of

the ablation zone. Corresponding pre- and post-ablation elevation maps obtained with the CTS are shown in Figure 8-20. Raw elevation profiles along a horizontal meridian through the apex were extracted from each map and are plotted in Figure 8-21. Here the dotted line represents the pre-ablation profile, and the solid line the post-ablation profile. The ablation protocol consisted of 500 pulses with a fixed 6 mm aperture. The expected ablation depth in this case is 100 μm.

The difference between the pre- and post-ablation profiles can be computed to obtain the actual achieved ablation depth, shown in Figure 8-22. This result reveals that the expected depth of 100 μm was obtained at the edges of the zone, but that the central depth was about 80 μm.

In addition to direct measurement of the post-PRK topography and verification that the desired ablation profile was achieved, elevation-based topography data can be used in a variety of other ways including:

- Measurement of beam uniformity and ablation rate via topographic analysis of test surfaces subjected to a predefined ablation protocol
- Simulation of a proposed ablation protocol, using the preoperative topography, the beam characteristics, and the predicted ablation profile to calculate the postoperative topography and refractive properties
- Measurement of ablation depth part way through a procedure to verify the ablation rate and adjust the treatment protocol if necessary
- Preoperative measurement of irregular corneas and definition of the optimal ablation protocol to attain the desired end effect.

Optometry

Optometric diagnostic applications of CTS are similar to the ophthalmic diagnostic uses described above, with perhaps a stronger emphasis on contact lens fitting. In addition, the increased sharing of patient care responsibilities between MDs and ODs in the managed care environment of the future will create a demand for highly flexible networking capabilities for topography systems, so that these two groups of caregivers can share data and more easily consult on individual cases. The powerful computing and communication capabilities incorporated into the CTS design and its implementation within a standard Windows® environment place it in an advantageous position to meet these future needs.

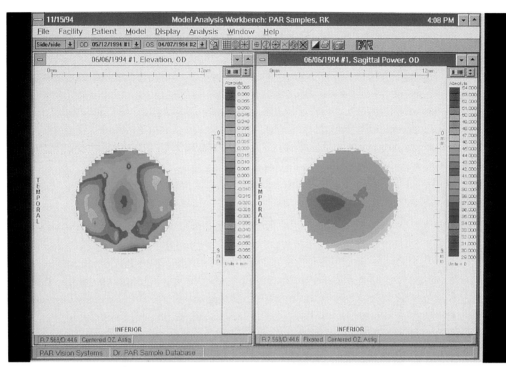

Figure 8-14. Elevation and curvature maps, post-RK. Central flattening is readily apparent in both maps.

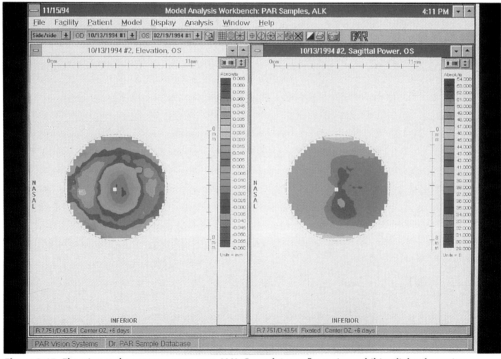

Figure 8-15. Elevation and curvature maps, post-ALK. Central 4 mm flat region exhibits slight elongation.

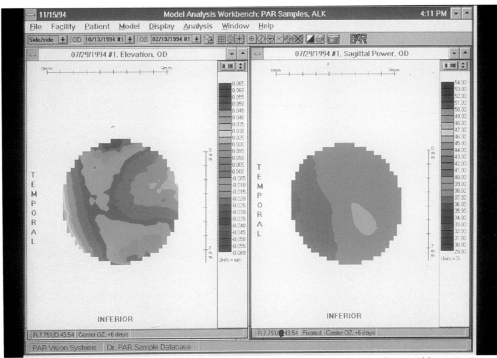

Figure 8-16. Preoperative elevation and curvature maps for ALK patient. *Courtesy of Jon Dishler, MD, Denver, CO.*

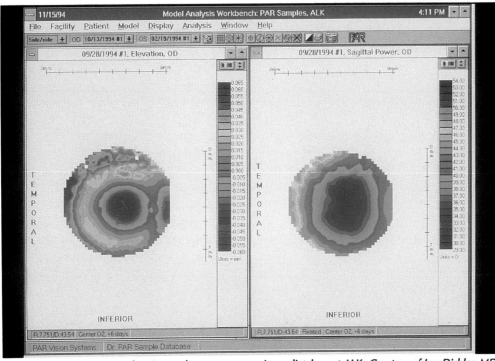

Figure 8-17. Intraoperative elevation and curvature maps immediately post-ALK. *Courtesy of Jon Dishler, MD, Denver, CO.*

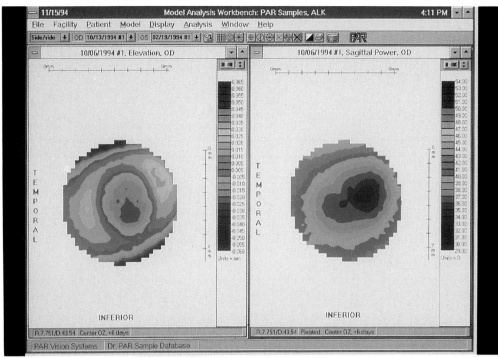

Figure 8-18. Elevation and curvature maps 1 week post-ALK. *Courtesy of Jon Dishler, MD, Denver, CO.*

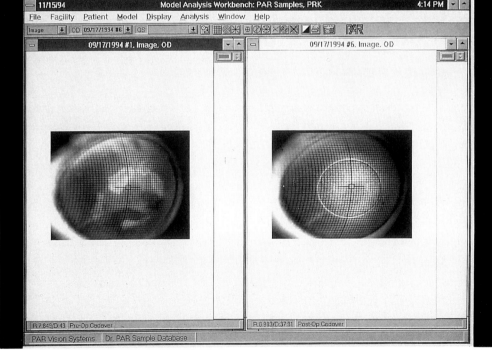

Figure 8-19. Fluorescence images, pre- and post-PRK.

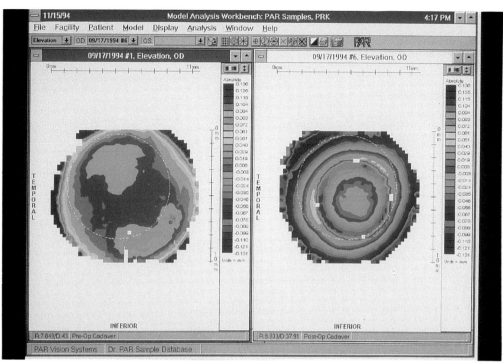

Figure 8-20. Elevation maps, pre- and post-PRK.

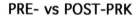

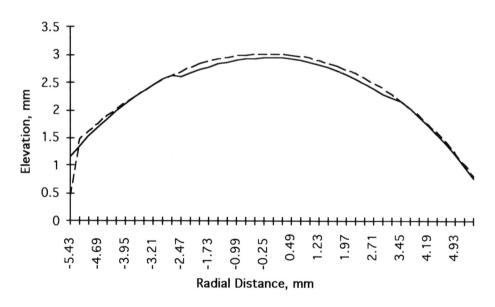

Figure 8-21. CTS elevation profiles, pre-ablation (dotted line) and post-ablation (solid line).

Figure 8-22. CTS ablation profile.

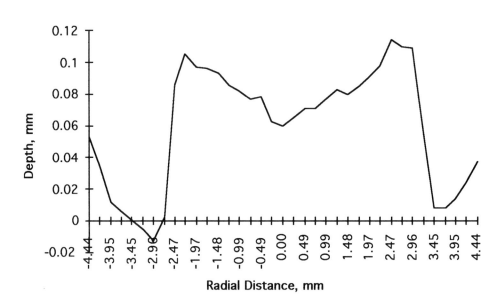

Ablation Profile

FUTURE GROWTH

The PAR Corneal Topography System is designed and implemented to permit easy growth and expansion as new functions are added and existing functions enhanced. The CTS is implemented within a state-of-the-art Object Oriented Program System, specifically designed to permit rapid and efficient implementation of new functions with minimal impact on existing software. PAR is committed to the ongoing support of CTS as new clinical applications are identified and existing functions are expanded and improved.

REFERENCES

1. Warnicki J, Rehkopf P, Curtin S, et al. Corneal topography using computer analyzed rasterstereographic images. *Appl Opt.* 1988;27:1135-1140.
2. Belin M, Litoff D, Strods S, et al. The PAR Technology Corneal Topography System. *Refract Corneal Surg.* 1992;8:88-96.
3. Arffa R, Warnicki J, Rehkopf P. Corneal topography using rasterstereography. *Refract Corneal Surg.* 1989;5:414-417.
4. Belin M, Zloty P. Accuracy of the PAR Corneal Topography System with spatial misalignment. *CLAO J.* 1993;19:64-68.
5. Applegate RA. Comment on "Characterization of the inherent error in a spherically-biased corneal topography system in mapping a radially aspheric surface." *Refract Corneal Surg.* 1994;10:113-114.
6. Mandell R. The enigma of the corneal contour. *CLAO J.* 1992;18:267-589.
7. Roberts C. The accuracy of "power" maps to display curvature data in corneal topography systems. *Invest Ophthalmol Vis Sci.* 1994;35:3525-3532.
8. Belin M. Intraoperative raster photogrammetry—the PAR Corneal Topography System. *J Cataract Refract Surg.* 1993;19(suppl):188-192.

THE TOMEY TECHNOLOGY/COMPUTED ANATOMY TMS-1 VIDEOKERATOSCOPE

Michael K. Smolek, PhD
Stephen D. Klyce, PhD

The Tomey Technology/Computed Anatomy TMS-1 topographic modeling system is an integrated videokeratoscope (VKS) and videokeratograph analysis instrument designed for clinical diagnosis and research. Its predecessor, the Corneal Modeling System,[1,2] was the first commercially available VKS and incorporated the color-coded contour map developed by Maguire et al.[3] The TMS instrument is composed of several hardware components, namely the VKS unit, the VKS Light Cone, the central computer (an IBM-compatible, tower-based personal computer), a high resolution color monitor, and a color printer. Version 1.6 of the software package is currently available for use with the instrument. As in previous versions of the software, an image is acquired from the VKS, analyzed, and a color-coded contour map is generated to show the relative distribution of dioptric powers across the cornea. Several display schemes are available to suit the needs or preferences of the user. The software also incorporates several new clinical applications of the information derived from the analysis, primarily to assist the corneal surgeon in planning or assessing the outcomes of various keratorefractive procedures.

HARDWARE

The main VKS unit contains the Light Cone illumination system, the video camera, the laser illumination system for the corneal rangefinder, and the operator's console. The unit is located atop a motorized ophthalmic examination table with an adjustable patient headrest. The operator's console has a 5-inch black and white monitor which provides the user with a view of the patient's cornea along the optical axis of the instrument for the purpose of alignment, focusing, and mire inspection. The operator's joystick, the VKS unit

vertical height adjustment, and the monitor contrast adjustment are easily controlled from the console position. The Light Cone is a patented, solid-state device that easily attaches to the VKS unit, and is available as two separate modules for either normal use or contact lens analysis. The DOS-based personal computer contains a high quality 80486 motherboard with an Intel CPU, floppy disk and hard disk drive, a mass storage device such as an Iomega Bernoulli® drive, and various I/O boards for controlling the TMS-1 video camera as well as the color monitor and printer. The storage components and memory of the computer are upgradable according to the needs of the user. The color monitor displays a 256-color SVGA image of the system software screens and images of the processed TMS-1 videokeratographs. The software provides drivers for IBM PaintJet-compatible printers.

THE PRINCIPLES OF VIDEOKERATOSCOPY

The basic principles of videokeratoscopy are illustrated by the physical laws of geometric optics for the formation of an image by a convex, spherical mirror (Figure 9-1). A diminished, erect, virtual image is formed behind the reflecting surface (ie, the anterior surface of the cornea), and the relative size and position of the image can be demonstrated through ray tracing. A light ray drawn from a point on the object toward the focal point of the mirror, F, is reflected from the mirror surface along a path parallel to the optic axis of the mirror. A second ray drawn from the same object point toward the center of curvature of the surface, C, is reflected back along the same path. The intersection of these ray paths in virtual space behind the mirror surface indicates the relative location of the image. "Steeper" surfaces of higher curvature (i.e., a shorter radius of curvature) form virtual

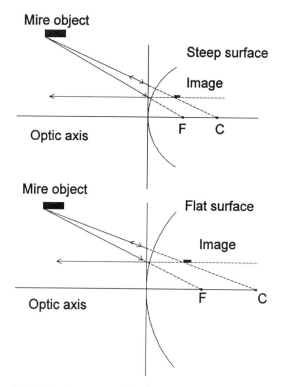

Figure 9-1. Reflection at a curved surface.

images that are smaller and closer to the optic axis, compared to "flatter" surfaces. Therefore, the mires of a keratometer (ophthalmoscope) or of a VKS will appear smaller and compressed toward the central cornea along the steep meridians of the cornea. It is the size and/or displacement of the image of the illuminated mires from the optic axis of the instrument that are the basis for corneal power calculation.[4]

It should be pointed out that the anterior corneal surface is not the surface being measured by reflected light. Rather, it is the air/tear film interface on the anterior corneal surface that acts as a polished, convex mirror surface (reflectance of approximately 2.5%). However, it is generally assumed that one can speak interchangeably of the anterior cornea surface as the surface being measured, and the calculation used to derive the corneal power is adjusted to account for the optical effects of the tear film. Also note that these devices have been designed to extrapolate total corneal power, rather than reporting only the anterior surface power of the cornea.[5]

THE VKS LIGHT CONE

In the Tomey/Computed Anatomy TMS-1 VKS, the back-illuminated mires are generated within a compact, truncated, cone-shaped projection system. This Light Cone also incorporates integrated lightguides for a laser rangefinder system (Figures 9-2 and 9-3). The bulk of the VKS cone is formed by a solid, transparent material with a central hollow tube lined with a series of black annular rings of specific width and spacing. Toward the camera end of the cone are several additional concentric rings on a flat plate, which project the mire pattern onto the most apical (ie, central) portions of the cornea. Early forms of the photokeratoscope and VKS were hampered by a lack of mire rings in the central region of the cornea. However the TMS-1 produces rings that are sufficient in covering the entire corneal surface.

Light produced by lamps within the VKS unit is directed into the base of the cone, which back-illuminates the mire targets. The diffusion coating on the interior of the cone and the translucent qualities of the central tube help provide even

Figure 9-2. Horizontal cross-section schematic of the TMS-1 Light Cone.® Patients are instructed to direct their sight into the truncated end of the cone and fixate a spot located in the center of a flat plate with additional annular rings. The operator of the TMS-1 aligns and focuses the video image by moving the entire optical system relative to the patient's cornea. Laser light travels along two lightguides oriented toward a point near the apex of the cone, and the operator adjusts the rangefinder system relative to the cornea to ensure proper focus of the mires.

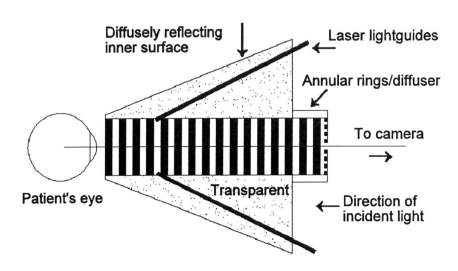

illumination from the most apical to the most limbal mires. A schematic representation of the mire image pattern on the corneal surface is shown in Figure 9-4. The most peripheral mire image is produced by the illuminated outer edge near the apex of the truncated cone, while the central point of the bull's eye pattern is the reflected image of the fixation point. Other VKSs utilize larger Placido imagers; peripheral portions of the mires of these units may be masked by the brow ridge or the nose of the patient. Two interchangeable Light Cones are available for the TMS-1: the "A" cone has 25 rings and is used for normal operation, while the optional "B" cone has 31 rings and is required when using the VKS for contact lens fitting. Two hundred fifty-six points around each ring are acquired during image processing and used for software analysis.

The integrated laser lightguides used for rangefinding are embedded in the transparent cone material along the horizontal plane, and are permanently oriented to converge two small light beams to a point in space located approximately 3.2 mm from the edge of the VKS cone and along the optical axis of the VKS (see Figure 9-3). It is important to note that the intersection of these two beams does not occur at the anterior surface of the cornea when the instrument is properly focused, but at a point located 0.165 mm within the cornea.[6] The focusing criterion employed by the TMS-1 system is the same optical sectioning principle found with the operation of a biomicroscope slit lamp. Thus, the rangefinder uses the smallest possible backscattered image of the cornea in cross-section as the criteria for the TMS-1 operator to determine the best focus of the instrument.

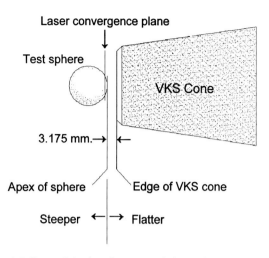

Figure 9-3. Determining best focus in a solid test sphere. The VKS laser rangefinder is designed to correctly focus the TMS-1 by taking advantage of the corneal tissue's light scattering ability and its relatively consistent stromal thickness. If incorrectly used with a solid, optically opaque, or highly transparent test surface, the laser convergence plane would be imaged at the anterior surface of the test surface, rather than within the material. If the test surface is mounted progressively further from the VKS cone, it will appear to become progressively more steep, particularly in the periphery. If the surface is mounted too close to the light cone, the surface will be analyzed as flatter than its true shape. By mounting the test sphere on a micrometer stage that can be adjusted along the length of the optical axis of the instrument, the operator can first focus (incorrectly) on the test surface. Then the surface can be retracted away from the cone by a distance of 0.165 mm to achieve correct focus. Alternatively, the test surface can be set to a distance of 3.175 mm from the plane defined by the edge of the VKS cone.

ALIGNMENT AND FOCUS OF THE TMS-1

The alignment and focus of a VKS are critical aspects of its operation. First, the patient's head must be aligned correctly with the VKS Light Cone to achieve acquisition of the maximum possible area of the cornea and to facilitate proper focusing of the mire image. A good approach is to have patients turn their head several degrees toward the direction of the eye not being imaged, so that their direction of gaze is slightly toward their temporal direction. For most individuals, the head is positioned fully forward in the headrest, with the chinrest adjusted until the patient's eyes are aligned with the red mark on the headrest frame. However, if a patient has deeply set orbits, the examination table must be raised so that the top of their head tilts back slightly from the forehead cushion.

Pressing the joystick button once turns on the illumination and video systems for 60 seconds. The central cornea should be clearly visible in the black and white monitor, and the image of the mires relatively centered on the cornea. The position of the TMS-1 unit or the patient's head may have to be adjusted until the mire image appears to be approximately centered within the area of the cornea. Next, the patient is instructed to carefully fixate the central spot of light in the bull's eye pattern while keeping the head motionless. Patients should be told to blink normally, but to open their eyelids as wide as possible between blinks. It is good practice to always acquire as large an area of the cornea as possible for analysis, because the percent of analyzed area is a useful corneal index when interpreting topography patterns. Precise alignment must now be performed by the operator superimposing the electronic crosshairs, the reflected image of the fixation source on the cornea, and the laser beams (Figures 9-4 through 9-6). Although the cornea now may be aligned properly with the instrument, correct analysis of the cornea's curvature requires proper focusing as well. If the crosshairs are well centered, but the laser beams are not coincident with the crosshairs, the captured image will be out of focus (Figure 9-5). The operator moves the joystick until the two laser scatter spot images are exactly coincident with the crosshairs,

Figure 9-4. Schematic illustration of the unaligned, unfocused view of the corneal mire image as seen in the monochrome console monitor. The anterior view of the eye and the iris are not illustrated for clarity. The operator must observe that the mire image rings are complete, and the fixation image is present in the center of the mire pattern.

Two images of the laser lightguides exits will be visible, but are not to be confused with the laser light spots caused by the backscatter of light from within the corneal stroma. Also, light scattered from the iris by the laser beams should not be confused with the stromal scatter. Electronically generated crosshairs within a small box will be visible at the center of the monitor, but are not visible to the patient.

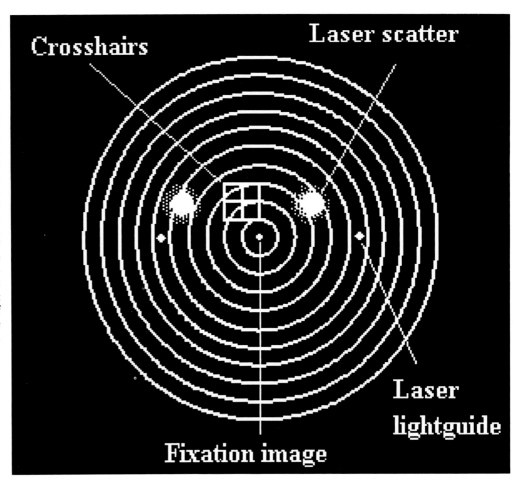

and are at their smallest diameter (Figure 9-6). This process is facilitated by proper instructions to the patient to fixate diligently, having the patient blink to refresh the tear film layer, and by a high level of expertise by the operator gained through practice. The key to high quality videokeratographs is in the hands of the operator; these individuals should be fully trained and always cognizant of the alignment and focus processes.

To improve the chances of capturing the best possible image, the TMS-1 software allows up to four videos of each exam to be taken and stored in succession. The operator can process all or select only the best image for processing. The operator should carefully examine the continuity and focus of the mire images; the rings should not touch one another, except in cases of extremely distorted corneal surfaces. Incomplete mire images occurring with otherwise apparently normal corneas are usually indicative of a tear film deposit, or the breakup of the tear film layer. Patients should blink fully before taking the picture to refresh the tear film. Accidental involuntary motion such as blinks or fixation nystagmus during the image capture should be guarded against; blurred images should be recaptured. The operator also should be

aware of the appearance of tear film pooling in the inferior margin of the cornea, and avoid using these images for analysis. For this reason, it is best to immediately process the mire images and examine the corneal curvature contour patterns while the patient remains seated for additional videos, if necessary.

Research applications of the TMS-1 with artificial corneal surfaces require more elaborate procedures to achieve proper focus. If the test surface is located too far from the VKS cone, the surface (particularly the peripheral margin) will tend to appear too steep, while a test surface located too close to the VKS cone appears too flat (see Figure 9-3). As most test surfaces will be composed of either opaque or highly transparent materials of various thicknesses, the appearance of best focus to the operator (ie, the point producing the smallest light scatter spot) will not occur at the proper distance of the surface from the VKS cone. *Thus, the image in the console monitor cannot be used to determine proper focus.* When test surfaces are used, best control over focus can be obtained by mounting the surface on a three-dimensional motion controller with micrometer resolution, particularly along the optic axis of the VKS. For

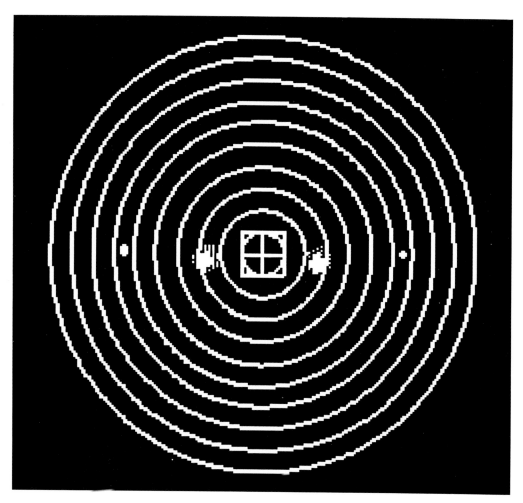

Figure 9-5. Aligned, but unfocused view of the corneal mire image. The fixation point and the mire image have been aligned by movement of the joystick and the vertical height adjustment of the VKS. However, the stromal scatter spots are not aligned to the crosshairs, indicating that the VKS remains unfocused. A photo acquired at this stage will not be properly analyzed.

example, one can focus the instrument based on the smallest spot size criterion, and then use the micrometer setting to move the test surface 0.165 mm closer to the VKS cone. As shown in Figure 9-3, the apical point of an in-focus, test surface should be located 3.175 mm from the edge of the VKS cone, regardless of the size of the laser spots to the operator.[7]

USE OF THE TMS-1 SOFTWARE

The main menu of the TMS-1 computer monitor display lists the basic selections for operation and data management. Version 1.6 of the Computed Anatomy software includes the following categories: History/Pictures, Single Displays, Multiple Displays, Process Photos, Utilities, File Handling, Applications, and Quick-Pix. The new Quick-Pix category is a macro utility to automate procedures ordinarily made by the operator. Access to all software features can be made by either use of a mouse pointing device or by the keyboard.

The first step for taking a video requires choosing item 1 of the opening menu: patient history and pictures. A window of blank input fields is displayed requiring keyboard input to fill in the empty data fields. This information includes in the order of their input: last name, first name, address (two lines), clinic ID#, date (automatically displayed), refraction, social security number, Snellen best-corrected visual acuity (BCVA), date of birth, exam number (automatically incremented), eye (OD or OS), sex, diagnosis, group, operator, and institution (automatically displayed).

Good data management and the best use of the instrument would suggest that most if not all of these inputs should be filled in by the operator prior to acquiring the videokeratograph; however, only the eye selection is mandatory. When performing exams of both eyes for the same patient, pressing the F5 function key redisplays the previous exam information. The operator then must make changes in only a few items, such as the eye, BCVA, etc., before proceeding to taking the picture. Pressing F9 completely deletes a field's input. Pressing F1, the Help function key, displays a brief description of entering and editing the patient history section fields.

After completing the history section, the software automatically opens the picture acquisition window. Up to

Figure 9-6. Aligned and focused view of the mire image. The crosshairs are aligned with the fixation point, and the corneal scatter spots of the two laser beams are aligned with the crosshairs and are at their minimum diameter. The operator should make a final check of mire image quality, and completeness of coverage into the periphery. A final full blink by the patient may be needed to refresh the tear film layer before taking the photo.

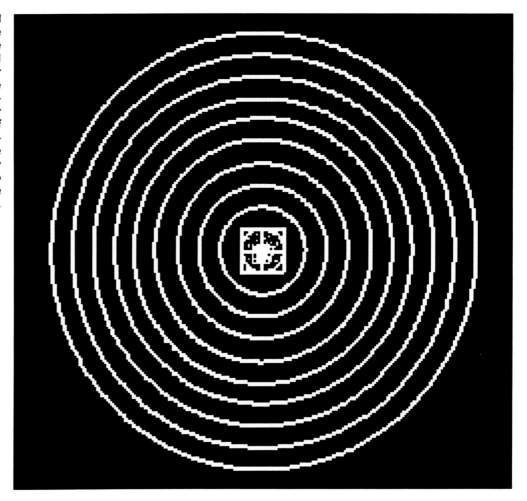

four videos can be taken for a given exam, and these are displayed in sequence across the central part of the screen. Below the video images is the indicator for the VKS cone that should be currently installed on that machine. If the incorrect cone is installed, or if the software setting (found in the Setup submenu of the TMS-1 Utilities category) is incorrect for the cone, the image will not be processed correctly.

Pressing the joystick button causes the monochrome monitor on the operating console of the VKS unit to display a real-time view through the video camera. On the computer color monitor, a 60-second countdown is displayed on the right-hand side of the screen. If a picture is not taken by depressing the joystick button a second time, the VKS illumination system will shut down to prevent deterioration of the lamps and the laser rangefinder system. After acquiring the desired image and checking focus and mire continuity, the image can be processed by following the instructions on the screen. After processing, the image can be displayed in any one of several display formats. These display options can be accessed at any later time through the main menu.

SINGLE MAP DISPLAYS

The second selection from the main menu of the TMS-1 is the single photo display, which allows the results to be presented using any one of three different dioptric scale options. Figure 9-7 shows the absolute scale which is the most clinically useful.[8] The central portion of the dioptric scale is divided into 1.5 D steps, and the extreme limits of the scale are divided into 5 D steps. The entire range of the absolute scale is from 9.0 to 101.5 D in 26 color-coded steps ranging from "cold" to "hot" colors of the spectrum. This range includes virtually all corneal powers ordinarily observed in a clinical situation.

Figure 9-8 shows the normalized scale that takes the extreme power limits of the cornea under test and subdivides this range into 10 steps with a minimum of 0.4 D of bin resolution. The example shown here has the corneal contours between 37.5 to 42.5 D divided into 0.5 D steps. The normalized scale enhances the small dioptric scale details on the contour map, but has certain limitations. For example, it is difficult to compare two maps, because the color bins no

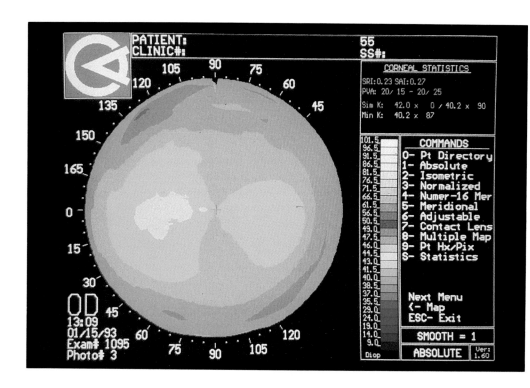

Figure 9-7. Single map—absolute scale display. A single photo TMS-1 display is dominated by the appearance of the corneal contour map visible in the central field. The absolute color-coded scale with "hot" to "cold" spectrally dispersed colors is seen to the immediate right of the contour map, while the applied scale can be confirmed by the label field shown in the lower right corner of the screen. The absolute scale ranges from 9.0 to 101.5 D with the central portion of the range in 1.5 D steps, and the extreme limits of the range in 6.0 D steps. The smoothness factor of the contour isobars is shown below the Help menu box. Note that the video image of the anterior aspect of the eye is switched on, with the contour map superimposed over it.

longer demarcate regions of specific powers. Second, it is difficult to communicate the power information to others without first explicitly pointing out and defining the color-coded dioptric scale in use on the map. Third, relevant information in the color-coded map may actually be lost in the complexity of the contour pattern.

Figure 9-9 further illustrates the difficulties associated with the normalized scale. If we were shown a daily temperature map of the United States, and we knew that the colors of each temperature isobar were absolutely fixed, we could easily appreciate the temperature differences across the nation at a glance, knowing that the scale has not changed from the previous day. On the other hand, if the temperature map used a normalized scale, the scale limits and step size would vary from day to day as the temperature extremes varied, and the bin coloration would also change. Not only is the normalized scale prone to misinterpretation, there is also a loss of convenience in using such a scale.

The final variation of single image displays is the adjustable scale. This display maintains 26 steps of equal intervals with a user adjustable lower starting limit of the dioptric powers and step size. For example, Figure 9-10 shows a starting power of 38 D with a step size of 0.4 D per contour. Application of this display requires some knowledge about the powers already present on the cornea, and usually some specific reason for choosing the starting power. One reason might be to graphically isolate all the high-powered

regions of a given cornea, since all corneal regions below the starting power would appear the same color. For example, one might wish to emphasize the area encompassed in keratoconus corneas for power-defined regions above a value of 50 D, and demonstrate how the area varies with the time course of the disease.

Figures 9-7, 9-8, and 9-10 also show other features of the single video TMS-1 display. Above the central map in Figure 9-10 is the header showing the patient name, institution name, clinical ID number, and patient social security number. In the lower left-hand corner of the video box is located the exam information for the eye (designated OS or OD), the time of the exam, the date of the exam, the exam number, and the photo number. In the upper right of the screen is a box showing either the corneal statistics (see Figure 9-10) or the current location and power information of the crosshair cursor, which is adjustable by mouse movement or keyboard control (see Figure 9-8). Note that the indices in the corneal statistics box are color-coded: green denotes a value in the normal range, yellow denotes a value between two and three standard deviations from the normal mean, and red indicates a value >3 standard deviations above the mean.

Below the statistics box is the Help menu window. The Help menu is always available in the displays by pressing the F1 function key. Pressing F1 once brings up the first Help menu that lists the function key path to various types of displays available for a single video. Pressing F1 a second

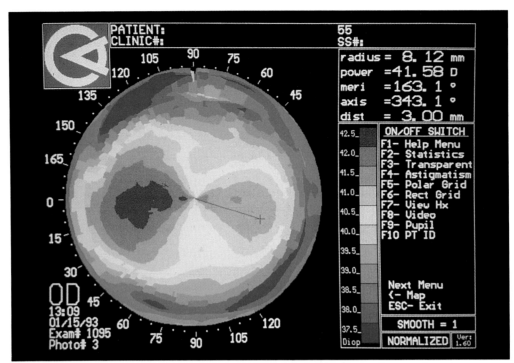

Figure 9-8. Single map—normalized scale display. The exam shown in this figure is the same shown in Figure 9-7, except the normalized scale is applied. Note the more complex appearance of the contour map. The normalized scale is automatically adjusted to show the range of powers present on the cornea in an eleven step, color-coded scale. Thus, if the range of powers is large, the steps will be necessarily large. The minimum step size that can be displayed is 0.4 D. In this figure, also note that the statistics box has been replaced with a cursor information or "score" box. The cursor crosshairs can be seen displaced along axis 343.1 at a distance of 3 mm from the central cornea in the map. Mouse movement or use of the keyboard arrows to move the cursor automatically updates the score box. The second menu of the Help function also is displayed.

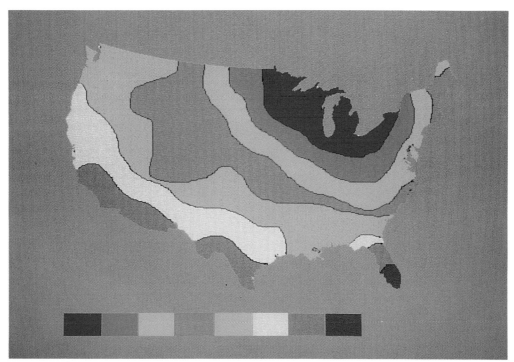

Figure 9-9. Absolute versus normalized scales. If the normalized scale were used with national weather maps, we would not know if the city of Chicago was suffering the effects of subzero cold, or enjoying a pleasantly warm day, unless we specifically examined the values associated with the color bins on the scale. On the other hand, the absolute scale never changes from day to day, and users would immediately know the temperature in Chicago or Miami without the need to refer to the color scale, daily. The same issue of scaling is a concern when deciding the best way to display and compare corneal topography maps.

Figure 9-10. Single map—adjustable scale display. The eye used in this figure is the same shown in Figures 9-7 and 9-8, although the exam number differs. The adjustable scale system is similar to the normalized scale, except that the starting power and the incremental step change of power are under the user's control. To the right of the contour map field, an input box is used to select the customized start and step parameters. Note the high level of contour detail that can be obtained in the map. The adjustable scale has the ability to reproduce the same exact scale for other exams, which facilitates comparisons. This figure also demonstrates the video background off option, and the patient header information has been turned off.

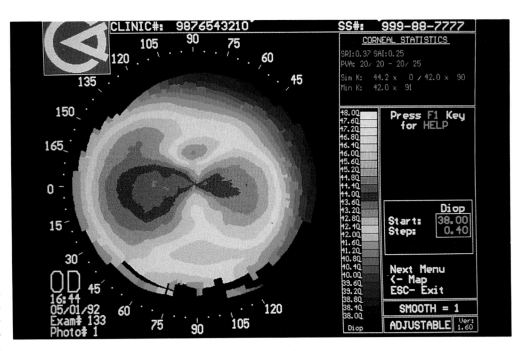

time brings up a Help menu of the function keys that switch options on and off within the display currently in view (see Figure 9-8). Pressing F1 a third time brings up a Help menu of additional functions that can be used to manipulate the display (Figure 9-11). In the lower right-hand corner of the single map display are indicators for the contour smoothness factor and the label of the diopter scale currently displayed.

The display option switches of the second Help menu control the following display features: F1 (Help menus), F2 (Statistics box), and F3 (Transparency view). With the transparency option, the video image of the cornea and the mires can be seen through a transparent image of the overlying contour colors (Figure 9-12). The F4 key controls the astigmatism axes option shown in Figures 9-13 through 9-15. Pressing F4 once draws orthogonal axis markers for the major and minor keratometry axes as determined by the TMS-1 software (see Figure 9-13). Pressing F4 a second time displays the instantaneously changing keratometry axes (see Figure 9-14). Pressing F4 a third time pulls up an overlay of the mean keratometry axes for a polar coordinate-based system centered on the fixation point for 3-, 5-, and 7-mm diameter zones (see Figure 9-15). Notice that the Help menu box changes to display detailed color-coded numerical information about power, meridian, and axis in each zone.

A similar polar coordinate system can be displayed without the keratometry axes by pressing F5 (Figure 9-16). If a Cartesian coordinate system is preferred, pressing F6 once overlays rectangular (X,Y) coordinate axes with a millimeter scale centered on the cornea (Figure 9-17). Pressing F6 a second time displays a complete X,Y grid. The F7 key returns the user to the patient history window, while the F8 key turns the background video on and off (see Figure 9-10). Pressing F9 displays an overlay of the machine interpreted location of the patient's pupil as determined from the pupil margin seen in the video image (see Figure 9-17). Users can confirm that the correct location of the pupil was made by the software interpretation by using the F8 key and the F3 key to view the video image. Finally, pressing F10 turns on and off the patient ID information located in the display header if patient confidentiality is needed.

The additional functions of the third Help window (see Figure 9-11) also include resetting the crosshair cursor (shift F5), adding a comment line to the display header (shift F10), printing a screen (ctrl-print screen), displaying a reversed map background (alt F3), and displaying a surgeon's inverted map (alt F1). Figure 9-18 shows both the reverse background and the surgeon's inverted view turned on. The inverted map displays the analogous view seen through a surgical micro-

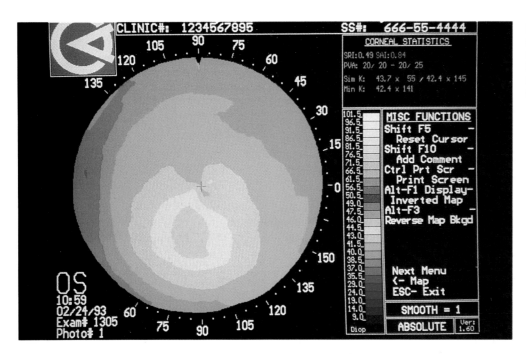

Figure 9-11. Single map—absolute scale display. The miscellaneous functions of the third Help menu are shown. Note the contour map indicative of the early stages of keratoconus.

scope from a surgeon's perspective, and has several fill boxes available for planning a surgical procedure. These boxes include the number of incisions and the optical zone for radial keratotomy (RK); the length, optical zone, and axis for astigmatic keratotomy (AK); and the pachymetry measurement (PAC) and blade setting (BLA).

Several additional single displays are available either via the single map selection menu, by the first Help menu, or by using the function keys. These include the isometric display in which the contour map is replaced by a color-coded relative power distribution plot (Figure 9-19). The 256 points in each ring are plotted against the meridian value, which shows the limits and median power tendency of the corneal power. A three-dimensional perspective display of this same data is also shown. The 16 meridian numeric display (Figure 9-20) replaces the contour map with representative color-coded corneal power values printed along 16 meridians of the cornea. A composite image display (Figure 9-21) incorporates the absolute scale isometric display, a color-coded absolute scale contour map, and an absolute color-coded wire mesh representation of the corneal surface. The meridional map display plots, in absolute scale, the dioptric power of the steep and flat keratometry meridians as a function of distance from the center of the cornea (Figure 9-22). The meridional display also plots the dioptric power difference of the steep and flat meridians versus the distance on the cornea in the lower half of the screen. The final single image display is the mean ring power table shown in Figure 9-23. The upper left-hand box displays the mean power for each ring, while the upper right-hand box displays patient information obtained from the patient history fields.

MULTIPLE MAP DISPLAYS

The TMS-1 also displays multiple images of either two, four, or six contour maps. This option can be very useful for comparing corneal topography from different patients with similar conditions, or topography from a single patient at different times. In the two-map display, (Figure 9-24), the contour plots are presented in the lower half of the screen, separated by a user selected absolute, normalized, or adjustable color-coded scale. In the upper left and upper right are the corneal statistics boxes for the two contour plots. Between the two statistics boxes is an information box for date of birth, refraction, diagnosis, and the group identity. This box is relevant only for the first eye image if maps from different individuals are displayed. Four and six map absolute color-coded displays are also available, but without corneal statistics (Figures 9-25 and 9-26, respectively).

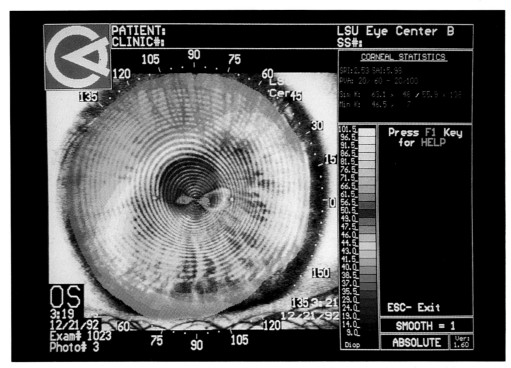

Figure 9-12. Single map—map transparency option. The underlying video image of an advanced keratoconus cornea and the VKS mire pattern can be seen with the overlying contour map colors displayed in a transparent mode. This option is useful for confirming the continuity of the mires associated with unusual powers seen in the contour map, or for examining the pupil location in the video image.

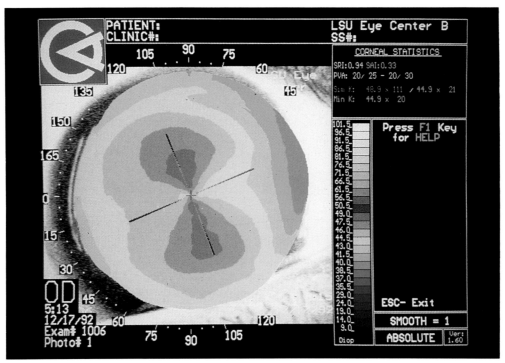

Figure 9-13. Single map—orthogonal astigmatism indicator. Pressing the F4 button once displays the a contour map overlay of the orthogonal major and minor keratometry cylinder axes determined from the TMS-1 analysis. The orthogonal axes will not be displayed if the cylinder power is < 0.2 D.

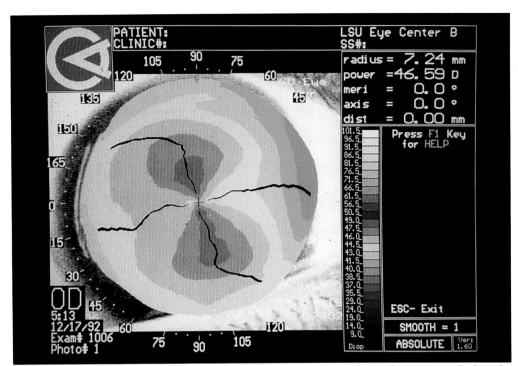

Figure 9-14. Single map—instantaneous astigmatism indicator. Pressing the F4 button twice displays the instantaneously changing contour map overlay of the major and minor keratometry cylinder axes. The cylinder axes are reanalyzed with increasing distance from the central cornea. If the keratometry cylinder is <1 D, the instantaneous axes will not be displayed. This display accentuates the lack of constant meridians for the keratometry axes.

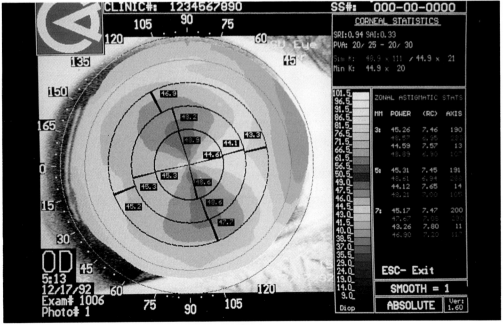

Figure 9-15. Single map—zonal axes astigmatism indicator.

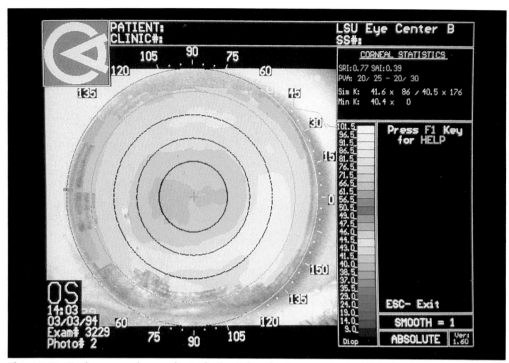

Figure 9-16. Single map—polar coordinate display. When the F5 button is pressed in the single photo display, a concentric polar coordinate ring pattern centered on the fixation point of the mire image will be displayed. The circles are set to 3, 5, 7, 9, and 11 mm in diameter. In this example, the axes are displayed on a contour map of a postoperative myopic photorefractive keratoplasty cornea.

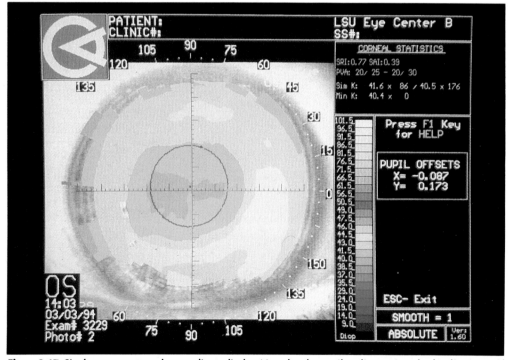

Figure 9-17. Single map—rectangular coordinate display. Note that the pupil outline option also has been turned on, and the pupil offset in millimeters of X and Y distance from the fixation center is shown in the Help box area.

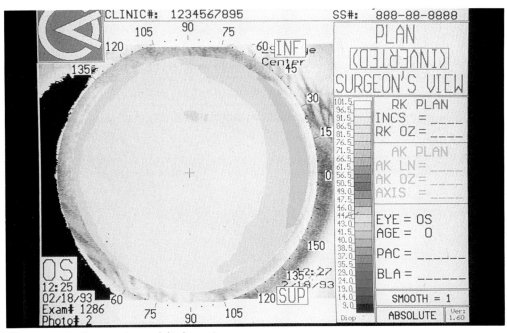

Figure 9-18. Single map—inverted display option.

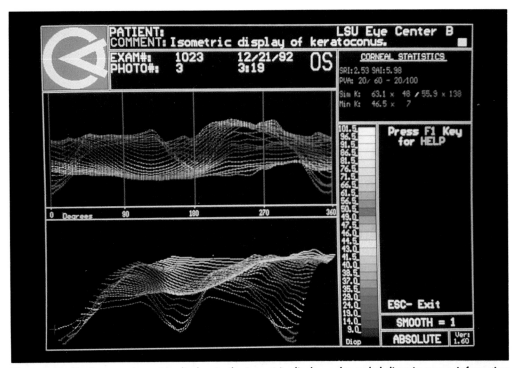

Figure 9-19. Single map—isometric display. In the isometric display, color-coded dioptric power information associated with 256 points along each ring of the VKS is plotted in a Cartesian coordinate system. This distorts the true physical relationships of the cornea, but emphasizes other aspects such as the limits and median value of corneal power, or the sinusoidal shape of the plot with cylinder power. In the upper graph, the power is plotted as a function of the meridian axis for all rings. In the lower plot, a perspective view of the same data is established to emphasize the spatial relationship of points among the rings, which is not evident in the first plot. In the example shown here, keratoconus is displayed. Note that the comment line for the header has been turned on.

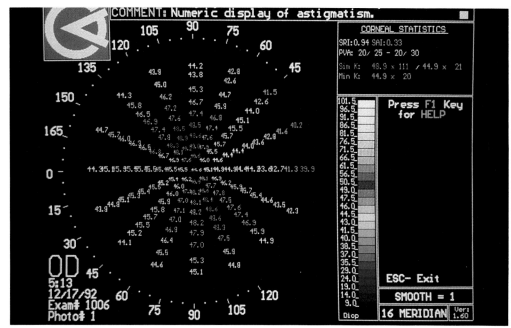

Figure 9-20. Single map—numeric format display. The power data in the color-coded contour map can be condensed into a numerical format. In version 1.6 of the TMS-1 software, 16 meridians are available. The numbers are color-coded according to the scale on the right, and the values represent power at that location to within one tenth of a diopter. If millimeters had been chosen in the TMS-1 setup menu, the values will be displayed as radii. This display is useful for making a permanent record of the power at numerous locations on the cornea with a better dioptric resolution than is possible with the contour map display.

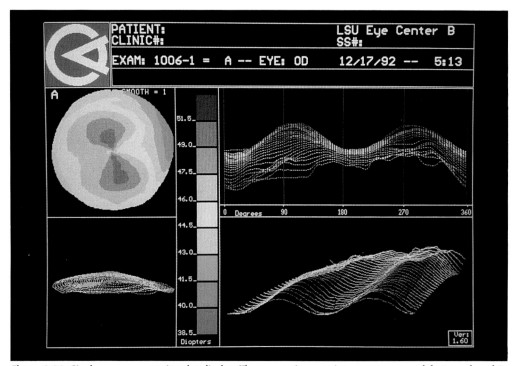

Figure 9-21. Single map—composite plot display. The composite map incorporates several features found in other TMS-1 displays. The color-coded wire frame mesh in the lower left corner of the screen is a three-dimensional perspective diagram of the absolute scale contour map above it. High powers are plotted up and low powers are plotted down in the wire mesh diagram. A true sphere would appear as a flat disk. An isometric display is shown on the right. The absolute color-coded scale is shown in the center of the screen. However the range of colors displayed is restricted to those actually found in the map.

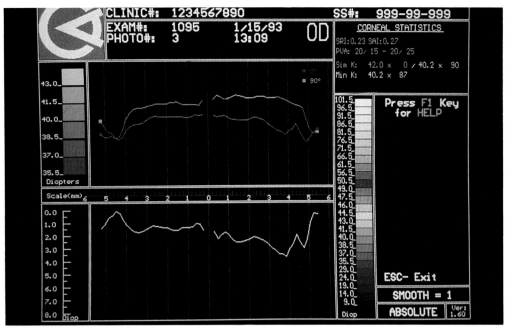

Figure 9-22. Single map—meridional display. The meridional display shows the change in curvature of the steep and flat meridians as a factor of distance from the central cornea in the upper plot box. The axes are distinguished by color-coded points at the ends of the two plots and a color-coded axis key. The plot lines are made up of a series of color-coded segments based on the range-limited absolute scale to the immediate left of the plot. A full range absolute scale is also provided on the right. The lower box shows the difference between the steep and flat meridians of the upper plot, using the difference scale to the left of the lower box.

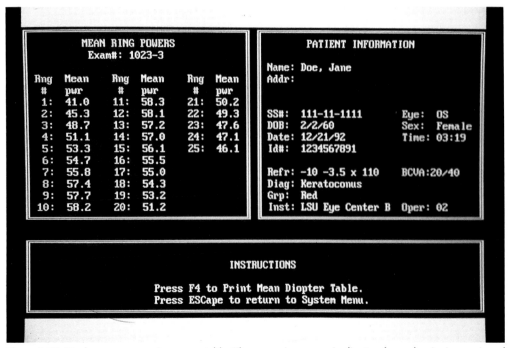

Figure 9-23. Single map—mean ring power table. The mean ring power in diopters for each mire image ring of the indicated exam is shown in a tabular format in the box on the left. To the right is a box with a summary of the patient history fields.

The differential map is an important feature of the multiple map display (Figure 9-27). An absolute scale is shown on the extreme left, adjacent to the two maps being compared (labeled A and B). On the right is the power difference contour map of the A and B maps. The color-coded difference scale is located near the top of the display. A supplemental screen is generated prior to displaying the differential map, and it shows the mean power difference in each ring for the two maps being compared (Figure 9-28). The differential map is most useful for comparing postsurgical changes in topography where the progression or remission of corneal surface power changes can have dramatic effects on the quality of visual acuity.

The TMS-1 software has numerous support utilities and file management capabilities accessible through the main menu. Of special interest to researchers is the data table utility that converts the binary data files of the TMS-1 into ASCII text files. Another useful utility is the TMS-1 personality setup. The system default settings can be altered to meet the needs of the user that do not ordinarily change between or during a given session, but may need to be changed for special tasks. These options are shown in Figure 9-29, and include the curvature display in either diopters or millimeters of radius, the degree scale as either an axis or a meridian measure, the cone type setting for normal or contact lens inclusive analysis, plus several additional options.

APPLICATIONS

Figure 9-30 shows the Casebeer keratorefractive surgery planning field entries. The Casebeer system is accessed through the Applications category of the TMS-1 main menu. Use of this system requires prior completion of formal training and total familiarization with the Casebeer system. The software first requires keyboard entry of a target postoperative refraction value between -5.00 and +0.25 D, and the age of the subject, which is typically obtained from the patient history. The spherical equivalent is then automatically calculated from the composite cycloplegic refraction which is also entered by the operator. Acceptable ranges for the refraction components are: -9.50 to +3.00 D for the sphere; -6.00 to +6.00 D for the cylinder; and between 0° and 180° for the axis. To assure that errors are not made, the input fields for the refraction data are blacked out, and the information is requested a second time. If there is an error between the two refraction fields, the operator is requested to determine the correct refraction.

After automatically calculating the spherical equivalent from the refraction, the program suggests a surgical plan based on the Casebeer nomograms. These nomograms are also directly viewable in tabular form from the menu screen.

The recommended plan is shown in terms of the number of RK incisions to be made, the RK optical zone, and the theoretical power residue which is the difference between the nomogram results and the calculated spherical equivalent. When there is more than one plan that meets the Casebeer system criterion, the first plan that is recommended is indicated by an asterisk. The map of either plan may be displayed by highlighting the entry.

The selected Casebeer system procedure is shown overlaid on the absolute scale contour map as a series of black lines indicating the incision sites and the extent of the optical zone (Figure 9-31). Additional information is provided to the right of the map, including the number of RK cuts and the diameter of the RK optical zone, as well as the length of the AK cuts and the AK optical zone, when astigmatism correction is needed. The box also displays the preexisting cylinder axis, the eye, the age of the patient, and two user fill-in fields for the pachymetry measurement and the blade setting. Up to two additional color-coded surgical enhancements can be computed for a given exam and overlaid on the contour map. The user should refer to the TMS-1 manual and to the Casebeer course materials for additional information.

The Applications category also provides access to the Rabinowitz[9] and the Klyce/Maeda[10] systems of keratoconus detection (Figure 9-32). The Rabinowitz method uses Sim K and I-S values to determine whether keratoconus may be present. The calculated values are displayed, and can be compared to their normal mean values and the two and three standard deviation values which are presented in a small table.

The Klyce/Maeda system detects keratoconus-like topography patterns by calculating a keratoconus prediction index (KPI) based on discriminant analysis of a wide population of normal, keratoconus, and keratoconus confounding topographies. The corneal indices used in the Klyce/Maeda system are: Average Corneal Power (ACP), Opposite Sector Index (OSI), Corneal Eccentricity Index (CEI), Center-Surround Index (CSI), Standard Deviation of Power (SDP), Irregular Astigmatism Index (IAI), Differential Sector Index (DSI), and the Analyzed Area (AA). The closer the KPI value is to 100%, the more likely the exam exhibits topography associated with keratoconus. Unlike the Rabinowitz method, which in practice should be used when the opposite eye's topography is available, the Klyce/Maeda system can always be used independently of the topography of the opposite eye. Also, the KPI value tends to be more accurate, sensitive, and more specific to keratoconus when presented with confounding pathological or postsurgical conditions.

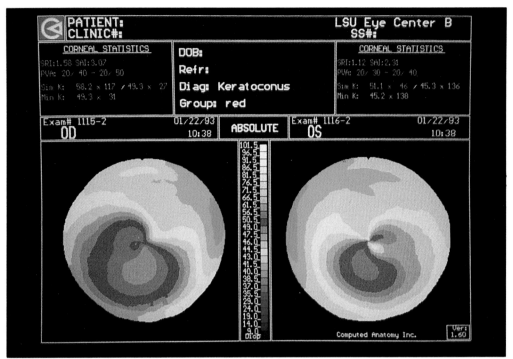

Figure 9-24. Multiple map—two photos. Two-photo displays can be produced with adjustable, normalized, or as shown here, absolute scales. The two photo display is an excellent way to show left and right, or pre- and postoperative corneas for a given patient. Movement of the crosshair cursor can be performed simultaneously in both maps, with individual score boxes for each map appearing in place of the statistics boxes.

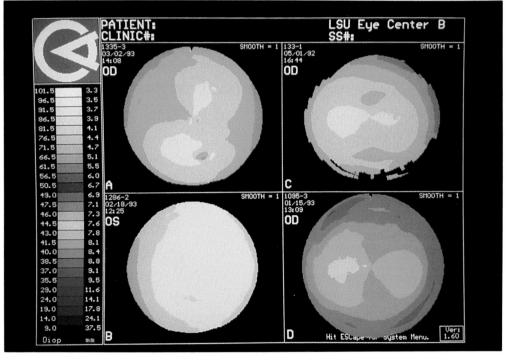

Figure 9-25. Multiple map—four photos. The four- photo display only has the absolute scale available. Exam data is provided in the upper left-hand corner of each photo, and the header provides a field for patient information. If the display is used to compare exams from four separate individuals with similar conditions, the patient header should be turned off to avoid confusion. If exams of a single subject are displayed, the header may be left on, and will display information obtained from the first selected exam.

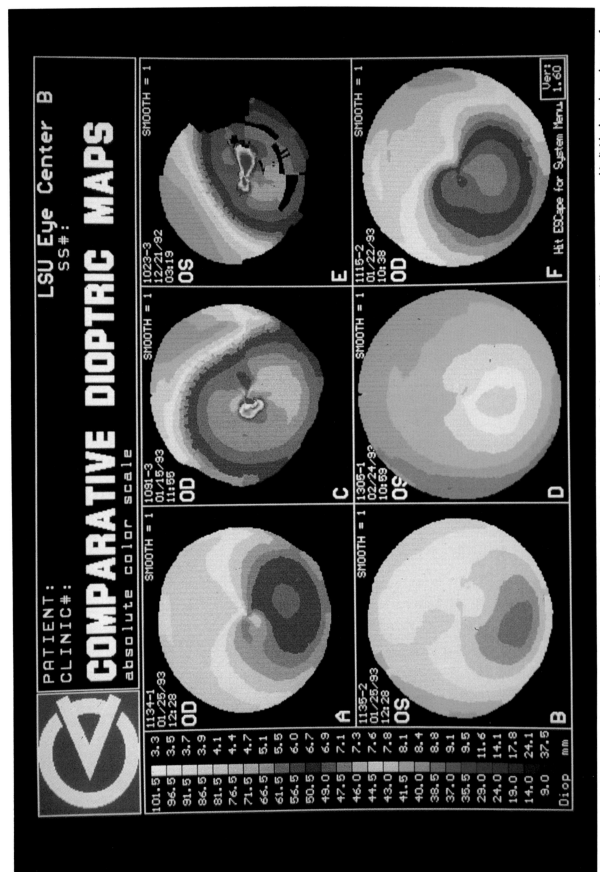

Figure 9-26. Multiple map—six photos. The six-photo map is similar to the four-photo map. It is suited for showing topography differences among several individuals as shown here, or for showing a time series of changing topography in a single individual.

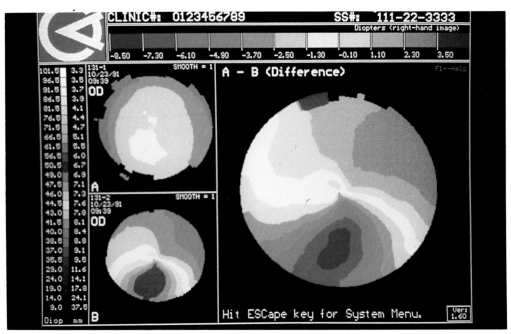

Figure 9-27. Multiple map—differential map.

DIFFERENTIAL FILE GENERATOR

Exam#1: 131   Exam#2: 131
Photo#: 1   Photo#: 2
Patient name: Patient name:

Ring# – d power	Ring# – d power	Ring# – d power
1 = –1.95	11 = –1.89	21 = –1.54
2 = –1.91	12 = –1.84	22 = –1.49
3 = –1.89	13 = –1.80	23 = –0.63
4 = –1.90	14 = –1.77	24 = –1.99
5 = –1.86	15 = –1.75	
6 = –1.83	16 = –1.73	
7 = –1.80	17 = –1.71	
8 = –1.82	18 = –1.69	
9 = –1.86	19 = –1.64	
10 = –1.89	20 = –1.59	

Hit ESCape to return to system menu.
To hold table on screen, hit [F1] key.

Figure 9-28. Multiple map—differential file generator. Before displaying the difference map shown in Figure 9-27, power differences in the two maps are first calculated and the mean difference in each ring shown in tabular form. Exam number, photo number, and patient name are provided for both exams at the top of the screen.

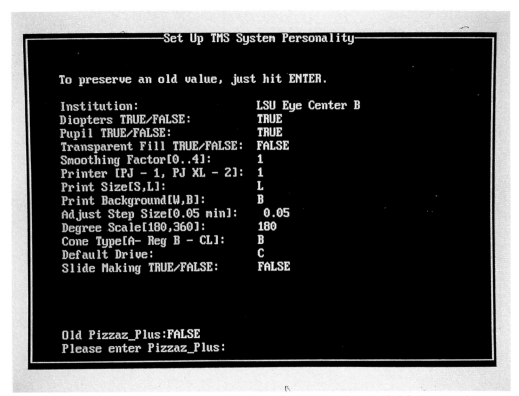

Figure 9-29. The TMS-1 personality setup menu. Prior to use, the TMS-1 can be set with default settings for several functions. For example, either diopters or millimeters of radius can be displayed with the color-coded scales, or the adjustable map step size setting can be set according to the user's preference. When changing the VKS Light Cone between the 25 and 31 ring types, the user must remember to change to the correct setting in the personality menu.

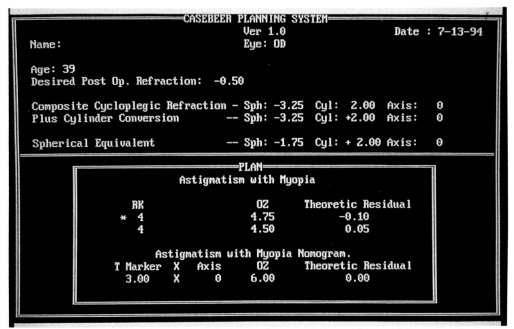

Figure 9-30. Casebeer Keratorefractive Surgical Planning System. The box at the top of the screen shows user input fields requesting patient information. Note the use of two composite cycloplegic refraction fields. Astigmatism correction is displayed when necessary.

The keratoconus screening display also includes an absolute scale contour map with the scale in diopters and millimeters, patient information including BCVA, and a video image of the eye with the mire pattern highlighted in color. Green mire points indicate continuously plotted ring images, while red areas indicate missing or noncontinuous regions that may not be processed accurately. Additional Help screens are available with the two keratoconus screening systems, which explains the indices used to formulate the results (Figure 9-33).

The Application menu also has the option of computing Klyce corneal statistics, which are a primary source of topographical data for clinical research purposes (Figure 9-34).[10-13] The corneal statistics are displayed in a box in the lower right-hand corner of the screen, and are color-coded in green, yellow, and red to allow the user to immediately notice abnormal values. An interpretation box is provided with a tutorial summary of each of the indices. The normal, suspect, and abnormal cutoff levels of each of the indices are shown along the bottom of the screen. At the top of the display screen are boxes for the video image, the contour map in the absolute scale, and a patient information box.

The final Application of the TMS-1 is the contact lens fitting system. Figure 9-35 shows the setup screen with the corneal statistics relevant for contact lens fitting, the lenses and lens material parameters incorporated into the TMS-1 software, and a box showing the recommended lens fit for the patient. As shown in the example, a warning may also be indicated on the right-hand side of the screen, if the residual astigmatism error remains significantly high. If the patient requires a custom lens, the operator should proceed to the contact lens fluorescein map display. The fluorescein map (Figure 9-36) displays a central video image of the cornea with a computer-simulated contact lens modeled on the cornea. The fluorescein pattern models the staining hues and patterns expected to be seen in the patient wearing the actual lens.[14] The computer-generated fluorescein pattern is thus based on predicted clearance measures of the corneal topography and the lens curvature. The contact lens clearance in a given meridian is plotted in the box to the right of the map, which can be adjusted by keyboard control to show the clearance for any meridian on the cornea. The hue scale is calibrated to a clearance range of 0 to 80 μm. An information box in the upper right displays current lens information, including the lens diameter, optical zone, edge lift, posterior curvature, and the Sim K value of the cornea. The box also provides the input fields for the custom lens design.

SUMMARY

The Tomey/Computed Anatomy TMS-1 Topographical Modeling System was the first widely used and accepted method of analyzing corneal topography. Since its inception, the capabilities of the instrument and the software have been improved to meet the needs of the user. Surgeons now can better prepare for surgical procedures. For example, the keratoconus detection application will undoubtedly reduce the number of patients with early keratoconus from undergoing keratorefractive procedures which may become problematic as their keratoconus worsens. Likewise, patient follow-up is more meaningful when serially acquired videokeratography is available. Issues involving a patient's declining or improving visual acuity should be clearly evident from the topography maps. Clinical researchers will be delighted to find the availability of corneal indices on the TMS-1, and will most likely suggest even more advanced measurement tools and clinical tests for future versions of the instrument. Clearly, the TMS-1 has set a standard by which all other VKSs are measured, and continues to provide state-of-the-art technology.

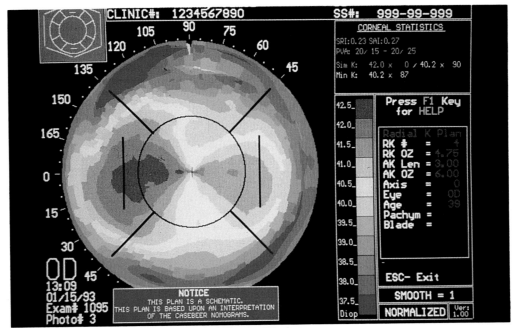

Figure 9-31. Casebeer Keratorefractive Surgical Planning Display.

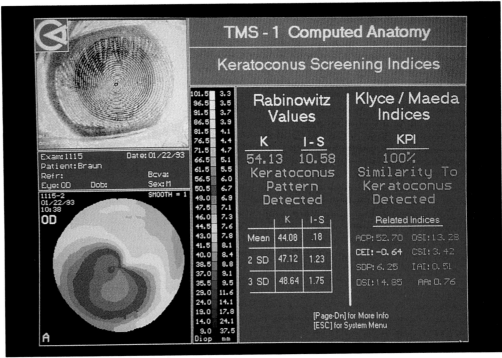

Figure 9-32. Automated keratoconus detection.

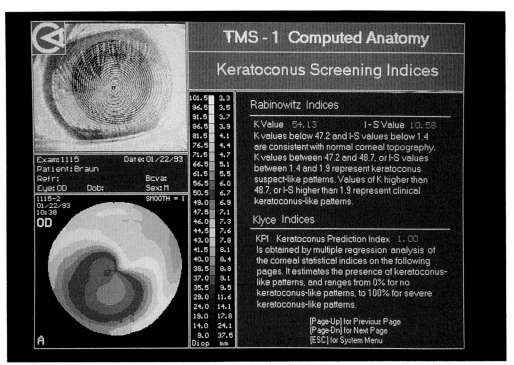

Figure 9-33. Keratoconus screening indices. The Sim K and I-S keratoconus screening indices of Rabinowitz and the corneal research indices of Klyce are described in greater detail by paging down from the screen shown in the previous figure. Several screens provide considerable information about the relationship between specific corneal indices and the topographical features of the cornea.

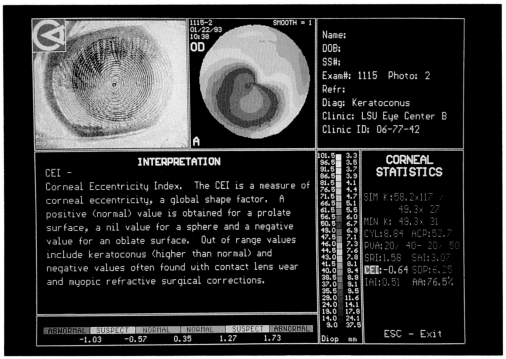

Figure 9-34. Klyce corneal statistics.

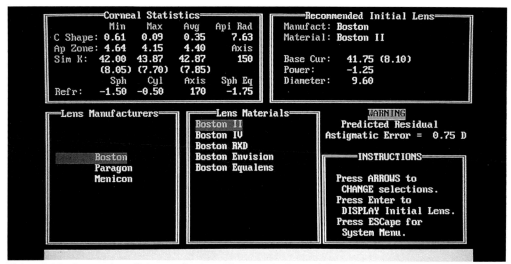

Figure 9-35. Contact lens fitting application. The suggested initial lens first requires a selection from a manufacturer listed in the box in the lower left, followed by a selection of the manufacturer's lens materials listed in the box in the bottom center of the screen. If a specific lens material is not chosen, custom lens settings can be made in the display screen shown in Figure 9-36.

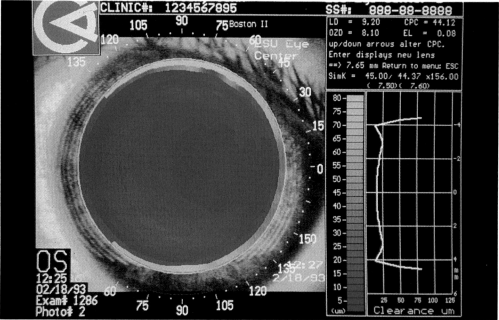

Figure 9-36. Contact lens fluorescein pattern.

REFERENCES

1. Gormley DJ, Gersten M, Koplin RS, Lubkin V. Corneal modeling. *Cornea* 1988;7:30-35.
2. Mammone RJ, Gersten M, Gormley DJ, et al. 3-D corneal modeling system. *IEEE Trans Biomed Engineer.* 1990;37:66-72.
3. Maguire LJ, Singer DE, Klyce SD. Graphic presentation of computer-analyzed keratoscope photographs. *Arch Ophthalmol.* 1987;105:223-230.
4. Klyce SD. Computer-assisted corneal topography: high resolution graphical presentation and analysis of keratoscopy. *Invest Ophthalmol Vis Sci.* 1984;25:1426-1435.
5. Dabezies OH, Holladay JT. Measurement of corneal curvature: keratometer (ophthalmometer). In: Dabezies OH, ed. *Contact Lenses. The CLAO Guide to Basic Science and Clinical Practice.* New York, NY: Grune and Stratton, Inc; 1984:17.1-17.27.
6. Application Note #34. Analyzing objects other than corneas with the TMS-1 Topographical Modeling System. New York, NY: Computed Anatomy, Inc.
7. TMS-1 Instruction and Operating Manual, Version 1.41. New York: Computed Anatomy, Inc.
8. Wilson SE, Klyce SD, Husseini ZM. Standardized color-coded maps for corneal topography. *Ophthalmology.* 1993;100:1723-1727.
9. Rabinowitz YS, Garbus JJ, McDonnell PJ. Computer-assisted corneal topography in family members of patients with keratoconus. *Arch Ophthalmol.* 1990;108:365-371.
10. Maeda N, Klyce SD, Smolek MK, Thompson HW. Automated keratoconus screening with corneal topography analysis. *Invest Ophthalmol Vis Sci.* 1994;35:2749-2757.
11. Dingeldein SA, Klyce SD, Wilson SE. Quantitative descriptors of corneal shape derived from computer-assisted analysis of photokeratographs. *Refract & Corneal Surg.* 1989;5:372-378.
12. Wilson SE, Klyce SD. Quantitative descriptors of corneal topography. A clinical study. *Arch Ophthalmol.* 1991;109:349-353.
13. Maeda N, Klyce SD, Hamano H. Alteration of corneal asphericity in RGP contact lens-induced warpage. *CLAO J.* 1994;20:27-31.
14. Klyce SD, Estopinal HA, Gersten M, et al. Fluorescein exam simulation for contact lens fitting. *Invest Ophthalmol Vis Sci Suppl.* 1992;33:697.

THE TOPCON COMPUTERIZED MAPPING SYSTEM CM-1000

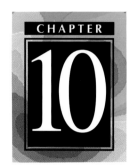

Kazuo Nunokawa

The TOPCON Computerized Mapping System CM-1000 (Figure 10-1) is a Placido ring-based corneal analysis system. The CM-1000 consists of an optical head, i486-based PC with control and analysis software, and a color LaserJet printer. The CM-1000 projects a 15-ring conical Placido disc which is positioned 73 mm in front of the cornea. The diameter of the measured region is 1 to 10 mm for a 42.2 D cornea. The Placido image reflected by a cornea is captured and stored along with a data set which includes patient information and analysis information. The CM-1000 provides various ways for evaluating cornea, such as a color-coded power map, 2UP, 4UP, 6UP, a difference map, etc (Figure 10-2).

FOCUS AND ALIGNMENT

The CM-1000 has an active focus sensing detector which is similar to the sensor used in 35 mm cameras. The control software processes a signal from it, displays a focus status on a monitor screen, and controls the image capturing function based on the focus status.

It also has an alignment decting system. The control software finds the position of reflected light from the cornea using the CCD video signal and controls the image capturing function based on the alignment status. Basically, the control software does not allow an image to be captured if the focus and alignment are out of range.

A corneal measurement result is influenced by the focusing and alignment. These unique and precise focus and alignment detecting systems prevent operation error when taking images. In other words, they eliminate the error factors of focusing and alignment and enhance repeatability. Also, a small aperture function in the capturing optics provides greater comfort for the patient and a greater depth of focus

when digitizing the image. A flash, which freezes any eye movements, makes the image sharp. A typical image captured by a CM-1000 is shown in Figure 10-3.

ALGORITHMS

A ring detecting program identifies each ring's position. Each of the 15 Placido rings in the image is searched at 1° intervals (360°) for a total of 5400 points. A pupil detecting program traces the pupil margin and finds the center of it.

Then, a number of highly sophisticated programs are applied to the above data in order to derive topographic data. The CM-1000 applies a differential geometric analysis method to precisely calculate the corneal shape. A corneal shape is expressed with an equation:

$$X = F(Y)$$

We know a height Ym, which is measured on the image, and a dX/dYm, which was predetermined for this apparatus. That is, we can determine $F'(Y) = dX/dY$ from the Placido image data. We assume a proper function F(Y) which has several undetermined coefficients. We apply a high order curve fitting of F'(Y) to the ring positions using the least squares method to determine the coefficients for F(Y).

Once each coefficient has been calculated, a radius at any position of the cornea is derived by the following equation:

$$R(Y) = [1 + \{F''(Y)\}2]3/2|F''(Y)|$$

where, F'(Y), F''(Y) are the first and second order differential coefficient of F(Y).

Then, a number of application programs convert the power (radius) data into a series of color graphics displays and numerical data displays.

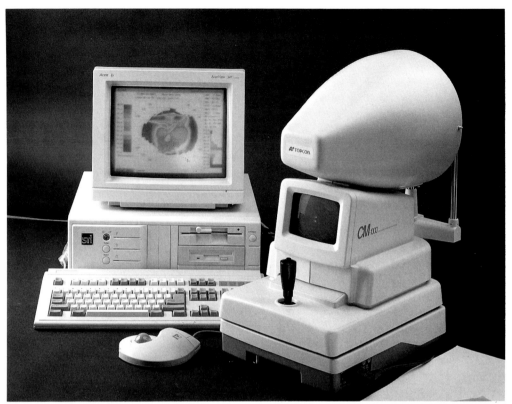

Figure 10-1. The TOPCON Computerized Mapping system CM-1000.

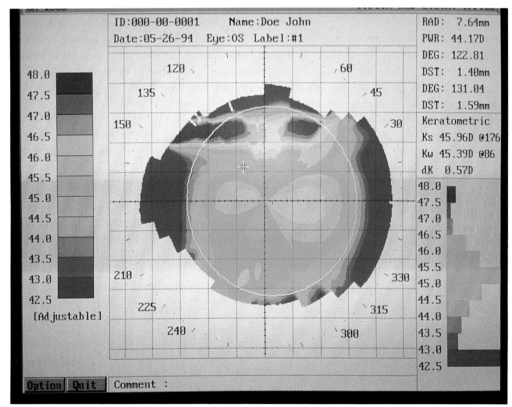

Figure 10-2. CM-1000 topographic color map.

SOFTWARE

The CM-1000 uses a standard pull-down style graphical user interface (GUI) with mouse control. It is easy to operate and enhances system navigation (Figure 10-4). Modular design allows for a variety of system configurations for installation. All data needed for recalculating are stored with each image, allowing editing and recalculation using the calibration that was in effect when the image was taken. An advantage of this feature is that images taken from different machines, which each have their unique calibration, can be compared. Also images on the same system may be compared even if the system has been recalibrated.

SPECIFICATIONS

- Methodology: Placido disk, 15 rings
- Corneal coverage: 1 to 10 mm (at 42.2 D)
- Working distance: 73 mm
- Field of view: 17.5 mm x 13.1 mm on alignment monitor, 13.1 mm x 13.1 mm on system monitor
- Number of data points: 5400 (analyzed), 10,440 (sampled)
- Semi-meridian range: 0° to 360°
- Dioptric range: 10 to 100 D (33.75 to 3.375 mm)
- Resolution: 0.1 D
- Reproducibility: ±0.25 D.

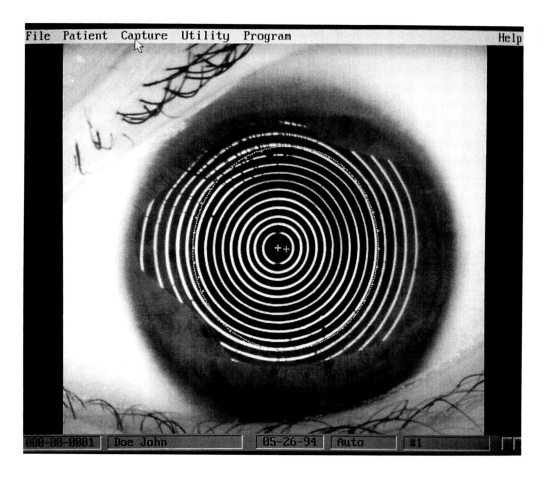

Figure 10-3. A typical image captured by the CM-1000.

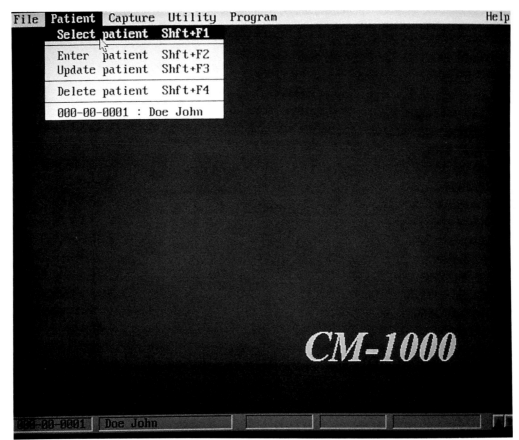

Figure 10-4. A software screen of the CM-1000.

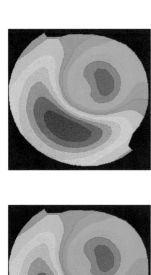
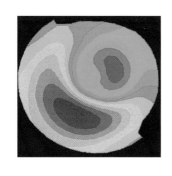
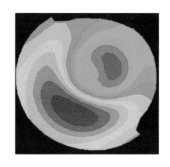
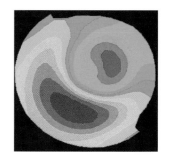

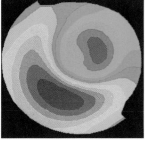

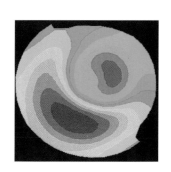

CLINICAL
APPLICATIONS

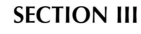

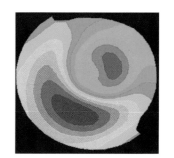

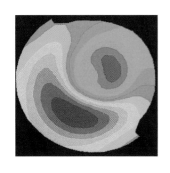

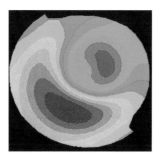

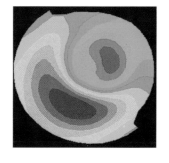

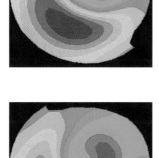

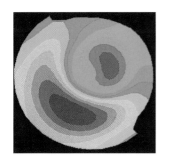

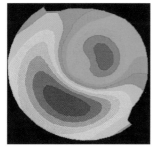

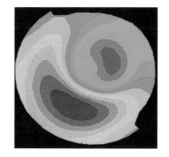

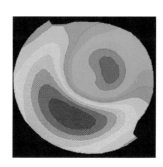

CORNEAL TOPOGRAPHY TO DETECT AND CHARACTERIZE CORNEAL PATHOLOGY

CHAPTER 11

Douglas D. Koch, MD

Syed E. Husain, MD

Computerized videokeratography (CVK), or computerized corneal topography, is the preferred methodology for detecting, diagnosing, and monitoring the management of keratoconus and related corneal topographic disorders. Maguire and Bourne first described nine eyes of seven patients in which keratoconus was diagnosed only by corneal topography, having previously eluded clinical detection.[1] In eyes with early keratoconus, slit lamp corneal changes are too subtle for detection or have not yet occurred, keratometry and retinoscopy may be normal, topographical keratometry may show only nonspecific peripheral steepening, and qualitative Placido systems may not reveal topographic abnormalities. The greater sensitivity of corneal topography is required to make the diagnosis (Figures 11-1A and B).

Corneal topography is increasingly considered to be a key component of the preoperative evaluation of refractive surgical patients. Nesburn and colleagues reported that 6 of 91 consecutive patients screened for excimer laser photorefractive keratectomy (PRK) had subclinical keratoconus.[2] Wilson and Klyce reported that keratoconus was detected in 5.7% of 53 patients who presented for an opinion regarding refractive surgery; interestingly, 33% of 106 eyes were found to have abnormal corneal topography.[3] Radial keratotomy, astigmatic keratotomy, and excimer laser PRK are currently contraindicated in patients with keratoconus. Although Mortensen and Öhrströ recently reported good results in four of five keratoconic eyes treated with excimer laser PRK,[4] it is generally felt that excimer laser PRK is also contraindicated in keratoconus, and preoperative diagnosis is presumably essential in order to appropriately assess the patient's eligibility and design the treatment pattern.

Corneal topography has been essential in developing a classification scheme for keratoconus and in establishing diagnostic criteria. Although the differential diagnosis of keratoconus is limited, other conditions that can demonstrate topographic features similar to keratoconus include other corneal thinning disorders, contact lens-induced corneal warpage, and irregular astigmatism following penetrating keratoplasty.

Using the Corneal Modeling System, Wilson and colleagues evaluated 85 eyes of 49 patients.[5] In the 61 eyes that could be accurately processed and had signs of keratoconus, two types of patterns were noted. Forty-four of the cones (72%) were peripheral, typically either inferiorly or inferotemporally (Figures 11-2A and B). The remainder of the cones were central with or without a superimposed asymmetric pattern of bowtie astigmatism (Figure 11-3).

In an earlier study, Rabinowitz and McDonnell similarly noted these two types of keratoconus, and they described three diagnostic topographic features of keratoconus:

1. Central corneal power > 47 D
2. A difference of 3 D or more in corneal power comparing points 3 mm inferior to the center to points 3 mm superior to the center (I-S)
3. Asymmetry between central corneal power of fellow eyes in excess of 1 D[6] (Figures 11-4A through C).

Because of the variability of the location of the cone, the above three diagnostic features should be used in concert and subjective interpretation may be required. For example, the central cone may yield a I-S value of <3 D but a central corneal power of >47 D. Conversely, we have on rare occasions seen apparently normal corneas with central curvatures >47 D.

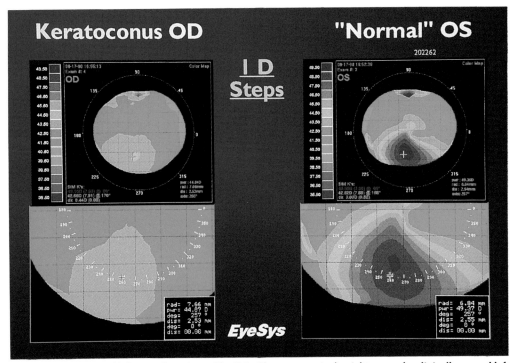

Figure 11-1A. Right and left eyes of a patient with clinical keratoconus in the right eye and a clinically normal left eye. There was no distortion of keratometer mires with keratometry of 42.5 x 43 at 90° in the left eye. The bottom images are magnified views of the inferior cornea. Topography scaled in 1 D steps to emphasize the obvious keratoconus in the right eye. There is a suspect area in the inferior cornea of the left eye but the power in that area is only 44 D.

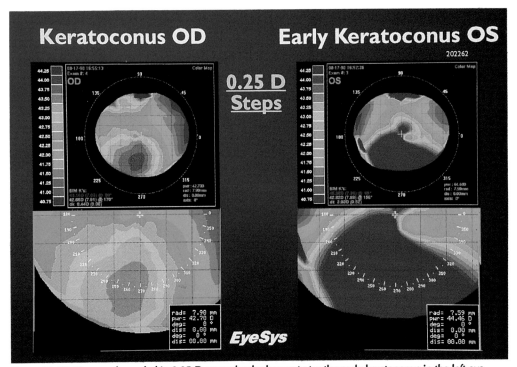

Figure 11-1B. Topography scaled in 0.25 D steps clearly demonstrates the early keratoconus in the left eye.

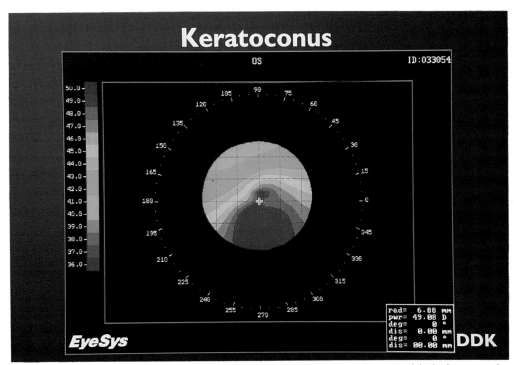

Figure 11-2A. Peripheral keratoconus left eye. There is inferior steepening extending toward the limbus. Note also the superonasal flattening. Normalized scale in 1 D steps.

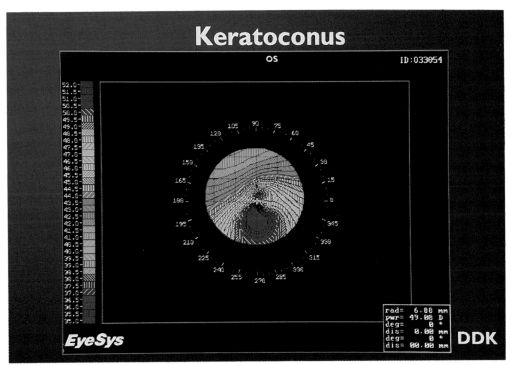

Figure 11-2B. Absolute scale in 0.5 D steps.

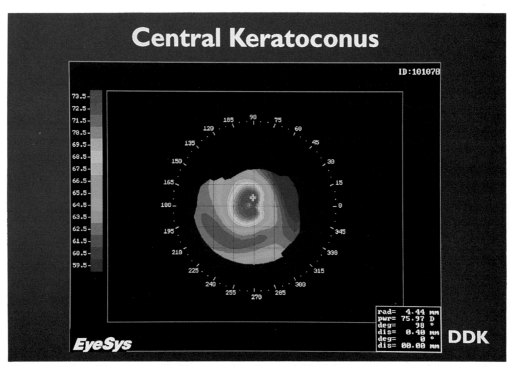

Figure 11-3. Central keratoconus. In this cornea there is remarkably little asymmetry around the apex of this nipple cone.

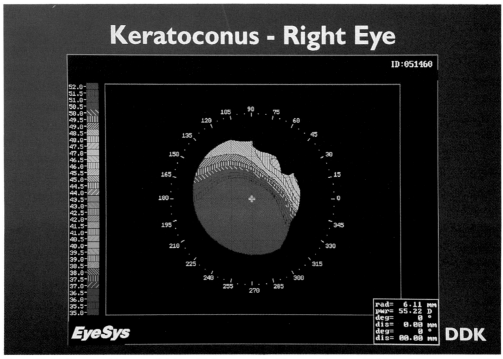

Figure 11-4A. Topographic maps of right and left corneas of a 31-year-old male with bilateral keratoconus. All of the diagnostic features of keratoconus described by Rabinowitz and McDonnell[4] are present. Note the marked central steepness OU (55.00 D OD and 51.00 D OS), the (I - S) disparity due to the greater inferior steepness, and the marked difference in central power between the two corneas. Right eye absolute scale.

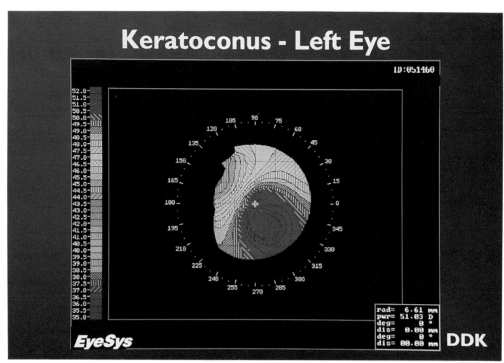

Figure 11-4B. Left eye absolute scale.

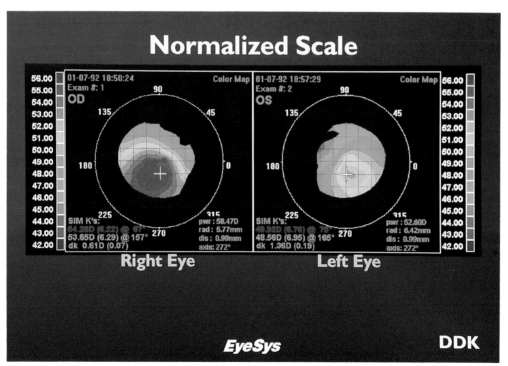

Figure 11-4C. Both eyes normalized scale (1 D steps).

Figure 11-5. Flattening of keratoconus by rigid gas permeable contact lens wear. Upper left, topographic map of cornea 30 minutes after removing contact lens. Lower left, after 3 days of contact lens abstinence, the cone has steepened 2 D. Right, difference map showing the steepening of the cone.

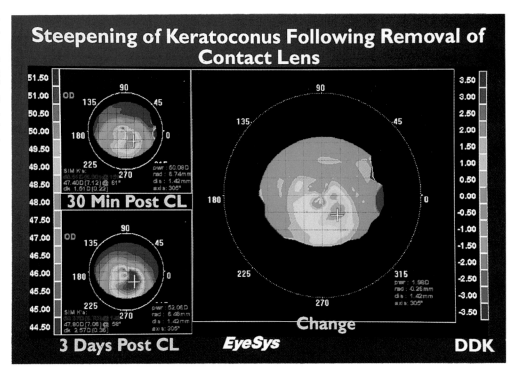

Recently, several investigators have described new approaches for increasing the ease and accuracy of diagnosing keratoconus using computerized quantitative and objective interpretation of topographical patterns. Using the TMS-1 (Computed Anatomy), Maeda, Klyce, et al developed a discriminant analysis classifier based on eight quantitative indices derived from corneal topography.[7] Carrying this process one step further, they developed an expert system classifier, which is a form of artificial intelligence that utilizes step-by-step decision rules. Their system used the value derived from the discriminant analysis and four quantitative topographic indices in the formulation of the decision tree. Evaluating the detection of keratoconus in a validation set of 100 corneas, the expert classifier has a sensitivity of 89%, specificity of 99%, and accuracy of 96%. The expert classifier system was superior to discriminate analysis in sensitivity and overall accuracy.

In a subsequent study, Maeda, Klyce, et al compared three keratoconus detection schemes:
1. SIMK: average simulated K readings >2 SD from the normal mean (45.7 D)
2. MRM: central corneal power >47.2 D or I-S value >1.4 D (Modified Rabinowitz method)
3. Expert system classifier (as described above).[8]

In an analysis of 176 corneas in 125 patients, they found the expert classifier system to be superior to the other two with a sensitivity of 97.7% and specificity of 98.5%.

Sarver, Padrick, et al described a new approach for automated analysis of corneal topographic maps.[9] Using the EyeSys Corneal Analysis System, they developed a hybrid transform for compression of computerized topographic data, in essence a set of computations that provides nearly full representation of corneal topography using only 32 coefficients in place of the original thousands of data points. Each cornea's topography is thus uniquely represented by these 32 coefficients. New corneas are analyzed by comparing them to a library of known images. Sarver's work indicates that this hybrid transform provides a highly accurate and reproducible shape classification for keratoconus and for the full spectrum of corneal topographic variations. This system will therefore be useful as a generalized system for the detection and classification of all types of corneal topographic disorders.

Computerized corneal topography is also helpful in evaluating progression of keratoconus,[10] in fitting contact lenses and monitoring their effects in keratoconus (Figure 11-5), in detecting unusual forms of keratoconus (Figure 11-6), and in diagnosing and evaluating related disorders such as keratoglobus (Figures 11-7 through 11-9B) and pellucid marginal degeneration. Other types of corneal pathology, such as pterygia (Figure 11-10), epithelial dysplasia (Figure 11-11), and epithelial basement membrane disease (Figure 11-12) can also be evaluated using corneal topography.

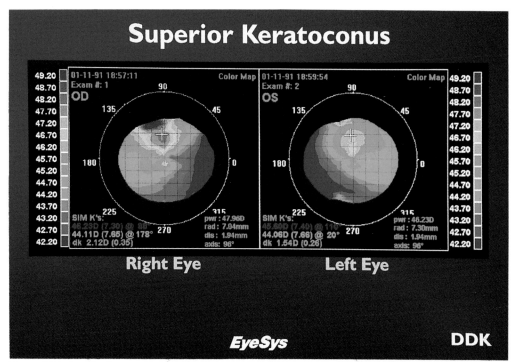

Figure 11-6. Superior keratoconus. This rare variant of peripheral keratoconus shows findings similar to standard inferior keratoconus, except the steepening is present superiorly and slightly temporally. Note the nasal flattening, which is classic for keratoconus, although in these corneas the flattening is centered below the horizontal meridian.

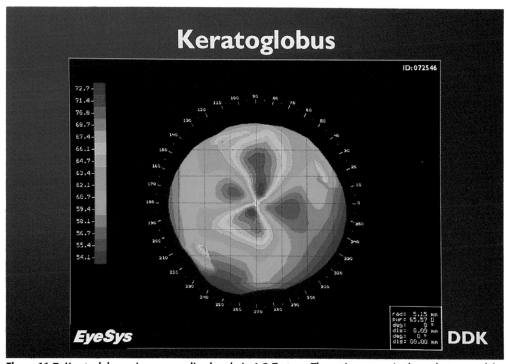

Figure 11-7. Keratoglobus using a normalized scale in 1.5 D steps. The entire cornea is above the range of the absolute scale (>52 D).

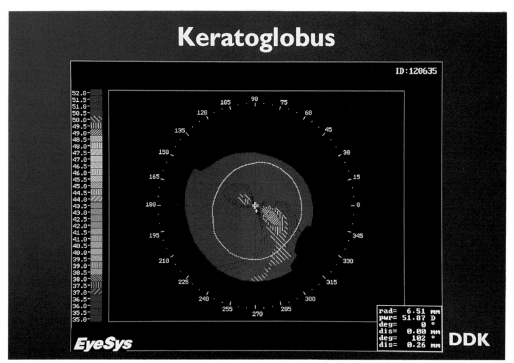

Figure 11-8A. Corneal topographic map of the right eye of a 56-year-old white male with keratoglobus. Note the steep overall curvature with negligible flattening towards the periphery; superimposed is an irregular bowtie pattern of astigmatism. Corneal ultrasonic pachymetry measured 0.47 mm centrally, and, adjacent to the limbus, 0.45 mm superiorly and 0.51 mm inferiorly. The fellow eye had corneal hydrops. Absolute scale. The whole cornea is at the most extreme end of this scale. Green and yellow ranges are normal.

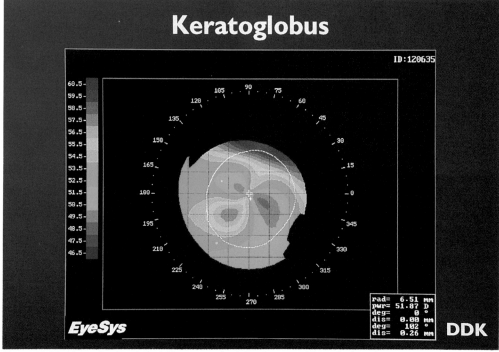

Figure 11-8B. Normalized scale in 1 D steps emphasizing the central irregular bowtie pattern.

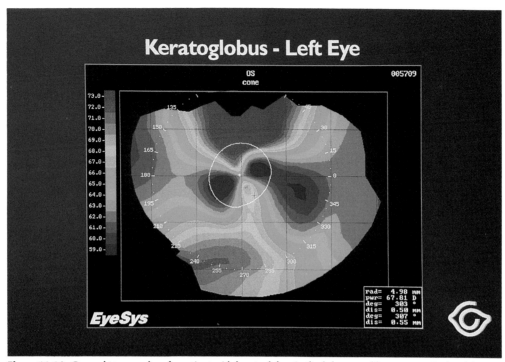

Figure 11-9A. Corneal topography of a patient with keratoglobus in the left eye and keratoconus in the right eye. Image taken without contact lens. The entire cornea ranges from 59 D to in excess of 73 D, with severe with-the-rule astigmatism.

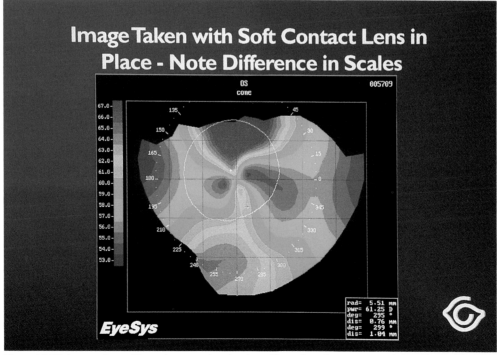

Figure 11-9B. Image taken with a soft contact lens in place. The astigmatic pattern remains unchanged, but 6 D of flattening has occurred across the entire cornea. *Courtesy of Johnny L. Gayton, MD.*

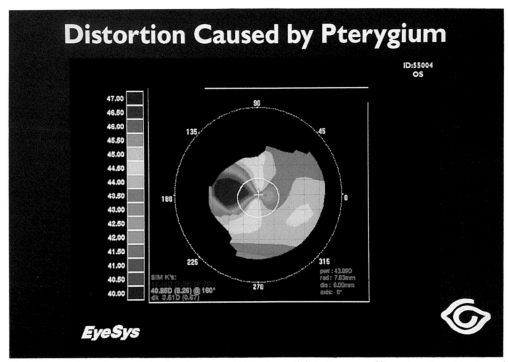

Figure 11-10. Corneal topography showing corneal flattening and distortion caused by a pterygium. *Courtesy of Johnny L. Gayton, MD.*

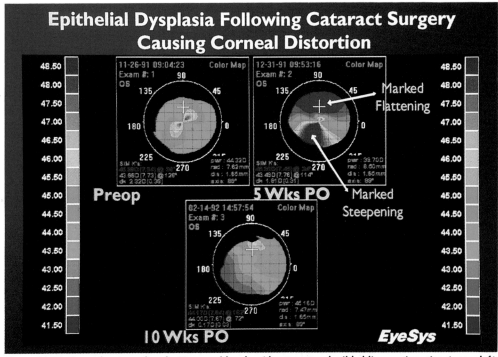

Figure 11-11. Corneal topography of a 71-year-old male with cataract and mild oblique astigmatism (upper left). Five weeks following cataract extraction, the corneal topography shows a large amount of superior flattening with inferior steepening along the 57° semi-meridian (upper right). The slit lamp examination revealed epithelial dysplasia superiorly extending nearly to the visual axis. The patient was treated with scraping of the epithelium and cryotherapy of the superior limbus. Three weeks following treatment (10 weeks post-cataract, bottom), there is minimal astigmatism and the corneal surface is quite regular.

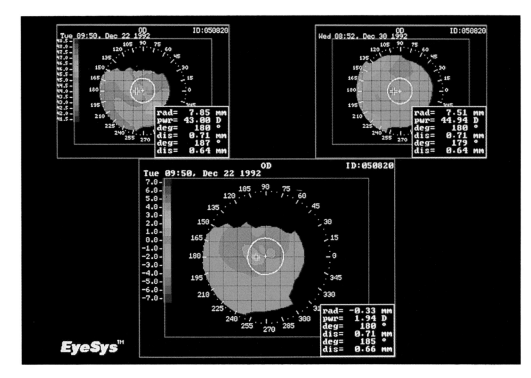

Figure 11-12. Corneal topographic changes induced by epithelial basement membrane disease. Upper left, corneal topographic map of a 72-year-old woman referred for consideration of AK 1 year following cataract surgery. Slit lamp examination revealed thickening of the epithelium with gray sheetlike intraepithelial opacities. Corneal map shows irregular astigmatism, especially centrally, with a bizarre pattern of steepness along the 115° meridian. Upper right, following epithelial debridement, the corneal topography is much more regular, and the central astigmatism has been eliminated. Below, the difference map shows the elimination of the central irregular area produced by the epithelial scraping. Best-corrected vision improved from 20/40 to 20/20.

REFERENCES

1. Maguire LJ, Bourne WM. Corneal topography of early keratoconus. *Amer J Ophthalmol.* 1989;108:107-112.
2. Nesburn AB, Bahri S, Berlin M, et al. Computer assisted corneal topography (CACT) to detect mild keratoconus (kc) in candidates for photorefractive keratectomy. *Invest Ophthalmol Vis Sci.* 1992;33/4(suppl):995.
3. Wilson SE, Klyce SD. Screening for corneal topographic abnormalities before refractive surgery. *Ophthalmology.* 1994;101:147-152.
4. Mortensen J, Öhrström A. Excimer laser photorefractive keratectomy for treatment of keratoconus. *J Refract Corneal Surg.* 1994;10:368-372.
5. Wilson SE, Lin DTC, Klyce SD. Corneal topography of keratoconus. *Cornea.* 1991;10:2-8.

6. Rabinowitz YS, McDonnell PJ. Computer-assisted corneal topography in keratoconus. *Refract & Corneal Surg.* 1989;5:400-408.
7. Maeda N, Klyce SK, Smolek MK, Thompson HW. Automated keratoconus screening with corneal topography analysis. *Invest Ophthalmol Vis Sci.* 194;35:2749-2757.
8. Maeda N, Klyce SK, Smolek MK, Rabinowitz YS. Comparison of three keratoconus detection schemes with videokeratography. *Invest Ophthalmol Vis Sci.* 1994;35-4(suppl):2078.
9. Sarver EJ, Padrick TD, Gadkari S, Soper B. A hybrid transform for use with corneal topography. *Invest Ophthalmol Vis Sci.* 1994;35-4(suppl):2107.
10. Maguire LJ, Lowry JC. Identifying progression of subclinical keratoconus by serial topography analysis. *Amer J Ophthalmol.* 1991;112:41-45.

THE CONTRIBUTION OF CORNEAL TOPOGRAPHY TO THE EVALUATION OF CATARACT SURGERY

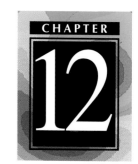

Robert G. Martin, MD
James P. Gills, MD
Johnny L. Gayton, MD

Corneal topography is a useful tool for monitoring the postoperative course of cataract removal and intraocular lens implantation. For the clinician, corneal topography may reveal problems not apparent on routine examination. For the researcher, it is an essential adjunct to the investigation of the relative merits of sutureless vs. sutured surgery, small- vs. large-incision surgery, temporal vs. superior surgery, and clear-corneal vs. scleral-tunnel surgery. Corneal topography makes important contributions to interpreting the visual rehabilitative results of these surgical options. The sequential image and change image display options are particularly useful for patient follow-up.

The sequential image option displays one preoperative and up to three postoperative images from the patient in the same scale. The resulting maps are directly comparable so postoperative changes in corneal shape can be monitored.

The change image, or delta map, option represents one of the most valuable features of computer-assisted video keratography: the ability to follow patients over time. The software will subtract point for point two maps from the same eye taken at different times. If the postoperative image is subtracted from the preoperative image, the change map visually demonstrates the surgically induced changes in corneal shape. The change map is analogous to vector analysis of keratometric measurements, but because it contains thousands of data points across the entire surface of the cornea, it is much more precise and detailed.

EFFECT OF SUTURES

The classic pattern of early with-the-rule astigmatism that regresses within the first 3 months postoperatively is a pattern well known to the cataract surgeon. Figure 12-1 shows preoperative, 1-week, 5-week, and 3-month postoperative images from a patient who received a foldable lens inserted through a 4-mm incision closed with a too-tight horizontal suture. The EyeSys system automatically uses the same scaling for all four images. Note that the preoperative cornea is fairly flat relative to the postoperative images and is fairly spherical.

At 1 week postoperatively the patient had asymmetrical with-the-rule astigmatism, steeper superiorly near the suture. The two lower images in this figure show the same patient at 5 weeks and 3 months postoperatively. Having all images on the same dioptric scale facilitates tracking the patient's progress. Figure 12-2 shows the change image display option for the same patient comparing preoperative to 1-week postoperative exams. The change image (bottom) clearly shows the substantial superior steepening (red) associated with the tight suture. At this time, the topographical image demonstrated that the superior cornea had been steepened by over 5 D. Figure 12-3A shows the change image 3 months postoperatively, clearly depicting over 2 D of residual steepness (orange) in the center of the cornea. Figure 12-3B is a magnified image of the central cornea at 3 months postoperatively. Two irregular areas of steepening can be seen within the central 2 mm of cornea, probably explaining the patient's persisting visual complaints.

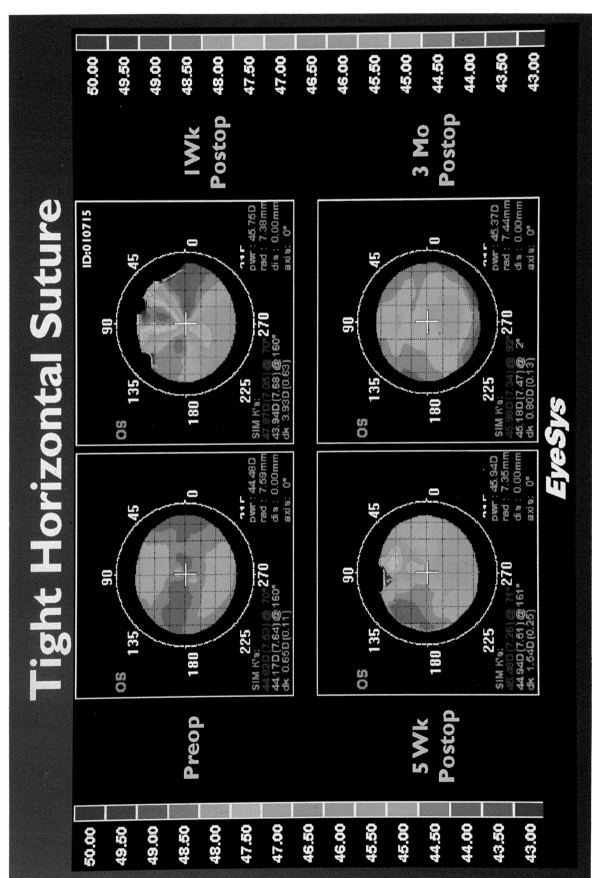

Figure 12-1. Preoperative and serial postoperative corneal topography of a case having a foldable IOL implantation, a 4-mm cataract incision and a too-tight horizontal suture in place.

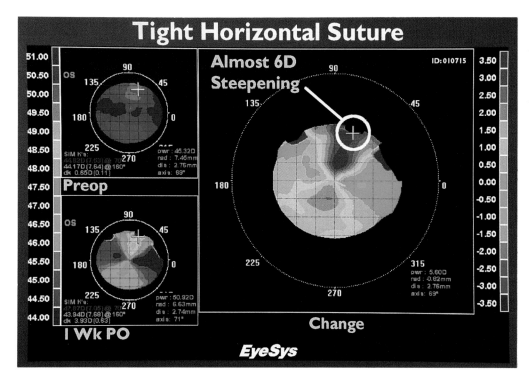

Figure 12-2. Preoperative, 1-week postoperative, and change or delta graph for the case shown in Figure 12-1, demonstrating superior steepening and with-the-rule astigmatism due to tight suture placement.

EFFECT OF INCISION SIZE—SUTURELESS SURGERY

Smaller incisions supposedly induce less astigmatism than larger incisions. However, with sutureless surgery, these differences may be too subtle to be picked up by keratometry, although significant visual acuity differences can be documented. We recently reported on a study comparing 3.2-, 5.0-, and 6.0-mm sutureless cataract incisions using visual acuity, keratometry, and corneal topography as efficacy variables.[1] The three groups did not differ significantly in mean keratometric cylinder preoperatively or at 1 to 2 days or at 3 to 6 months postoperatively, nor did they differ significantly in surgically induced cylinder at either postoperative time period. At 1 to 2 days postoperatively, significantly more patients receiving 3.2-mm incisions had uncorrected visual acuity of 20/40 or better: 75% in the 3.2-mm group vs. 50% and 47% in the 5.0-mm and 6.0-mm incision size groups, respectively.

Corneal topography, with its ability to show changes across the entire cornea, can demonstrate the actual differences between groups that keratometry may miss. Figure 12-4 shows the preoperative, 1-day postoperative, and change images for a patient receiving a Staar model AA-4203 foldable silicone lens through a 3.2-mm incision. The postoperative image closely resembles the preoperative image. Green areas on the change image indicate no difference

between the preoperative and postoperative images. In general, topographic images from patients receiving 3.2-mm incisions were rated as having fewer corneal changes than images from patients receiving 5.0-mm or 6.0-mm incisions (Figures 12-5A and B).

The most dramatic examples of flattening at the wound site are shown in Figures 12-6A and B, while milder cases are illustrated in Figures 12-7A and B. Central corneal changes were also noted. Figure 12-8 shows the change images from a patient who received a foldable silicone lens through a 3.2-mm incision. This patient exhibited slightly less than 3 D of central corneal flattening at 1 day postoperatively, shown in dark blue. Because this flattening was largely confined to the central 2 mm of the cornea, keratometry failed to detect it. This flattening, unusual in a recipient of a foldable lens, was transient, and by 2 weeks postoperatively regression had begun and by 6 weeks postoperatively the flattening had largely disappeared. Figures 12-9A and B show an example of extreme central corneal flattening, between 5 and 6 D, in a patient who received an unsutured 6-mm incision. Again, because the flattening is only in the very center of the cornea, keratometry failed to detect it. There was only a 0.2 D change in average keratometry. The applanation tension was 21 mmHg, so this change could not be due to hypotony. We also observed some mixed patterns: Figures 12-10A and B show peripheral flattening at the wound site (blue) and central

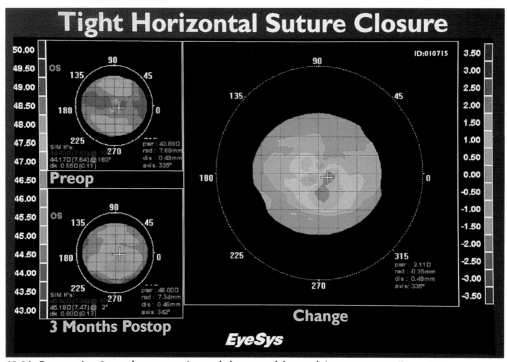

12-3A. Preoperative, 3-month postoperative, and change or delta graph in same case as Figure 12-1 demonstrating residual central corneal steepening.

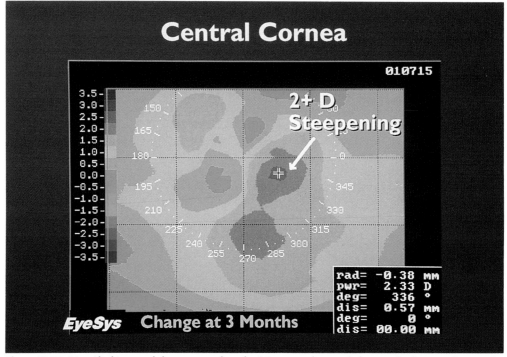

Figure 12-3B. Magnified image of change map of emphasizing central corneal changes. Each square is 1 mm by 1 mm.

steepening (yellow and orange). The concurrent flattening at the wound site in one upper quadrant with steepening in the opposite upper quadrant of the cornea was noted in four patients receiving 5.0-mm incisions and in three patients receiving 6.0-mm incisions, but not in any patient receiving a 3.2-mm incision. This pattern can be seen in Figures 12-11A and B.

In our study, keratometry indicated that fourteen patients experienced surgically induced astigmatism of 1 D or more. However, the topographic images from twelve of these patients did not indicate a true astigmatic pattern. Examples of the phenomenon are illustrated in Chapter 3.

EFFECT OF WOUND CONSTRUCTION AND LOCATION—CLEAR-CORNEAL INCISIONS

Many surgeons who previously used self-sealing scleral-tunnel incisions are now using a new technique in many of their cataract patients, the self-sealing clear-corneal incision. This technique involves making a small incision at the edge of clear cornea. When beginning this technique, many surgeons operated at their usual superior location and found the early visual results somewhat disappointing. Corneal topography enabled investigators to visualize the corneal changes caused by the surgery and appropriately modify their techniques.

Figure 12-12 demonstrates the induced changes of a superotemporal clear-corneal wound 4 days postoperatively. Note the marked flattening at the wound site. This flattening generally regresses over time, although visual rehabilitation is delayed. Figure 12-13 demonstrates the induced flattening at 1 day in a superotemporal clear-corneal patient and the subsequent early postoperative course. By 3 weeks, the flattening has markedly regressed. The surgeon who first reported the technique, I. Howard Fine, MD, did not observe this marked flattening in his patients. He used a temporal approach, theorizing that the temporal location is further from the visual axis, thus impacting less on vision if flattening occurs, and the incision is parallel to the effect of lid blink and gravity, thus experiencing less drag.[2,3] The change image shown in Figure 12-14 demonstrates the effect of a temporal clear-corneal incision. The overall green indicates no clinically significant induced corneal changes.

Do clear-corneal incisions compare favorably with scleral-tunnel incisions? Corneal topography allows direct comparison of these two techniques. A randomized, prospective study was conducted comparing topographic images of temporal clear-corneal and superior scleral-tunnel incisions.[4] Both techniques evidenced either no induced corneal changes (Figure 12-15A) or mild flattening at the wound site (Figure 12-15B). There were no significant differences between

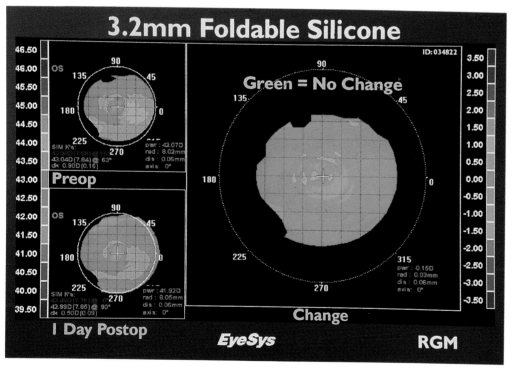

Figure 12-4. Preoperative, 1-day postoperative, and change or delta graph of a patient receiving a 3.2 mm foldable silicone IOL with little change in corneal power due to surgery.

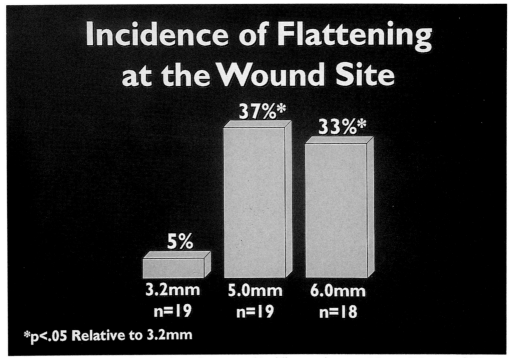

Figure 12-5A. Histograms showing the major topographic differences between 3.2 mm, 5.0 mm and 6.0 mm sutureless incisions. Incidence of flattening at the wound site.

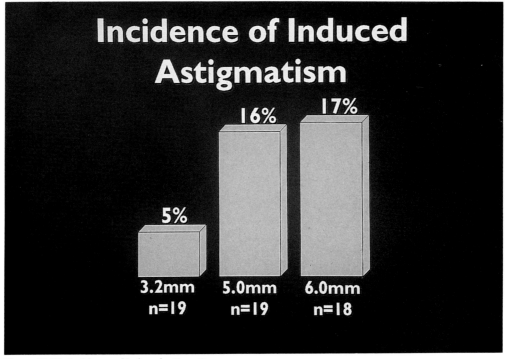

Figure 12-5B. Incidence of induced astigmatism.

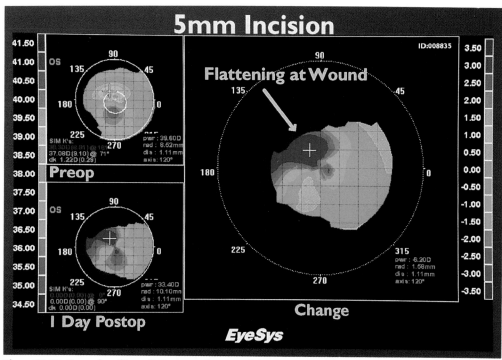

Figure 12-6A. Examples of large flattening at the wound site. Over 5 D of flattening were seen in these cases. 5.0 D incision.

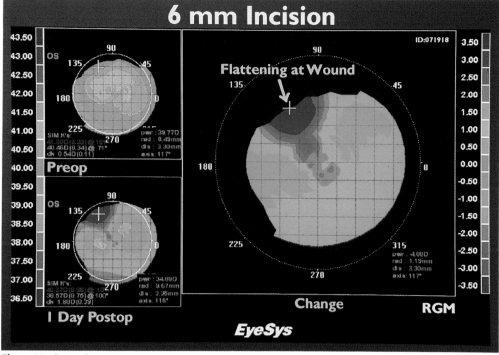

Figure 12-6B. 6.0 D incision.

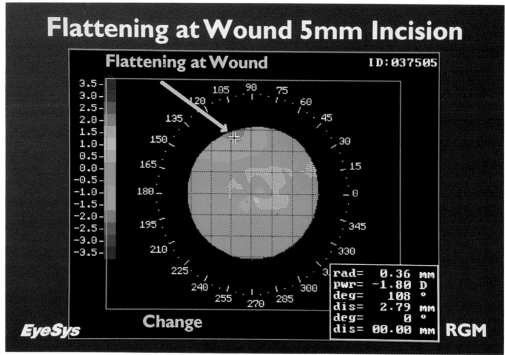

Figure 12-7A. Examples of mild flattening at the wound site, change or delta maps only. 5.0 D incision.

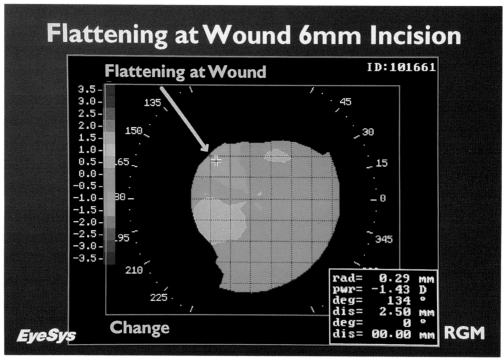

Figure 12-7B. 6.0 D incision.

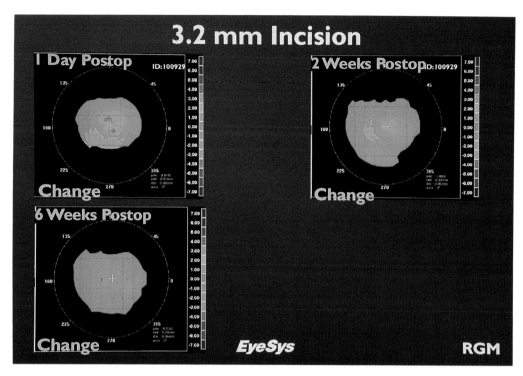

Figure 12-8. Corneal topography of a patient with a 3.2-mm incision. Upper left shows 1-day postoperative change map with area of central flattening of about 3 D. Upper right shows change map of same patient 2 weeks later, demonstrating marked regression. Bottom left, change map of same patient at 6 weeks postoperatively demonstrates resolution of flattening.

groups in incidence of flattening at the wound site, and this mild corneal change generally regressed. Under topographic analysis, both techniques appear to be essentially astigmatically neutral.

EVALUATING WOUND MANAGEMENT TECHNIQUES

Experience with temporal cataract surgery has enabled some surgeons to rotate the cataract incision to the steep axis, using an incision designed to flatten at the incision site, in an attempt to reduce preexisting astigmatism. One can monitor the effects of wound manipulation on resultant astigmatism using corneal topography. Figure 12-16 demonstrates a good result with a larger temporal clear-corneal incision. Preoperatively, the patient had approximately 1.5 D of against-the-rule astigmatism. One day postoperatively, the flattening at the wound site had markedly reduced the central astigmatism. By 3 weeks postoperatively, the peripheral flatness at the wound site had regressed, with an essentially spherical cornea.

Rotated scleral-tunnel incisions can also be used for astigmatism management. We conducted a prospective study of a series of scleral-tunnel incisions performed at the steep axis to reduce preexisting astigmatism. Figure 12-17 shows a with-the-rule astigmatism case, receiving a superior incision, that experienced some regression of effect. The first change image (bottom left) illustrates the flattening induced by the incision. Three weeks postoperatively, the cornea is essen-

tially spherical (top middle). However, at 7 months (top right) there is some return of the astigmatism. The second change image (bottom right) shows the steepening that has occurred between the two postoperative exams.

Another wound management technique has recently been reported: the use of a long limbal relaxing cataract incision.[5] This technique uses a relaxing incision at the limbus of 60° to 120° of arc, with a small scleral tunnel made at the center. Figure 12-18 shows topography of a patient with over 2 D of with-the-rule astigmatism preoperatively. After a limbal relaxing cataract incision at the steep axis, the astigmatism has been reduced by 1.25 D. The change image (bottom) shows the flattening that has occurred in the incision meridian and the steepening 90° away, known as the coupling effect. Figure 12-19 shows another patient with almost 3.5 D of against-the-rule astigmatism (top left). After the patient received a 120° limbal incision, the astigmatism was reduced to less than 1 D (top middle). The first change image (bottom left) indicates a large amount of flattening in the incision meridian, but no steepening 90° away, perhaps because of the large length of the incision. One month postoperatively, there has been some regression with a return of the astigmatic pattern (top right).

EVALUATING COMBINED PROCEDURES

Cataract surgery is often combined with other procedures, such as trabeculotomy. It can be difficult to separate the effects of each procedure on the cornea. Figures 12-20A

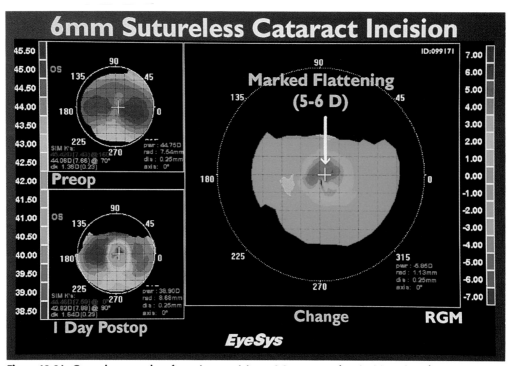

Figure 12-9A. Corneal topography of a patient receiving a 6.0-mm sutureless incision. One-day postoperative change map indicates a large area of central flattening of 5 to 6 D.

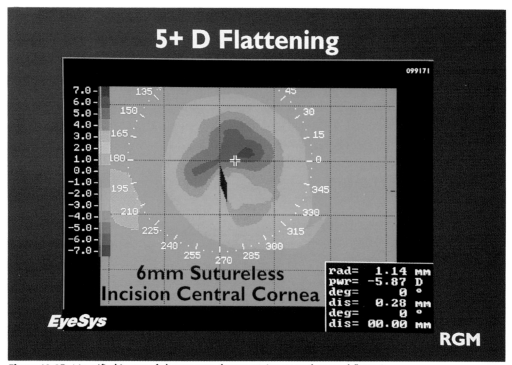

Figure 12-9B. Magnified image of change map demonstrating central corneal flattening.

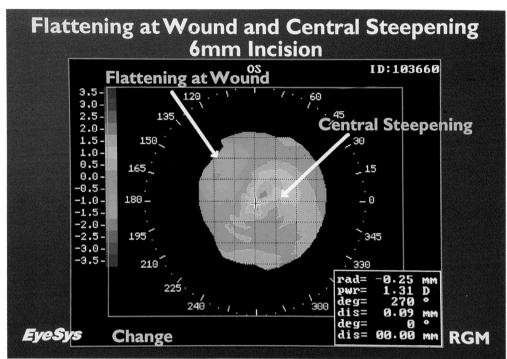

Figure 12-10A. Corneal topography change map with mixed pattern of peripheral flattening at the wound site with central steepening.

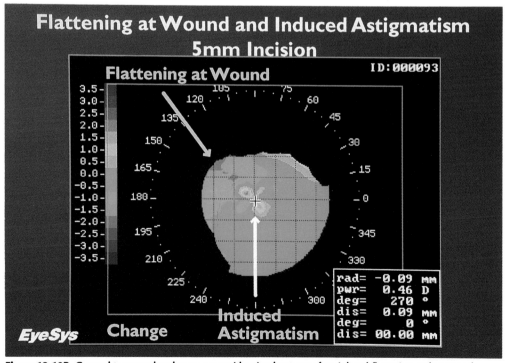

Figure 12-10B. Corneal topography change map with mixed pattern of peripheral flattening at the wound site with induced astigmatism.

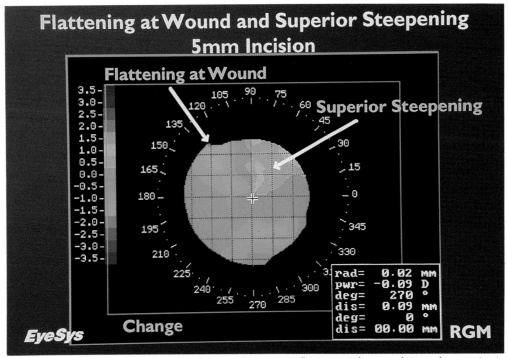

12-11A. Corneal topography change maps in cases of concurrent flattening at the wound site and steepening in the superior peripheral cornea.

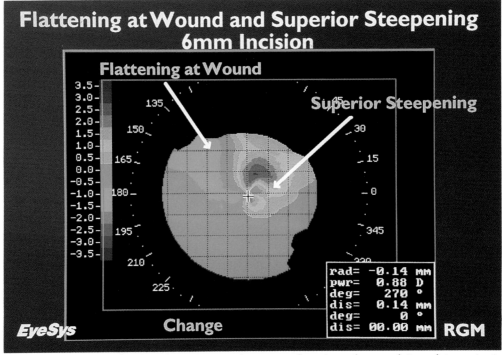

12-11B. Corneal topography change maps in cases of concurrent flattening at the wound site and steepening in the superior peripheral cornea.

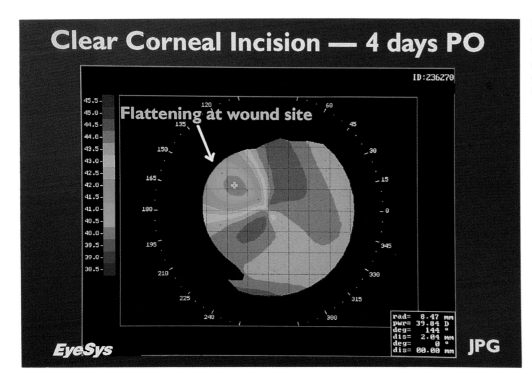

Figure 12-12. Change image of a superotemporal clear-corneal incision demonstrating induced corneal changes 4 days postoperatively. There is marked flattening at the wound site (blue).

and B show the topography of a patient receiving a temporal sutureless cataract incision and a sutured superonasal trabeculotomy. Preoperatively the patient's cornea was spherical. Three weeks postoperatively, the patient had with-the-rule cylinder. The change image showed overall steepening except in the meridian of the cataract incision. This steepening was caused by the tension from the trabeculotomy suture. Figure 12-20B shows the corneal appearance before and after this suture was cut to relieve the tension. After the suture was cut, the cornea returned to spherical.

CONCLUSION

Corneal topography permits the very precise visualization of surgical effect in cataract patients. Some apparent paradoxes in postoperative visual rehabilitation may be resolved with reference to topographic data. For example, patients may have poor postoperative visual acuity in spite of apparently normal clinical examinations and keratometric readings. This and other chapters have demonstrated that keratometry does not always adequately describe surgically induced effects. Furthermore, topography allows the clinician to monitor the effect of his surgical interventions and evaluate new techniques.

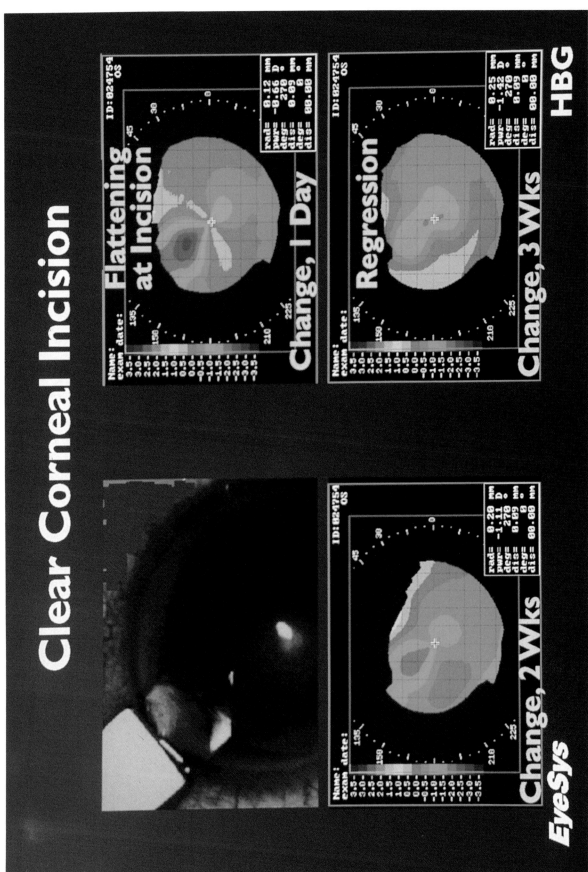

Figure 12-13. Topography of a superotemporal clear-corneal incision. Upper left shows location of incision. Upper right is the change image at 1 day, demonstrating marked flattening at the wound site. Bottom left and right are the 2-week and 3-week change images, respectively, indicating regression of the flattening. *Courtesy of Harry B. Grabow, MD.*

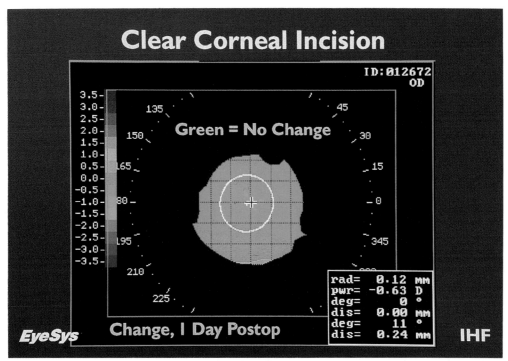

Figure 12-14. Change image 1 day postoperatively of a temporal clear-corneal incision. There are essentially no induced corneal changes. *Courtesy of I. Howard Fine, MD.*

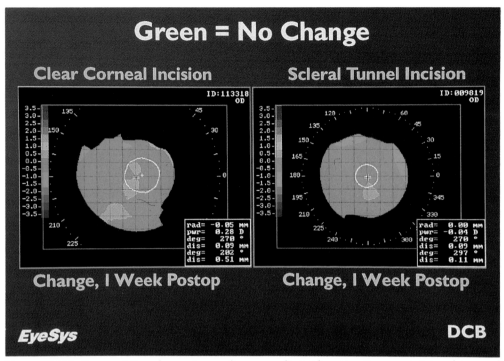

Figure 12-15A. Representative change images from a randomized, prospective comparison of temporal clear-corneal incisions and superior scleral-tunnel incisions. Most cases in both groups showed minimal corneal changes. *Courtesy of David C. Brown, MD.*

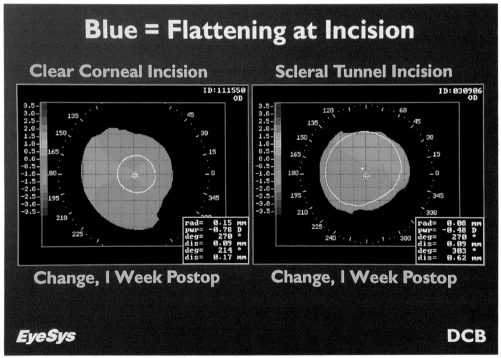

Figure 12-15B. Some cases in both groups evidenced mild flattening at the wound site.

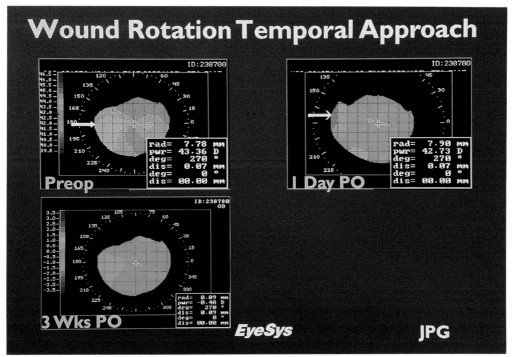

Figure 12-16. Corneal topography of a patient receiving a larger clear-corneal incision at the steep axis designed to flatten at the wound site. Preoperatively, the patient has over 1 D of against-the-rule astigmatism (upper left). The 1-day postoperative image indicates flatness at the wound site and mild residual central corneal astigmatism (upper right). The 3-week postoperative image indicates resolution of both the peripheral flatness and the central astigmatism, leaving an essentially spherical cornea (bottom left).

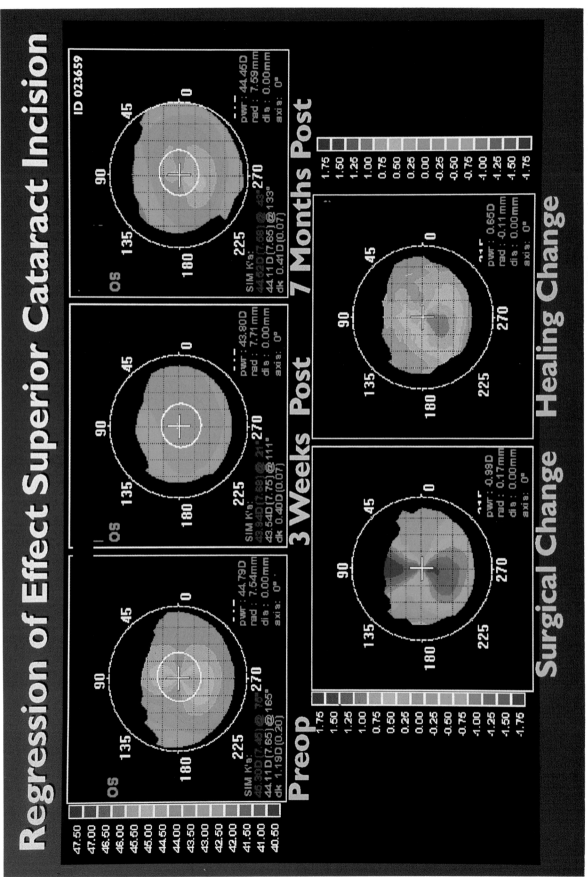

Figure 12-17. STARS view of a patient receiving a superior scleral-tunnel incision. Top left shows preoperative appearance, top middle shows 3-week postoperative appearance, and top right shows 7-month postoperative appearance. The surgical change image (bottom left) demonstrates the surgically induced corneal changes and the healing change image (bottom right) demonstrates the regression of effect between the two postoperative visits.

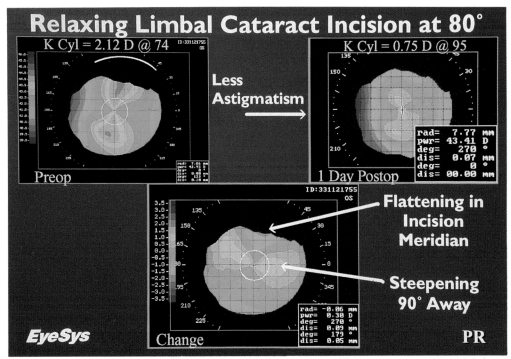

Figure 12-18. Case receiving a limbal relaxing incision with a scleral tunnel for cataract surgery. Upper left shows preoperative appearance and placement of incision. One day postoperatively (upper right) there is demonstrable reduction in astigmatism. The change image (bottom) indicates a coupling effect. *Courtesy of Patrick Rowan, MD.*

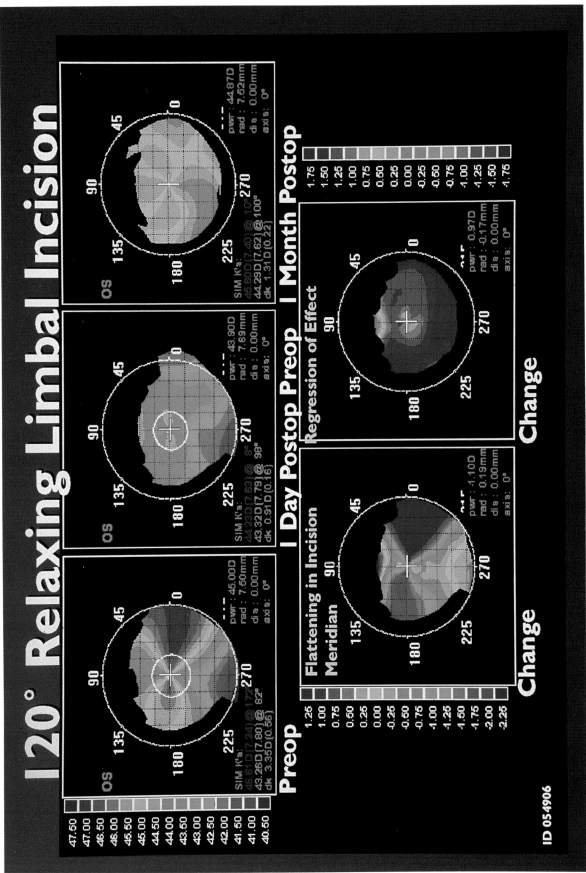

Figure 12-19. STARS display of a case receiving a 120° temporal limbal relaxing incision with a scleral tunnel for cataract surgery. Top left shows preoperative appearance, top middle shows 1-day postoperative appearance, and the first change image demonstrates the induced corneal changes. There is marked reduction of astigmatism produced by flattening in the incision meridian. Top right shows 1-month postoperative image and bottom right shows corneal changes between the two postoperative exams. There has been regression of effect, although there is still a reduction in astigmatism from preoperative. *Courtesy of Patrick Rowan, MD.*

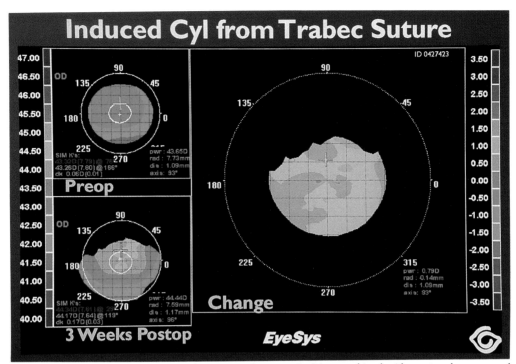

Figure 12-20A. Case receiving a sutureless temporal cataract incision combined with a sutured superonasal trabeculotomy. Upper left shows preoperative appearance, lower left shows 3-week postoperative appearance, and right shows induced corneal changes. The corneal steepening is caused by the trabeculotomy suture.

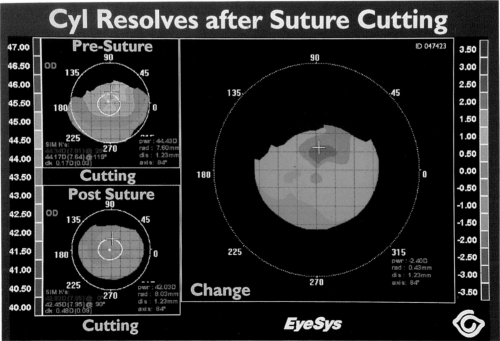

Figure 12-20B. After cutting the trabeculotomy suture, the induced cylinder resolves.

REFERENCES

1. Martin RG, Sanders DR, Miller JD, et al. Effect of cataract wound incision size on acute changes in corneal topography. *J Cataract and Refract Surg.* 1993;19:170-177.
2. Williamson CH, Fine IH. Foldable IOLs, topical anesthesia, and clear-corneal incisions. In: Martin RG, Gills JP, Sanders DR, eds. *Foldable Intraocular Lenses.* Thorofare, NJ: SLACK, Inc; 1993.
3. Fine IH, Sichman RA, Grabow HB, eds. *Clear Corneal Cataract Surgery and Topical Anesthesia.*, Thorofare, NJ: SLACK, Inc; 1993.
4. Utrata PJ, Brown DC. STAAR elastimide three-piece silicone IOL. In: Martin RG, Gills JP, Sanders DR, eds. *Foldable Intraocular Lenses.* Thorofare, NJ: SLACK, Inc; 1993.
5. Gayton JL, Rowan P, Van Der Karr MA. Cataract incisions at the steep axis. In: Gills JP, Martin RG, Thornton SP, Sanders DR, eds. *Surgical Treatment of Astigmatism.*, Thorofare, NJ: SLACK, Inc; 1994.

CORNEAL TOPOGRAPHY IN REFRACTIVE SURGICAL PROCEDURES

Johnny L. Gayton, MD
David Dulaney, MD
Spencer P. Thornton, MD, FACS
Robert G. Martin, MD

The results of refractive surgery for myopia and astigmatism are not as predictable as clinicians or patients would like. While many patients are highly satisfied with the correction achieved by surgery, a substantial minority experience undercorrection, overcorrection, and/or some degree of corneal and visual distortion. The use of corneal topography provides the potential to improve the predictability of refractive procedures, as well as being a useful tool in monitoring and evaluating results.

RADIAL KERATOTOMY

Figures 13-1A and B show the right and left eyes of a patient with 3 D of myopia bilaterally. The image in the upper left corner of each slide is preoperative. The corneas have a typical prolate appearance, being steeper centrally. The image in the lower left corner of both figures was made 1 week postoperatively. As expected, the central cornea in both eyes is now flatter than the periphery, which is referred to as an oblate-shaped cornea. Surgery resulted in refractions of +0.25 D in the right eye and -0.25 D in the left eye at 1 week. In the change images (right side), the darkest blue in the center of the corneas indicates 3 to 3.6 D of flattening. This flattening is fairly symmetrical and well centralized around the videokeratographic (VK) axis, indicating a successful radial keratotomy (RK). Note that the pupil was localized in the postoperative image in the left eye (Figure 13-1B, lower left), and in this case the center of the pupil is coincident to the corneal vertex. Notice also that while the postoperative flattened zone is not completely symmetrical, especially in the right eye (Figure 13-1A, lower left), the surgically induced change is symmetrical (right). This result is probably due to the corneal asymmetry in power that can be observed preoperatively.

Figures 13-2A and B are the right and left eyes of an RK case with 7 D of myopia bilaterally, plus 1 D of refractive astigmatism in the left eye. The patient received eight radials in each eye plus a short T-cut in the left eye. Note the obvious central flattening in both eyes, indicated by blue in the postoperative and change images. In the right eye, the flattening is very symmetrical and well centered, as expected from simple RK. In the left eye, the flattening is again well-centered, but somewhat less symmetrical, possibly because of the T-cut used in addition to the radial incisions. Note that the scale of the change graphs (right) is in 1 D steps as compared to 1/2 D steps for Figure 13-1. This scaling is in order to better visualize the greater degree of corneal flattening in this case.

Figures 13-3A and B show another bilateral RK case with moderate myopia and astigmatism. In the right eye, the astigmatism is clearly steeper inferiorly, while in the left eye it is more symmetrical. The patient received eight radials and a T-cut in each eye. The patient has no residual astigmatism in the right eye, as shown in the postoperative image. Notice how the blue area in the change image, representing 2.5 to 3.5 D of change, can be virtually superimposed on the corresponding steep area represented by orange in the preoperative image. The results were nearly as good in the left eye. Again notice how the change image corresponds to the location of the shape of the preoperative astigmatism.

Figure 13-4 shows the right and left eyes of a patient who has undergone bilateral RK. In this particular case, the patient sees well with the right eye but is complaining of visual distortion and discomfort using the left eye. The

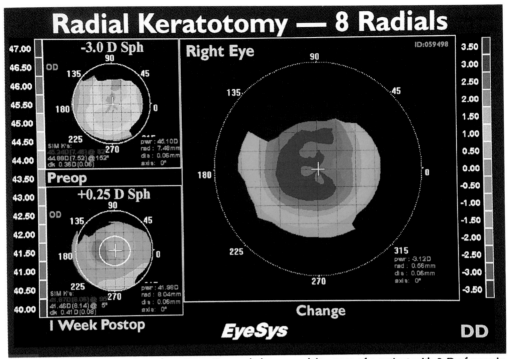

Figure 13-1A. Preoperative, 1-week postoperative, and change or delta maps of a patient with 3 D of myopia bilaterally. Note the large area of symmetrical flattening of 3 - 3.6 D shown in the change maps (right). Right eye.

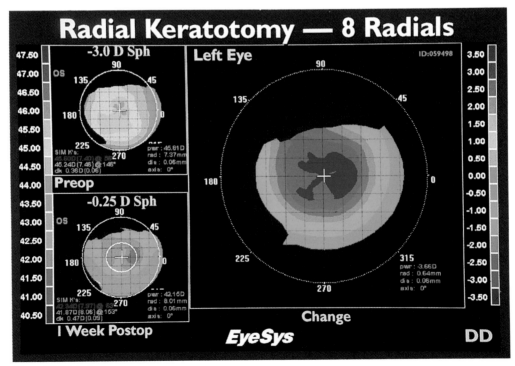

Figure 13-1B. Left eye.

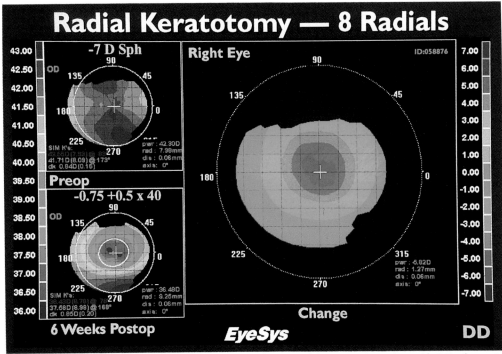

Figure 13-2A. Preoperative, 6-week postoperative, and change or delta maps of a patient with 7 D of myopia bilaterally. Right eye.

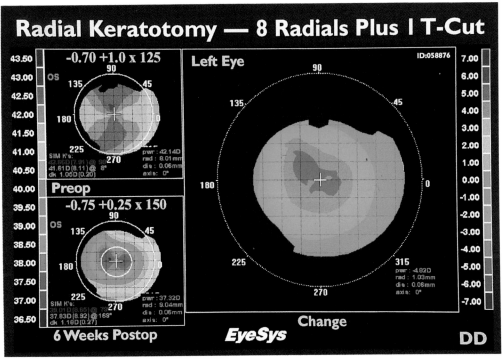

Figure 13-2B. Left eye.

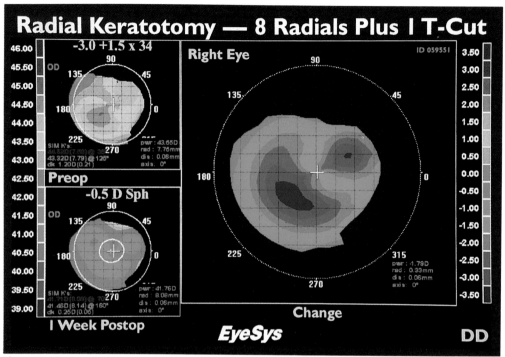

Figure 13-3A. Preoperative, 1-week postoperative, and change or delta maps of a patient with moderate myopia and astigmatism preoperatively. T-incisions resulted in a marked decrease in astigmatism postoperatively. Right eye.

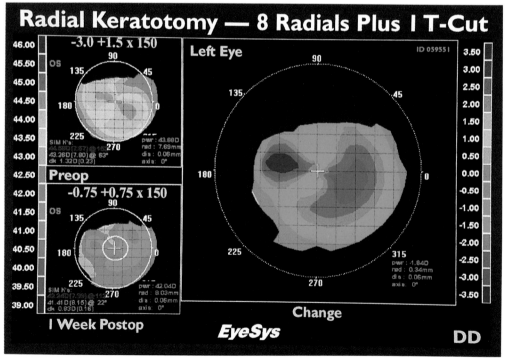

Figure 13-3B. Left eye.

pattern of flattening in the left eye appears to be heart-shaped. From the scale it is apparent that each color encompasses a 1/2 D interval. Figure 13-5 shows a zoom image of the central cornea. Keep in mind that each square on the grid outline is 1 mm by 1 mm. Within the central 2-mm optical zone, there is a range of 4 D of power represented. Within a 4-mm optical zone, there is a 5 D range. Thus the most probable cause for the patient's visual complaints is this multifocal central cornea. Only the corneal topographical mapping would suggest a possible surgical solution to this problem: a single or double T-cut only done superiorly, or possibly deepening or redoing the superior radial cut.

ASTIGMATIC KERATOTOMY

As we have seen in Figures 13-3A and B transverse incisions can be successfully combined with RK to correct astigmatism. One major value of corneal topography in this situation would be to detect asymmetric astigmatism which might benefit from asymmetric surgery.

Figure 13-6 demonstrates a case where most of the astigmatic power is present superiorly in the cornea. A four-incision RK with asymmetric arcuate T-incisions (35° of arc superiorly and only 25° of arc inferiorly) was performed. The postoperative image demonstrates a fairly symmetrical flattening.

Figure 13-7 shows a case that received four-incision RK with two pairs of arcuate incisions to correct 4 D of myopia and 2.75 D of with-the-rule astigmatism. Postoperatively, the patient was plano. The change map demonstrates the greater flattening in the meridian of the arcuate incisions.

Astigmatic Keratotomy Post Cataract Surgery

Figure 13-8 shows topography of an 89-year-old woman who had astigmatic keratotomy (AK) 7 years post cataract surgery. Her refraction was +2.25 -4.50 x 95 with 20/30⁻ best-corrected acuity and 20/200 uncorrected acuity. Two pairs of relaxing incisions were performed at the 6- and 8-mm optical zones. Each incision was 43° of arc.

Preoperatively, the topography demonstrated against-the-rule astigmatism. Two weeks postoperatively, there appears to be an overcorrection, with some oblique astigmatism. However, the refraction was only -0.50 -0.75 x 45 with 20/30⁻ uncorrected vision and 20/25⁻ best-corrected vision. The change map demonstrates the coupling effect, with flattening in the incision meridian and steepening 90° away.

Figure 13-9 is the topography of an 89-year-old woman receiving AK 10 years post cataract surgery. Refraction was +1.00 -4.00 x 90. Due to slight asymmetry in the cylinder power noted on the preoperative topography, two 35° arcuate relaxing incisions were placed nasally and one temporally. The resulting postoperative refraction at 3 months was -0.25 -0.75 x 155. The central pupillary area within the white circle in the postoperative image on the right in Figure 13-9 demonstrates a marked reduction in astigmatism. The change

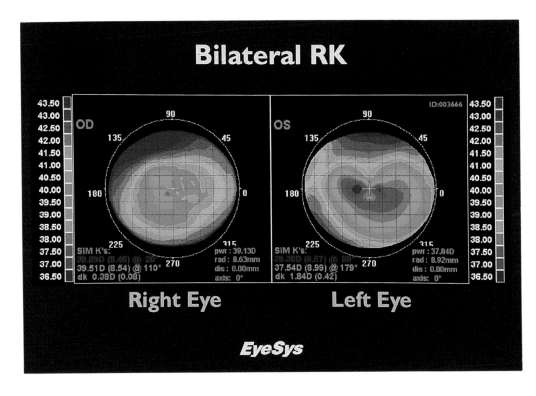

Figure 13-4. Late postoperative corneal topography maps of a patient who underwent bilateral RK. Patient complains of visual distortion and discomfort using the left eye.

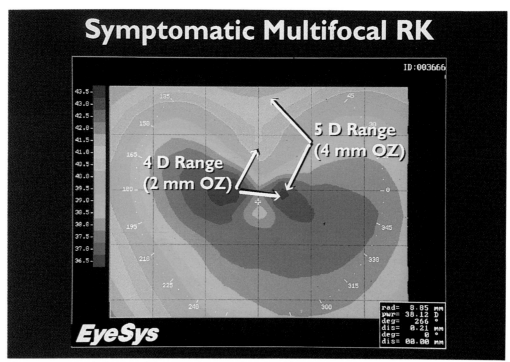

Figure 13-5. Magnified image of the corneal topography map of the patient's left eye emphasizing the central area demonstrating a multifocal central cornea, probably causing the patient's visual symptoms.

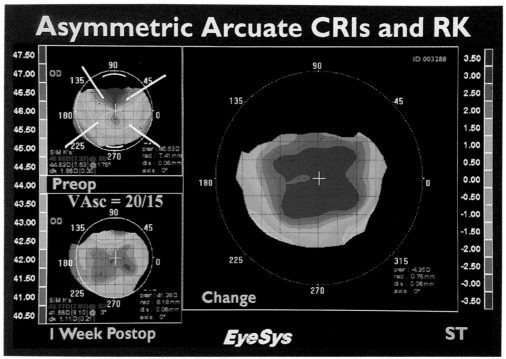

Figure 13-6. Asymmetric astigmatism in a case scheduled for radial and astigmatic keratotomy. Arcuate incisions of unequal length were chosen to treat the asymmetric astigmatism in addition to four-radial sutures. The postoperative image demonstrates improved symmetry of astigmatism postoperatively due to the use of asymmetric astigmatism surgery.

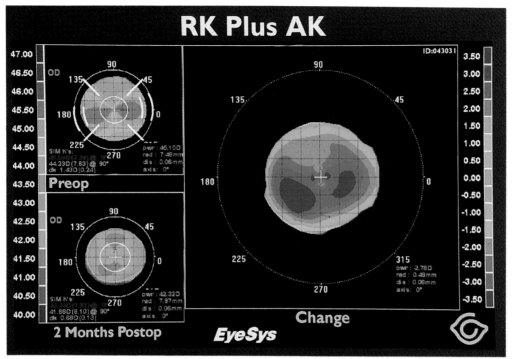

Figure 13-7. Combined radial and astigmatic keratotomy to correct against-the-rule astigmatism. The use of radials prevents the coupling effect caused by transverse relaxing incisions, that is, there is no steepening 90° away from the relaxing incisions. Indeed, the change map (right) for this case demonstrates flattening in the meridian of the relaxing incisions without steepening elsewhere. The 2-month postoperative image (lower left) indicates a relatively spherical cornea.

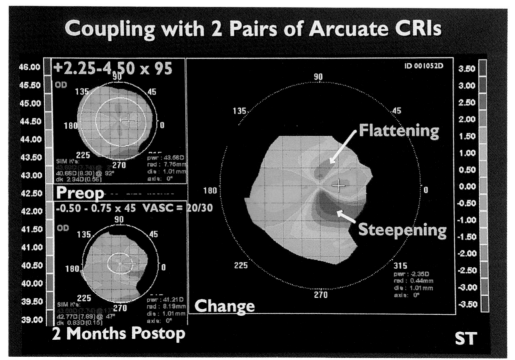

Figure 13-8. Corneal topography of a post-cataract case receiving two pairs of arcuate relaxing incisions. Upper left shows preoperative corneal appearance, lower left shows 2-month postoperative appearance, and right demonstrates the induced surgical changes. Note the coupling in this case, that is, flattening in the incision meridian combined with steepening 90° away.

Figure 13-9. Corneal topography of a post-cataract case receiving two relaxing incisions nasally and one temporally. Upper left shows preoperative corneal appearance, lower left shows 3-month postoperative appearance, and right shows surgically induced corneal changes. Note the greater flattening nasally in the change image.

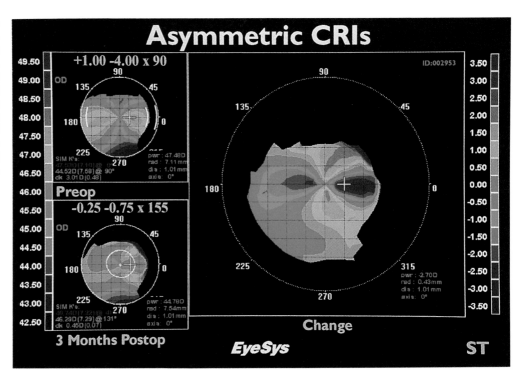

graph on the right demonstrates more effect nasally (a deeper blue color) where the two incisions were placed.

The 77-year-old male shown in Figure 13-10 received AK 2 years post cataract surgery. He presented with 3.75 D of refractive cylinder. An undercorrection was planned to match the refraction in the fellow eye. Two relaxing incisions were performed at the 7-mm optical zone. The nasal incision was 40° of arc while the temporal incision was slightly longer, 50° of arc, because the astigmatism was steeper temporally as shown by topography.

Postoperatively the patient had 1.5 D of residual refractive cylinder. Uncorrected visual acuity improved from 20/200 preoperatively to 20/50 postoperatively, with 20/20 best-corrected visual acuity.

Astigmatic Keratotomy Post Penetrating Keratoplasty

Figure 13-11A demonstrates the power of corneal relaxing incisions in corneal transplant cases. This case had over 11 D of against-the-rule astigmatism preoperatively, and by 4 weeks postoperatively demonstrated 5 D of with-the-rule astigmatism. This 16 D shift is so gross that it is obvious on the corneoscopic pictures shown in Figures 13-11B and C.

REFRACTIVE SURGERY ENHANCEMENTS

Many refractive surgeons take a conservative approach toward incisional keratotomy procedures to avoid overcorrections. Inevitably, some patients require enhancement of the original procedure to achieve their optimal result. Corneal topography can aid the surgeon in tracking the postoperative course, illustrating residual refractive errors and regression, and can be used in designing a surgical enhancement plan.

Figure 13-12 illustrates the corneal topography of an RK enhancement case with 7.5 D of myopia who received eight-incision RK with a 3-mm optical zone, with redeepening at the 5- and 7-mm optical zones at the time of the original surgery. Postoperatively, the patient had -1.75 D of residual myopia. The image on the upper left is before the enhancement and the image on the lower left shows topography following redeepening of the incisions at the 3-, 4-, 5-, 6-, and 7-mm optical zones. The change image (right) illustrates the additional flattening caused by the enhancement. One month post-enhancement, the refraction was -0.50 sphere, which has remained stable through 8 months post-enhancement.

Figure 13-13 demonstrates the corneal topography of a case receiving eight-incision RK with a 4.5-mm optical zone.

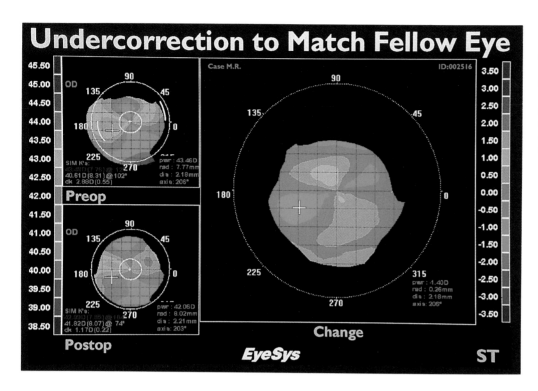

Figure 13-10. Corneal topography of a post-cataract case receiving a pair of relaxing incisions. The surgical plan called for an undercorrection. Upper left shows preoperative corneal appearance, lower left shows postoperative appearance, and right shows surgically induced corneal changes.

Preoperatively the refraction was -3.75 sph. Prior to enhancement the refraction was -3.25 +0.50 x 2. The pre-enhancement topography shows an unusual "island" of steepness, accounting for the residual myopia. The RK was enhanced by reducing the optical zone to 4 mm. One month post-enhancement, the refraction was -2 sph. The post-enhancement topography indicates a more spherical cornea, and the change image demonstrates the additional central flattening.

Figure 13-14 illustrates an RK and AK case initially receiving four radials and a single arcuate incision at the location of greatest corneal steepening. Preoperatively, the refraction was -6.50 +0.75 x 100 with uncorrected vision of count fingers. Postoperatively, the refraction was -2.50 sph, but the vision only improved to 20/100. After adding four more radials, the refraction 3 months after enhancement was -0.75 sph, with uncorrected vision of 20/25.

Figure 13-15 illustrates a patient who had refraction of -4.00 +2.75 x 5 preoperatively and received four radial incisions at the 4-mm optical zone and two pairs of arcuate incisions at the 6- and 8-mm optical zones of 35° of arc each. The first change view (bottom left) indicates the additional flattening caused by the arcuate incisions. Because there were also radial incisions, there is no coupling. Some residual

against-the-rule astigmatism remained (top middle), so the arcuates were lengthened, causing flattening in the incision meridian (second change image, bottom right). This time coupling is evident.

EPIKERATOPHAKIA

Corneal topography plays a vital role in all phases of the management of patients undergoing epikeratophakia. For myopic epikeratophakia, computer-generated topographic images are important tools for assessing the baseline corneal topography of the eye, particularly to check for the presence of asymmetric astigmatism or occult topographic disorders such as early keratoconus. For epikeratophakia for keratoconus, preoperative topography is extremely useful for analyzing the type of cone, since the success rate of epikeratophakia tends to be higher in corneas with small central cones. It is also useful in documenting cone flattening with epikeratophakia, and documenting suture effects (Figure 13-16).

Topography is also a key component in the postoperative follow-up and management of epikeratophakia patients. It can assist in selective suture removal (Figure 13-17), and is essential in the evaluation of the centration, size, and uniformity of the optical zone (Figures 13-18 and 13-19). It

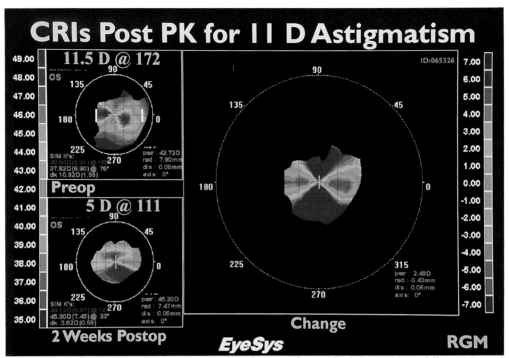

Figure 13-11A. Case with marked overcorrection which received corneal relaxing incisions following corneal transplantation. Preoperative, 1-week postoperative, and change or delta map demonstrating the marked overcorrection.

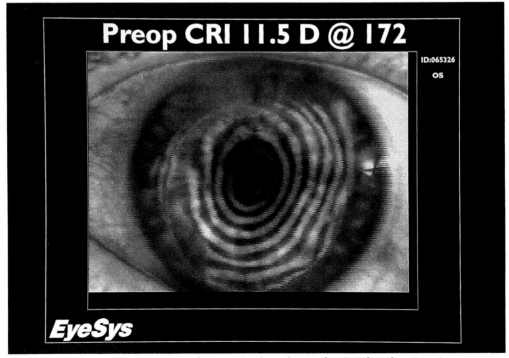

Figure 13-11B. Preoperative corneoscopy demonstrating large degree of against-the-rule astigmatism.

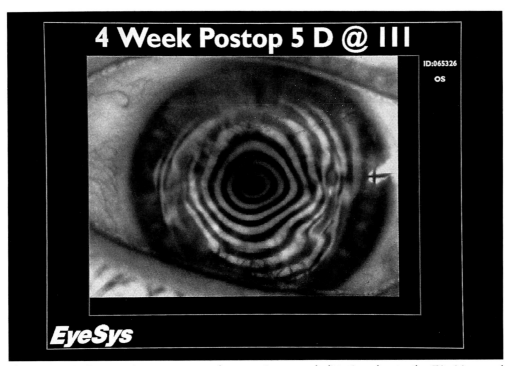

Figure 13-11C. Postoperative corneoscopy demonstrating corneal distortion due to the T-incisions and with-the-rule astigmatism.

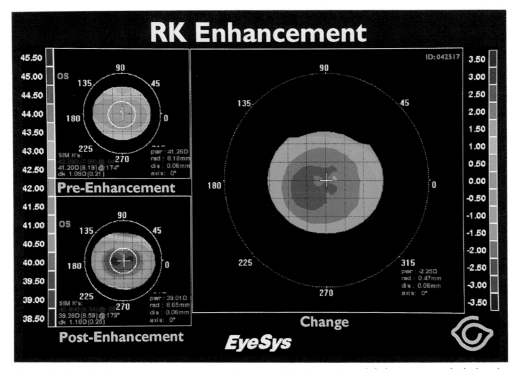

Figure 13-12. Radial keratotomy case receiving redeepening of incisions. Upper left shows topography before the redeepening, lower left shows post-enhancement topography, and right shows induced corneal changes.

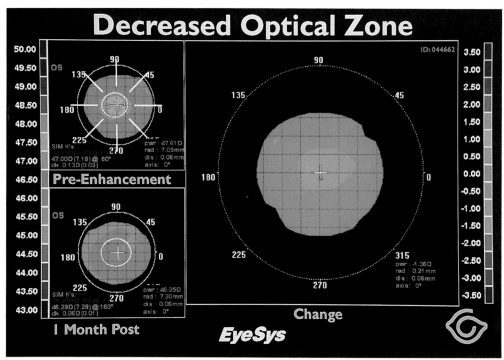

Figure 13-13. Radial keratotomy case exhibiting a rare "central island" postoperatively (upper left). Reducing the optical zone eliminated the problem (lower left). The right image demonstrates the additional central flattening produced by the enhancement.

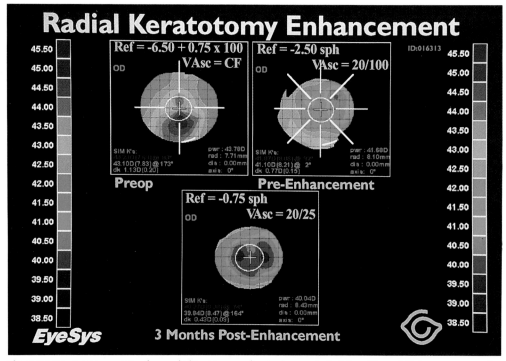

Figure 13-14. A case receiving four radial incisions and a single arcuate incision. Upper left shows preoperative appearance and placement of the incisions. Postoperatively the astigmatism was well corrected, but there remained 2.5 D of myopia, so four radials were added. Upper right shows pre-enhancement appearance and placement of all incisions received by the patient. The bottom image shows the post-enhancement appearance. The patient achieved excellent uncorrected visual acuity.

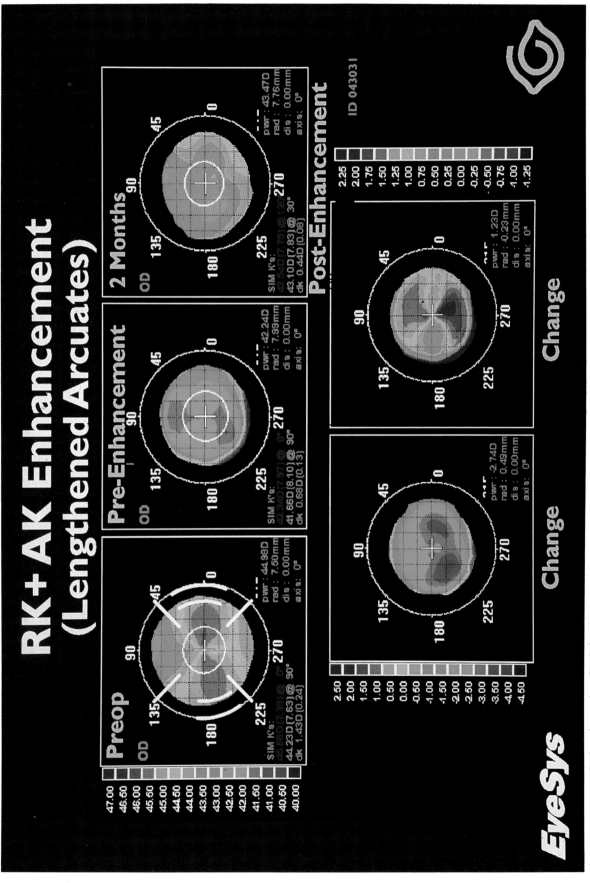

Figure 13-15. STARS display of a combined radial and astigmatic keratotomy case receiving four radials and two pairs of arcuate incisions (top left). Postoperatively (top middle), the patient has good correction of myopia but some residual against-the-rule astigmatism. The first change map (bottom left), shows the flattening caused by the combined incisions, with no evidence of coupling due to the presence of radial incisions. The arcuate incisions were then lengthened. Post-enhancement (top right), there is no evidence of central astigmatism. The second change map (bottom right), indicates coupling caused by the enhancement.

Figure 13-16. Preoperative, 3-day postoperative, and change corneal topography maps of the right eye of a keratoconus case that received a planar epikeratophakia to flatten the cone. Tight sutures were responsible for the nasal steepening observed. Later removal of these sutures evened out the topographic picture. *Courtesy of Dr. S. Ganem, Paris, France.*

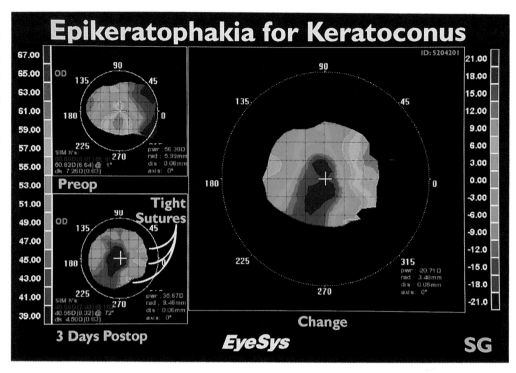

is also useful in managing any complications should they occur (Figure 13-20).

HEXAGONAL KERATOTOMY

Figure 13-21 is an example of an eye undergoing hexagonal keratotomy and later secondary AK. The patient received a 4.5-mm spiral hex for the correction of 4 D of hyperopia (Figure 13-21A). Approximately 3 D of symmetric steepening was achieved with uncorrected acuity improving from 20/200 to 20/80, with corrected acuity remaining unchanged at 20/30. The patient had approximately 2 D of postoperative cylinder and underwent secondary AK 7 months following primary hexagonal surgery. At that time the patient received a pair of arcuate transverse incisions at the 6.5-mm optical zone, resulting in a 1.5 D reduction in cylinder (Figure 13-21B). Following secondary AK, uncor-

rected acuity improved to 20/25 and corrected acuity improved to 20/20.

SUMMARY

The survey of the corneal topographic findings with the refractive procedures discussed above demonstrates the usefulness of videokeratography in understanding the effect of these procedures upon the cornea. It is clear that by relying upon keratometry alone the refractive surgeon is literally "flying blind."

All refractive surgeons have experienced the disappointment of apparently well-planned refractive surgery that produced negligible, incomplete, or unexpected results. The consideration of corneal topographic data in the planning of surgery may improve the predictability of results, and may begin to explain the occasional treatment failure.

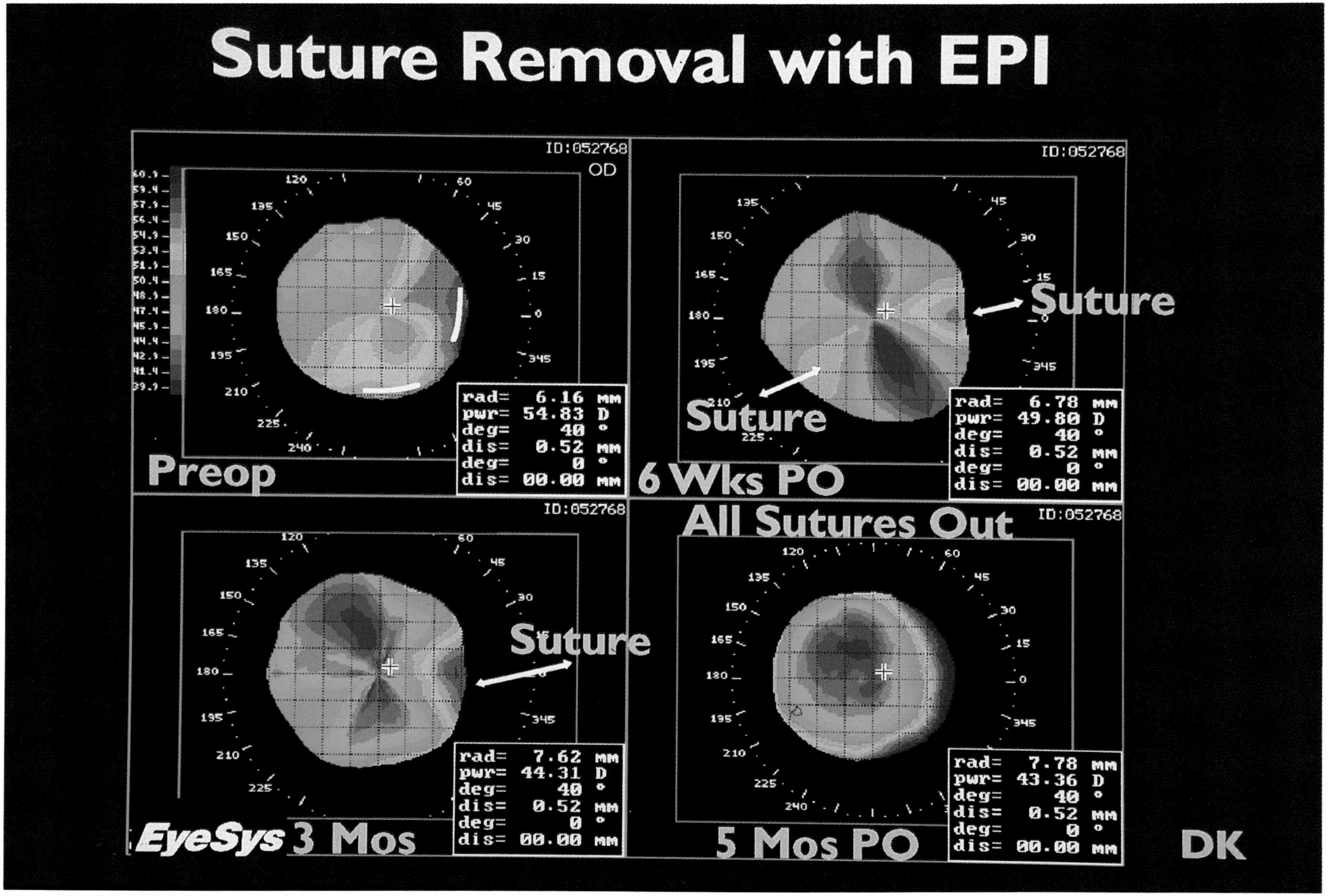

Figure 13-17. Upper left, right cornea of 24-year-old female who had undergone penetrating keratoplasty 2 years previously for herpetic corneal scarring. Refraction was -13.00 +5.75 x 30, with VAcc of 20/200. With a contact lens, she could see 20/80, but she was contact lens intolerant. Arcuate 45° incisions were placed just inside the graft-host junction along the two steep semi-meridians, and a myopic epikeratophakia was placed over the entire graft. Upper right, at 6 weeks postoperatively, there is moderate astigmatism at 5° and 230° due to the presence of interrupted sutures. Lower left, 3 months postoperatively, following removal of all but the 3:00 sutures, much of the astigmatism has been resolved. Lower right, 5 months postoperatively, all sutures are out. Keratometric astigmatism is 1.75 D, and refraction is -2.00 +1.50 x 25 with VAcc of 20/25. Note the mild temporal centration of the optical zone, paralleling the location of the flat region preoperatively. *Courtesy of Douglas Koch, MD.*

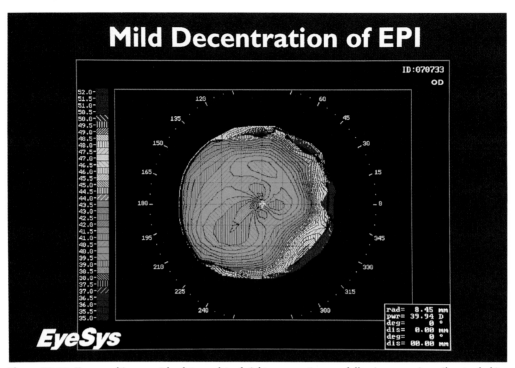

Figure 13-18. Topographic map (absolute scale) of right cornea 4 years following myopic epikeratophakia. Preoperative refraction was -16.00 +4.75 x 120 with VAcc of 20/40, and postoperative refraction was -0.50 +1.75 x 120 with VAcc of 20/40. Note the mild (approximately 1 mm) temporal decentration and the variable zones of power in the central cornea.

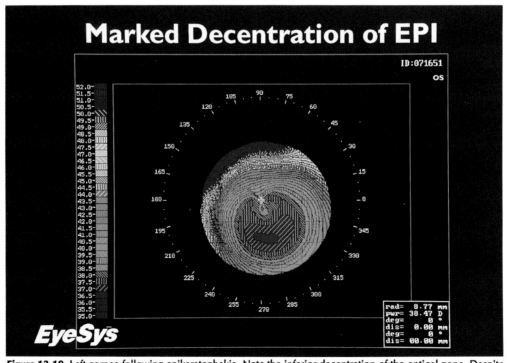

Figure 13-19. Left cornea following epikeratophakia. Note the inferior decentration of the optical zone. Despite best-corrected vision of 20/20 to 20/25, the patient complained of halos, especially at night.

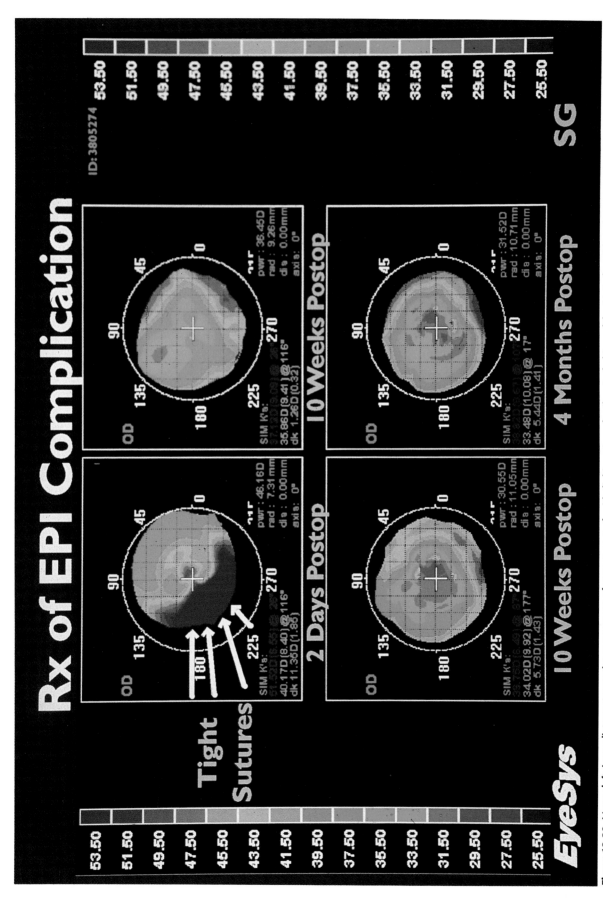

Figure 13-20. Upper left, immediate postoperative appearance after treatment of epithelial invasion of epikeratophakia graft-host interface. There is asymmetric astigmatism with a biphasic cornea due to four interrupted sutures at 190,° 200,° 210,° and 220° responsible for the steep curvature of this hemi-meridian. Upper right, 6 weeks postoperative. The optical zone is reappearing, but is decentered after cutting the sutures. Lower images, result after recentering the epikeratoplasty lens. *Courtesy of Dr. S. Ganem, Paris, France.*

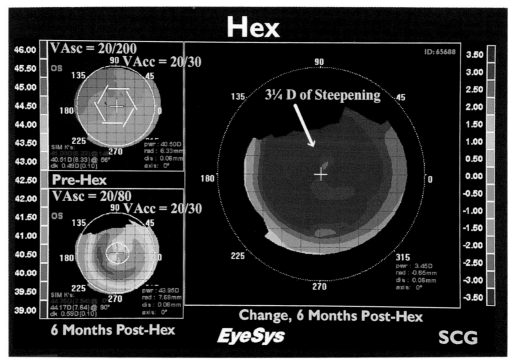

Figure 13-21A. Corneal topography of an eye undergoing hexagonal keratotomy and later secondary AK. The patient received a 4.5-mm spiral hex for the correction of 4 D of hyperopia. Upper left shows preoperative appearance and placement of incisions. Lower left shows 6-month postoperative appearance. The change map (right) demonstrates the induced steepening. *Courtesy of Stanley Grandon, MD.*

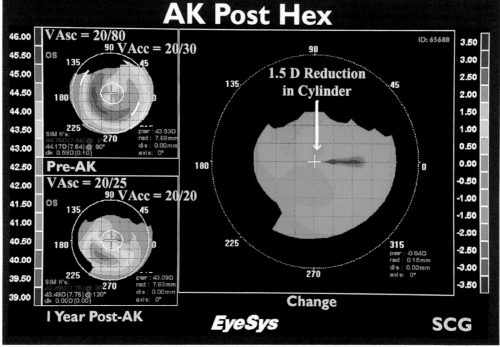

Figure 13-21B. The patient had approximately 2 D of postoperative cylinder and underwent secondary AK 7 months following primary hexagonal surgery. At that time she received a pair of arcuate transverse incisions at the 6.5-mm optical zone. Upper left shows appearance prior to AK and placement of all incisions, lower left shows appearance 1 year after AK, and right demonstrates the induced corneal changes. The AK resulted in a 1.5 D reduction in cylinder. *Courtesy of Stanley Grandon, MD.*

CATARACT SURGERY COMBINED WITH ASTIGMATIC KERATOTOMY

James P. Gills, MD
Robert G. Martin, MD

With the advent of truly small-incision cataract surgery utilizing foldable IOLs and sutureless surgery, significant surgically induced astigmatism has been largely eliminated. The surgeon can now concentrate on treating a patient's preexisting astigmatism without being concerned with large iatrogenic changes. In a recent survey of American Society of Cataract and Refractive Surgery (ASCRS) members, 8.7% of surgeons report using corneal relaxing incisions (CRIs) as an adjunct to cataract surgery and 68% consider it a viable option even though they may not personally utilize it. A number of studies on the efficacy of the procedure with cataract extraction have been reported.[1-7] In general, the efficacy variable has been changes in keratometric cylinder. As has been demonstrated in Chapter 3, keratometry may give incomplete information at best and at worst be misleading. We will show through a number of illustrations how corneal topography provides much more information and gives the surgeon a greater feel for the effect of the surgical procedure upon the cornea.

SCREENING

As with any refractive surgery candidate, cataract patients should be screened to determine their eligibility for astigmatic keratotomy. The importance of corneal topography in screening cataract patients was borne out in a study by one of the authors (RGM). The preoperative topographies from 100 consecutive patients presenting with cataracts were evaluated by an independent topography expert.

Four percent of the maps were found to be grossly abnormal, possibly indicating corneal pathology. Figure 14-1 shows an unusual pattern of marked superior steepness and inferior flatness. Since the cause of this pattern is unknown, refractive surgery would not be advisable in such a case. Figure 14-2 demonstrates inferior steepness in the topography. This pattern is sometimes indicative of corneal warpage due to long-term contact lens wear. However, it can also be indicative of incipient keratoconus.

Evaluating preoperative topographies is also important for determining surgical plans. In the Martin study, 7% of patients were found to have asymmetric astigmatism. Figure 14-3 shows a case of asymmetric astigmatism, with greater steepness inferiorly, of which the surgeon would wish to be aware in determining the surgical plan. Asymmetric surgery with more or longer relaxing incisions inferiorly would probably be more effective. Figure 14-4 demonstrates astigmatism that is not exactly orthogonal. A surgeon attempting to correct this astigmatism might wish to use the topography to place the incisions precisely in the steepest regions, and not exactly 180° apart.

TOPOGRAPHICAL RESULTS

Figure 14-5 illustrates the topography of a 77-year-old man who received a 3.2-mm sutureless scleral-tunnel incision and a pair of CRIs to counteract large with-the-rule astigmatism. Both the inferior and superior incision had a chord length of 3 mm.

Preoperatively, the patient had over 8 D of keratometric cylinder. The topography showed severely asymmetric astigmatism, with the cornea steepest inferiorly. Postoperatively, the topography showed the same astigmatic pattern, with a reduction in the steepness. The keratometric cylinder has been reduced by over 3 D, leaving 5 D of residual cylinder. The patient achieved reasonably good visual acuity, seeing

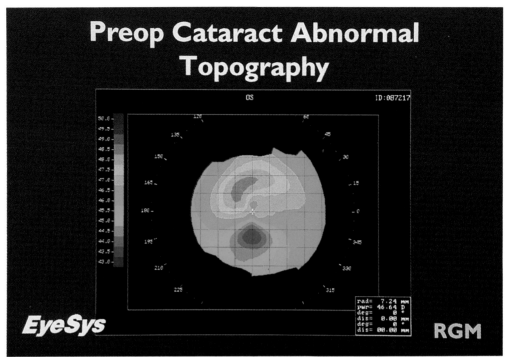

Figure 14-1. Preoperative topography of a patient presenting for cataract surgery. The cornea has an unusual pattern of marked superior steepness and inferior flatness.

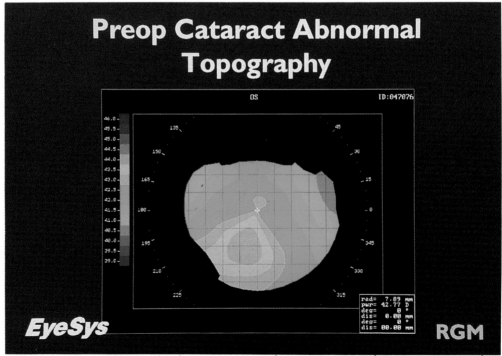

Figure 14-2. Preoperative topography of a patient presenting for cataract surgery. Inferior steepness as seen here can be indicative of corneal warpage due to long-term contact lens wear. In the absence of a history of contact lens wear, this pattern could signify incipient keratoconus.

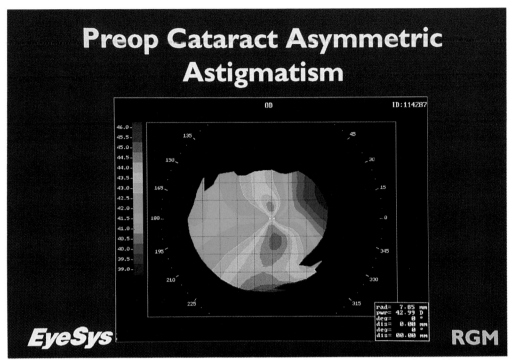

Figure 14-3. Preoperative topography of a patient presenting for cataract surgery and possible astigmatic keratotomy. The topography shows greater steepness inferiorly, which might be best corrected with an asymmetric surgical plan calling for more or longer relaxing incisions in that area.

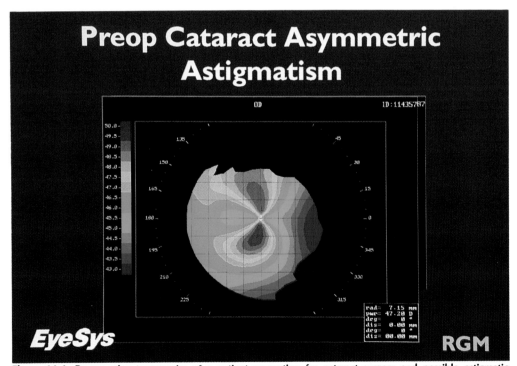

Figure 14-4. Preoperative topography of a patient presenting for cataract surgery and possible astigmatic keratotomy. The steep areas of the cornea are not exactly orthogonal. The preoperative topography could be used to precisely guide placement of the relaxing incisions to the steepest regions.

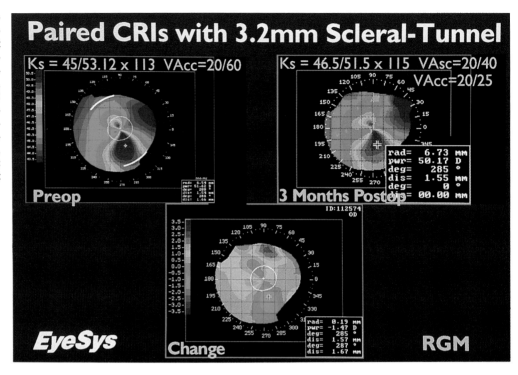

20/40 uncorrected and 20/20 corrected.

Figures 14-6A and 14-6B show a patient who underwent sutureless cataract surgery and CRIs to treat a little over 4 D of preoperative corneal astigmatism by keratometry. Three weeks following small-incision sutureless surgery, the cornea does not demonstrate a normal topographic configuration as shown in the postoperative topographical map in Figure 14-6A. There is only 20/40 best-corrected visual acuity which is probably explained by the corneal distortion as shown in Figure 14-6B. All we know from keratometry is that the astigmatism has decreased by 2.5 D. The change graph at the right side of Figure 14-6A shows that the deep blue areas of corneal flattening are in the axis of the preoperative astigmatism and in the axis of the CRIs.

Figure 14-7 demonstrates topography of a case receiving a temporal clear-corneal incision with an adjacent CRI. The change map (right image) demonstrates asymmetric flattening at the incision site, with some flattening 180° away and steepening 90° away. The postoperative image (lower left) shows the astigmatic pattern effectively broken up, and keratometry indicated sphericity.

The case shown in Figure 14-8 received a temporal clear-corneal incision with an adjacent CRI to correct asymmetric astigmatism. The change map indicates flattening in the location of the incisions with inferior steepening. Postoperative keratometry indicated only 0.25 D of cylinder. The patient achieved excellent visual acuity, seeing 20/25 uncorrected and 20/20 corrected.

Figure 14-9 shows topography of a case that received a small astigmatism correction. A temporal clear-corneal incision and adjacent CRI were performed to correct 1 D of keratometric cylinder. Two months postoperatively, the cylinder was well corrected. Keratometry was 42.75/43.25 x 143, and refraction was plano, with 20/25 uncorrected vision.

The case in Figure 14-10 received a longer sutureless incision, a 6-mm superior, arcuate scleral-tunnel incision for with-the-rule astigmatism. The cornea was steepest inferiorly, so the CRI was placed opposing the cataract incision. The change image demonstrates a coupling effect, with flattening in the meridian of the incisions and steepening 90° away. The astigmatism pattern is effectively broken up, as shown in the postoperative image.

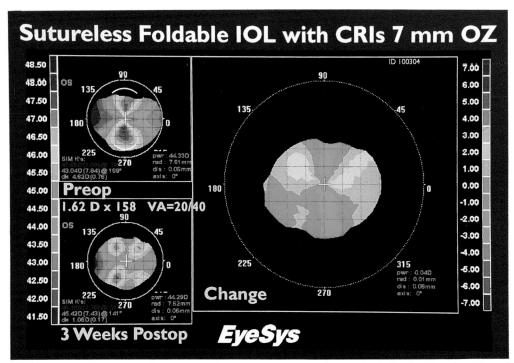

Figure 14-6A. Patient who underwent sutureless cataract surgery and corneal relaxing incisions for 4.0 D of corneal astigmatism. Preoperative, 3-week postoperative, and change or delta maps. The postoperative corneal map demonstrates disruption of the astigmatic pattern while the change map demonstrates surgically induced flattening in the axis of preoperative corneal steepness.

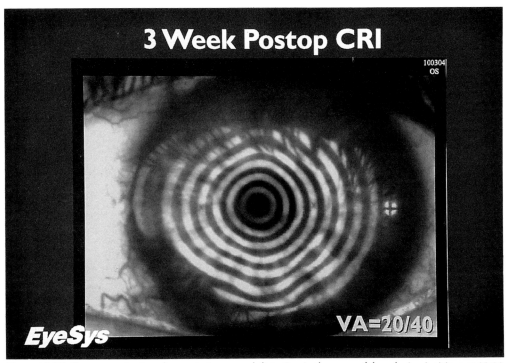

Figure 14-6B. Corneoscopic view demonstrates corneal distortion in the areas of the relaxing incisions at 12:00 and 6:00.

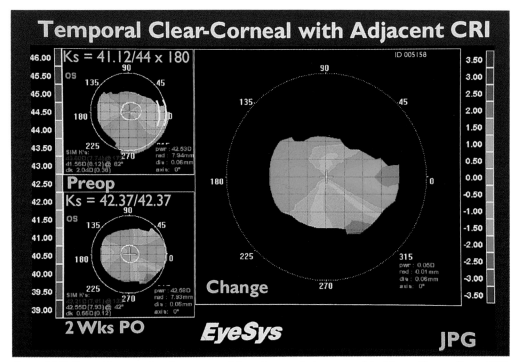

Figure 14-7. Corneal topography of a case receiving a temporal clear-corneal incision with an adjacent CRI. Upper left shows preoperative corneal appearance, lower left shows 2-week postoperative appearance, and right shows surgically induced corneal changes. The change image demonstrates asymmetrical flattening at the wound site, with steepening 90° away. Although the postoperative topography shows steep and flat peripheral regions, the keratometry indicates sphericity. The patient has 20/30 uncorrected acuity postoperatively.

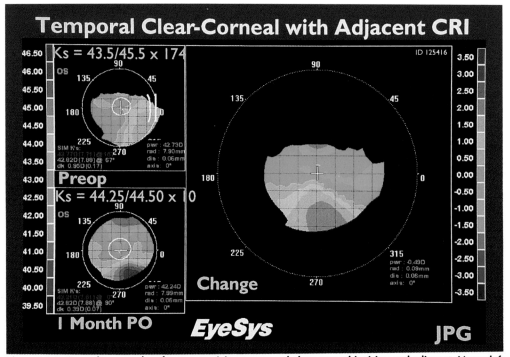

Figure 14-8. Corneal topography of a case receiving a temporal clear-corneal incision and adjacent. Upper left shows preoperative corneal appearance, lower left shows 1-month postoperative appearance, and right shows surgically induced corneal changes. The change image indicates some flattening at the wound site with significant steepening inferiorly. This pattern of induced change produced the steep inferior region seen on the postoperative image. However, since this region is mostly peripheral, it does not seem to adversely affect vision. The patient can see 20/25 uncorrected.

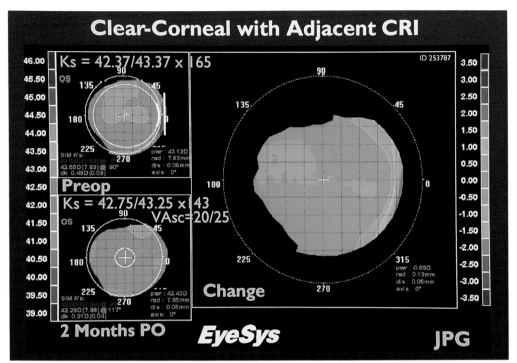

Figure 14-9. Corneal topography of case with 1 D of keratometric cylinder receiving a temporal clear-corneal incision and adjacent. Upper left shows preoperative corneal appearance, lower left shows 2-month postoperative appearance, and right shows surgically induced corneal changes. Note the relatively spherical corneal surface postoperatively.

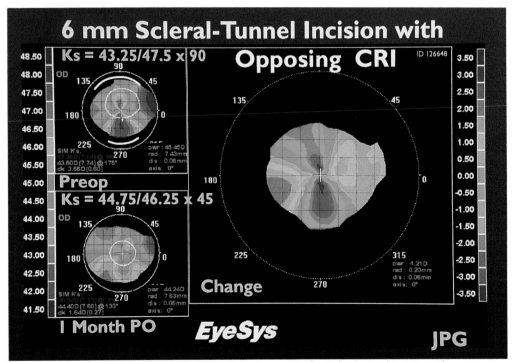

Figure 14-10. Corneal topography of a case receiving a 6-mm sutureless scleral-tunnel incision with an opposing, to correct 4.25 D of with-the-rule cylinder. Upper left shows preoperative corneal appearance, lower left shows 1-month postoperative appearance, and right shows surgically induced corneal changes. The change image demonstrates significant flattening in the incision meridian with steepening 90° away. As demonstrated by the postoperative image, the astigmatic pattern has been effectively broken up.

SUMMARY

As with any refractive surgery, proper screening, good centration, accurate placement, and ability to track postoperative progress are essential. These keys to surgical success are even more important when dealing with the complexities introduced by combining refractive surgery with cataract surgery. Keratometry can be inadequate to provide the detailed information demanded by combined surgery. Corneal topography provides cataract and refractive surgeons with the accurate information they need about the total corneal surface.

REFERENCES

1. Thornton SP, Sanders DR. Graded nonintersecting transverse incisions for correction of idiopathic astigmatism. *J Cataract Refract Surg.* 1987;13:27-31.
2. Osher RH. Paired transverse relaxing keratotomy: a combined technique for reducing astigmatism. *J Cataract Refract Surg.* 1989;15:32-37.
3. Davison JA. Transverse astigmatic keratotomy combined with phacoemulsification and intraocular lens implantation. *J Cataract Refract Surg.* 1989;15:38-44.
4. Maloney WF, Grindle L, Sanders DR, et al. Astigmatism control for the cataract surgeon: a comprehensive review of surgically tailored astigmatism reduction (STAR). *J Cataract Refract Surg.* 1989;15:45-54.
5. Shepherd JR. Correction of preexisting astigmatism at the time of small incision cataract surgery. *J Cataract Refract Surg.* 1989;15:55-57.
6. Agapitos PJ, Lindstrom RL, Williams PA, et al. Analysis of astigmatic keratotomy. *J Cataract Refract Surg.* 1989;15:13-18.
7. Maloney WF, Sanders DR, Pearcy DE. Astigmatic keratotomy to correct preexisting astigmatism in cataract patients. *J Cataract Refract Surg.* 1990;16:297-304.

CORNEAL RELAXING INCISIONS, MULTIFOCAL CORNEAS, AND "OMNIMMETROPIA"

CHAPTER
15

James P. Gills, MD

Our strategy for managing astigmatism in the cataract patient is dictated by the amount of cylinder present and the nature of the astigmatism. Figure 15-1 depicts the distribution of preexisting keratometric cylinder in a cohort of 356 patients presenting at St. Luke's Cataract and Laser Institute for cataract surgery. Twenty percent of patients typically have less than 0.75 D of cylinder (Group I). These patients with minimal amounts of cylinder receive only an astigmatically neutral cataract incision. The vast majority of patients generally present with between 0.75 and 3.0 D of keratometric cylinder (Group II). In these cases with moderate amounts of cylinder, only a single, arcuate corneal relaxing incision (CRI) is employed in addition to the cataract incision. Our experience with these moderate astigmats was that paired CRIs result in too much correction, and we believed that a single CRI used in conjunction with the cataract incision would be more appropriate. In our hands, paired CRIs are typically reserved for cases with high preexisting astigmatism, that is, greater than 3 D of cylinder (Group III). In general, our approach to managing astigmatism in the cataract patient has become more conservative in order to avoid overcorrections, particularly in cases having with-the-rule astigmatism.

With-the-rule cases receive a superior, scleral cataract incision, while cases having against-the-rule astigmatism receive a temporal, clear-corneal cataract incision. What is novel about our approach is the placement of a single CRI adjacent to, that is, in the same semi-meridian as, the cataract incision in moderate astigmats (Figures 15-2 and 15-3). The CRI is placed at the 8-mm optical zone and is 2 mm in length per diopter of correction desired.

CLINICAL RESULTS

Two hundred sixty-one eyes receiving CRIs and 95 control eyes undergoing cataract surgery, but receiving no CRIs, have been included in this retrospective cohort analysis. The mean follow-up is 1.5 months. Corneal topography was taken using the EyeSys Windows Workstation.

The Coupling Effect

While the idea of a single CRI adjacent to the cataract incision may seem counter intuitive, it is effective in reducing preexisting cylinder while maintaining the coupling effect, which is flattening in the incision meridian and steepening 90° away. As demonstrated in Figure 15-4, mean keratometric cylinder is reduced by more than half, from 1.9 D preoperatively to 0.9 D postoperatively. Figure 15-5 shows a left eye that received a temporal clear-corneal cataract incision and a single adjacent CRI for the correction of 3 D of against-the-rule astigmatism. The difference map demonstrates not only horizontal flattening (blue regions), but steepening of the vertical meridian (yellow regions).

The importance of coupling in the management of preexisting astigmatism in the cataract patient has been emphasized by Thornton.[1] Basically, if coupling is not maintained, average corneal power will change, mitigating against an optimal choice of IOL power.

Figure 15-6 represents the right eye of a high astigmatism patient who received two pairs of arcuate CRIs in the horizontal meridian for the correction of 4 D of preexisting cylinder. The difference map shows 2 D of steepening vertically, as well as 2 D of horizontal flattening, as determined via corneal topography. At 2 weeks postoperatively, this patient saw 20/30 unaided. Figure 15-7 is a case

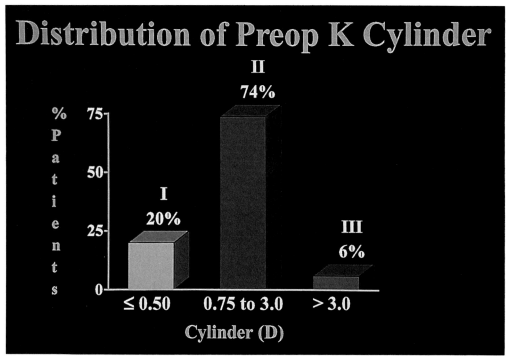

Figure 15-1. Distribution of preexisting keratometric cylinder. At the time of cataract surgery, Group I receives no CRIs, Group II a single CRI, and Group III paired CRIs.

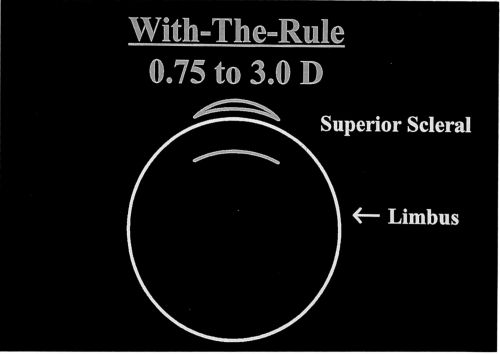

Figure 15-2. Patients presenting with 0.75 to 3.0 D of with-the-rule cylinder receive a superior scleral cataract incision and a single CRI.

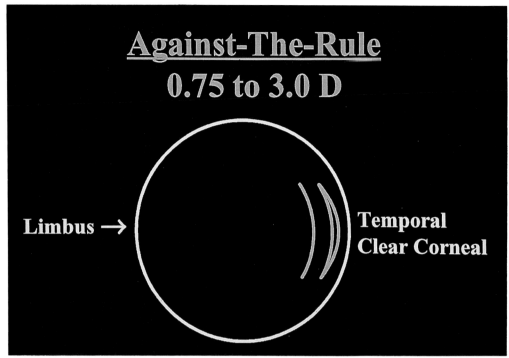

Figure 15-3. Patients presenting with 0.75 to 3.0 D of against-the-rule cylinder receive a temporal clear-corneal cataract incision and a single CRI.

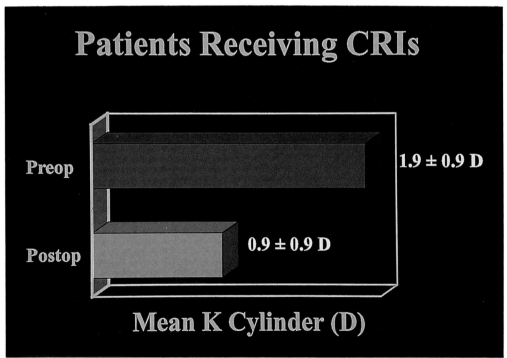

Figure 15-4. Comparison of pre and postoperative keratometric cylinder in patients receiving CRIs.

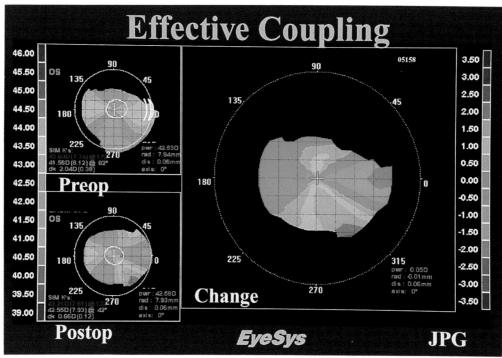

Figure 15-5. Effective coupling is achieved with a single CRI. The change map indicates not only horizontal flattening, but also steepening of the vertical meridian.

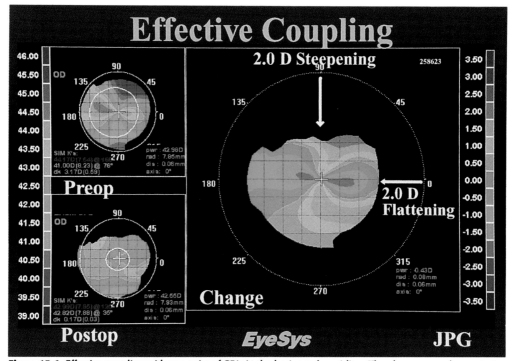

Figure 15-6. Effective coupling with two pairs of CRIs in the horizontal meridian. The change map demonstrates approximately 2.0 D of horizontal flattening as well as approximately 2.0 D of vertical steepening.

presenting with 2 D of asymmetrical against-the-rule astigmatism, who received three CRIs (1 mm in length) in conjunction with a temporal clear-corneal cataract incision. At 2 weeks postoperatively, she was plano-sphere with 20/20 vision.

Figures 15-8A and B demonstrate the effectiveness of this surgical approach to cataract with astigmatism in the form of a vector plot for a subset of against-the-rule cases. The length of each arrow represents the amount of cylinder for each patient, while its orientation depicts the axis of the cylinder. Each concentric ring represents 0.5 D of cylinder. The postoperative plot of Figure 15-8B indicates a dramatic reduction in against-the-rule preexisting astigmatism, which is indicative of our aggressive approach towards this type of astigmatism.

Increased Depth of Focus

We have come to notice that our CRI patients not only have excellent unaided distance acuity after surgery but often can read without the assistance of any spectacle addition. In more technical terms, these patients often display greater depth of focus following surgery than our typical cataract patients. For the purpose of quantifying depth of focus, we define it to be unaided distance acuity of 20/40 or better combined with unaided near acuity of J3 or better. A comparison of the prevalence of this level of depth of focus is shown in Figure 15-9 among three groups of patients:

1. Control eyes undergoing cataract surgery but receiving no CRIs
2. Eyes receiving a single CRI for the correction of less than 2.5 D of cylinder
3. Eyes receiving a single CRI for the correction of 2.5 D or more of preexisting cylinder.

There is a dramatic increase in the prevalence of depth of focus from 24% among control eyes to as much as 54% among the higher astigmatism cases receiving a single CRI.

In order to better understand this phenomenon, we have analyzed several clinical parameters that are known to influence depth of focus. Comparison is made among CRI patients who exhibit depth of focus and those who do not. As shown in the figures, neither postoperative spherical equivalent (Figure 15-10A), refractive cylinder (Figure 15-10B), nor pupil diameter (Figure 15-10C) is associated with increased depth of focus, as both groups have very similar levels of each parameter. Clinical trials of multifocal IOLs have taught us the importance of other parameters when studying increased depth of focus, such as best-corrected acuity, glare acuity, and contrast acuity. However, Figures 15-11A through C demonstrate no difference among eyes exhibiting depth of focus and those who do not in best-corrected acuity (Figure 15-11A), glare acuity (Figure 15-11B), or contrast acuity (Figure 15-11C).

While none of the traditional parameters which we might expect to explain the increased depth of focus do, such

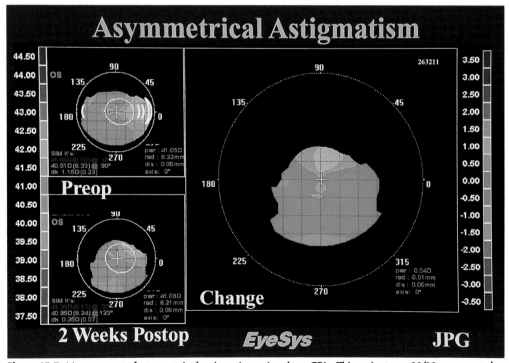

Figure 15-7. Management of asymmetrical astigmatism using three CRIs. This patient was 20/20 uncorrected at 2 weeks postoperatively.

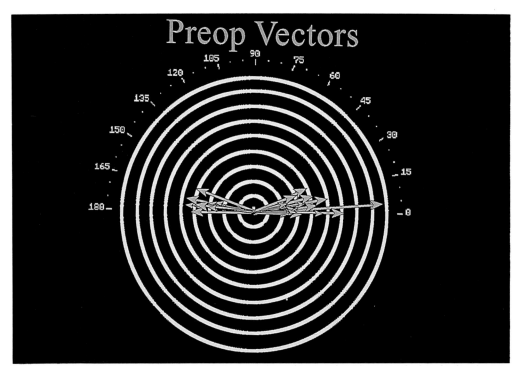

Figure 15-8A. Vector plots of preoperative cylinder in a subset of against-the-rule cases. The length of each arrow indicates the magnitude of cylinder for each patient, while its orientation depicts the axis of cylinder. Each concentric ring represents 0.5 D of cylinder. Visual comparison of A and B demonstrates a dramatic reduction in the against-the-rule nature of the preexisting astigmatism, which is indicative of our aggressive approach towards this type of astigmatism.

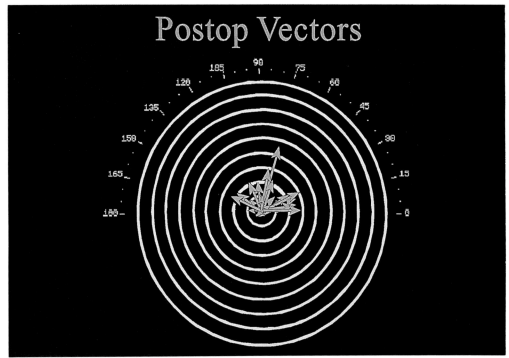

Figure 15-8B. Vector plots of postoperative cylinder in a subset of against-the-rule cases.

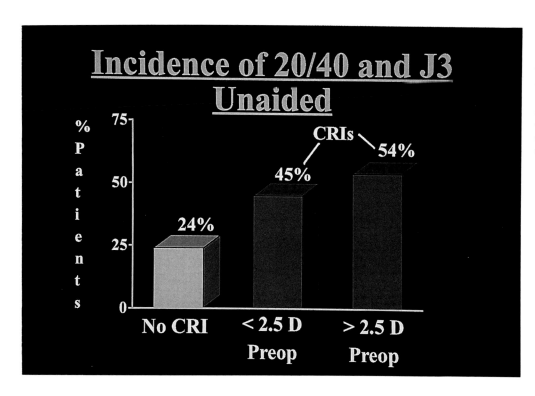

Figure 15-9. Incidence of unaided acuities of 20/40 for distance and J3 for near vision. There is a dramatic increase in the prevalence of 20/40 combined with J3 from 24% among control eyes receiving no CRIs to 54% among higher astigmatism cases receiving a single CRI.

as spherical equivalent, refractive cylinder, and pupil diameter, corneal topography does lend some clues. What we have observed is that eyes exhibiting increased depth of focus often have corneal regions that differ by as much as 3 to 5 D of optical power, as determined by the color maps.

Figure 15-12 is an example of such a postoperative image, showing a 3 D variation in corneal power. The magnitude of this additional steepening would be enough to allow for good near acuity, just as a 3 D spectacle addition does. Although the pupil diameter as seen on the topography map encompasses only portions of the flat and steep corneal regions, this patient sees 20/25 and J1+ unaided at 2 weeks postoperatively. The case demonstrated in Figure 15-13 received a single CRI opposite to a temporal clear-corneal cataract incision in the horizontal meridian. At 2 weeks postoperatively, he had achieved a 1.25 D reduction in cylinder with unaided acuities of 20/20 for distance and J2 for near. A 3.5 D variation in corneal power can be seen in the postoperative color map.

Figure 15-14 shows a left eye with unaided postoperative acuities of 20/30 and J1, with the postoperative color map showing as much as a 7 D inferior-superior variation in corneal power. This eye received a 3-mm temporal clear-corneal cataract incision with a single adjacent CRI at the 3:00 position for the correction of 2 D of preexisting astigmatism. This patient achieved a best-corrected acuity of 20/25 with refraction of +0.25 D sphere. It is possible with these topographic results that the flat regions of the cornea

contribute to distance vision and the steep regions contribute to near vision.

Figure 15-15 is another example of the effect of a single CRI adjacent to a temporal clear-corneal cataract incision. At 2 weeks postoperatively, this patient achieved a 2 D reduction in cylinder with a 3.5 mm CRI. Unaided vision was 20/25 and J3, and this patient required a minimal correction of -0.25 D sphere. Figure 15-16 shows the effect of a single adjacent CRI for the correction of 2.25 D of keratometric cylinder. At 2 weeks postoperatively, this case experienced a 1.25 D reduction in cylinder with 20/30 distance and J2 near vision unaided, and required a minimal correction of -0.50 -0.25 × 90°.

Defocus Testing

We have employed defocus testing, in a manner similar to that used in clinical trials of multifocal IOLs, in order to further quantify the enhanced depth of focus we have observed. This procedure involves neutralizing the spherocylindrical refractive error with trial frames, adding plus and minus sphere in 0.25 to 0.50 D increments over the range from +6 to -6 D, and measuring the Snellen acuity at each increment.[2] Of particular interest is the region between 0 and -3 D of defocus, which details the patient's distance, intermediate, and near vision. Figure 15-17 presents schematic representations of typical defocus curves for a pseudophake with a monofocal IOL and for a pseudophake with a multifocal IOL. As expected with a monofocal IOL, the best

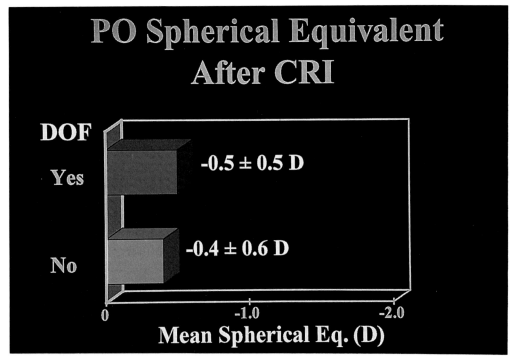

Figure 15-10A. Comparison of postoperative clinical parameters between CRI patients having 20/40 combined with J3 vision unaided (DOF = YES) with CRI patients who do not (DOF = NO). Both groups are very similar with respect to each parameter. Spherical equivalent.

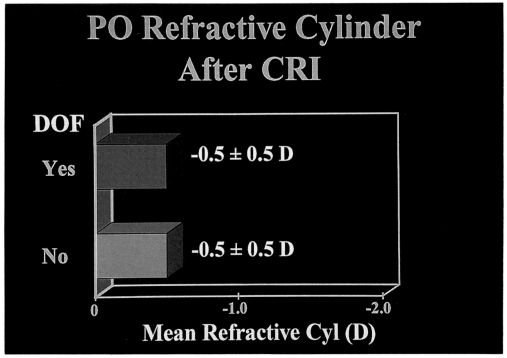

Figure 15-10B. Refractive cylinder.

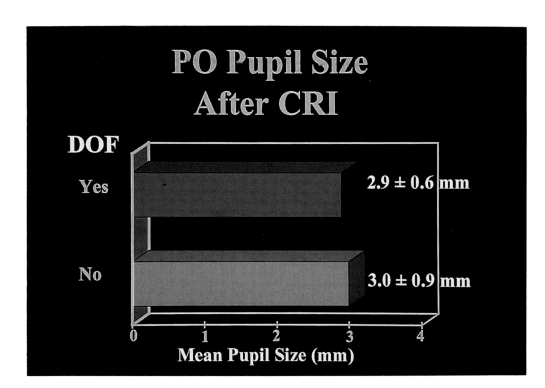

Figure 15-10C. Pupil size in ambient lighting.

distance vision occurs at 0 D of defocus. Overminusing by 1 to 2 D measures intermediate range vision, while overminusing by as much as 2.5 to 3.5 D measures near vision. Usually, the cutoff of functional vision is defined to be 20/40 (which is equivalent to J3 on a Jaeger reading scale). A typical monofocal IOL will then provide about 1.25 D of usable vision at that level.

Most multifocal IOLs under investigation today have defocus curves which exhibit two characteristic peaks, one at 0 D defocus corresponding to best distance vision, and another at about -3 D corresponding to best near vision (see Figure 15-17). However, because of the two-peak nature of these curves, there is a reduction in contrast of the image focused at the retina.

The defocus curves for 10 patients from our current investigation are shown in Figure 15-18. The average defocus curve for four patients with poor near vision is shown in magenta, while the average curve for six patients with excellent near vision is shown in yellow. The average defocus curves were calculated using the common logarithm of the decimal equivalent of the Snellen acuity, according to Holladay and Prager.[3] Interestingly, the magenta defocus

curve for patients with poor near vision resembles a typical monofocal curve, providing approximately 1.5 D of functional vision. However, the yellow curve for patients with good near vision looks nothing at all like the two-peak multifocal IOL curve, but rather is broadened substantially, and is associated with greater than 3 D of functional vision.

To prove that this effect is, in some way, influenced by corneal topography and not by some other means, we have undertaken a study of the effect of a rigid gas-permeable contact lens on near and distance vision in our CRI patients. If the increased depth of focus is caused by the cornea, one would expect the rigid contact lens to reduce it, or eliminate it, by confining the cornea to a symmetrical surface. Eyes were neutralized to plano for distance with the contact lens, and distance and near acuity were measured and compared with patients' unaided acuities.

In one eye, vision changed from 20/30 and J1 unaided to 20/30 and J10 with the contact lens in place, representing virtually a complete elimination of near acuity, thus implicating corneal shape in the phenomenon of increased depth of focus following cataract surgery with CRIs.

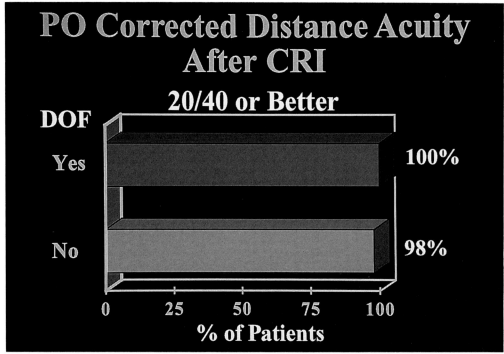

Figure 15-11A. Comparison of additional postoperative clinical parameters between CRI patients having 20/40 combined with J3 vision unaided (DOF = YES) with CRI patients who do not (DOF = NO). Both groups are very similar with respect to each parameter. Best-corrected acuity.

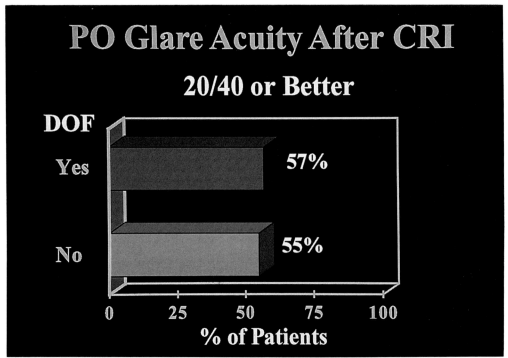

Figure 15-11B. Glare acuity.

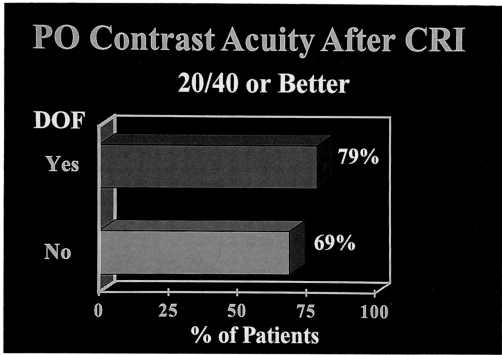

Figure 15-11C. Contrast acuity.

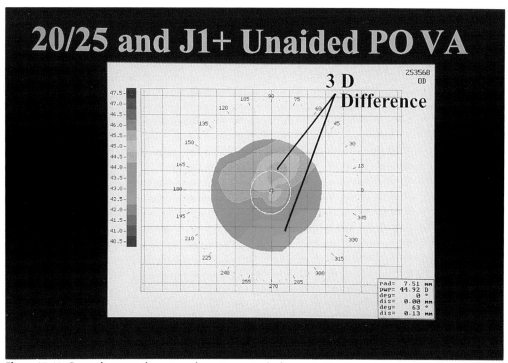

Figure 15-12. Corneal topography at 2 weeks postoperatively demonstrating as much as a 3 D variation in corneal power. This patient sees 20/25 and J1 + unaided.

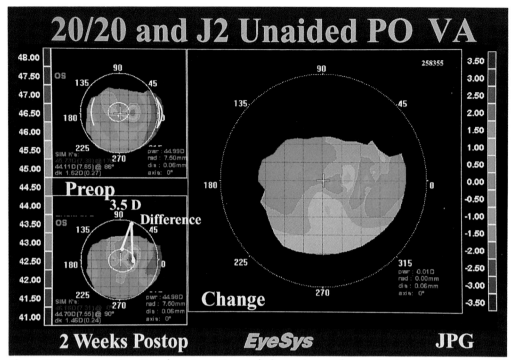

Figure 15-13. Preoperative, 2-week postoperative, and change images for a patient receiving a single CRI opposite to a clear-corneal cataract incision. The postoperative image demonstrates a 3.5 D variation in corneal power. This patient sees 20/20 and J2 unaided.

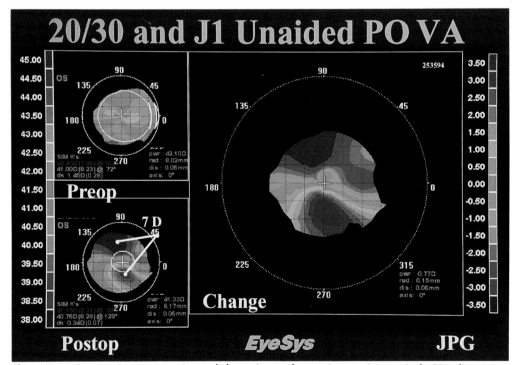

Figure 15-14. Preoperative, postoperative, and change images for a patient receiving a single CRI adjacent to a clear-corneal cataract incision. The postoperative image demonstrates as much as a 7 D variation in corneal power. This patient sees 20/30 and J1 unaided, with a best-corrected distance acuity of 20/25.

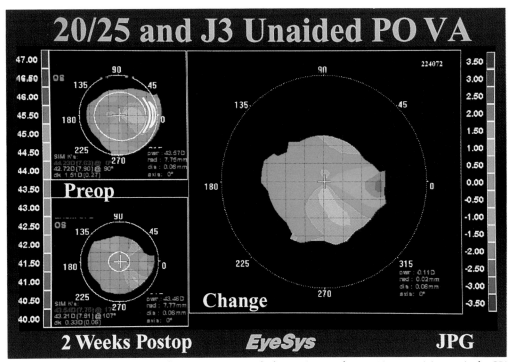

Figure 15-15. Preoperative, 2-week postoperative, and change images for a patient receiving a single CRI adjacent to a clear-corneal cataract incision. This patient sees 20/25 and J3 unaided.

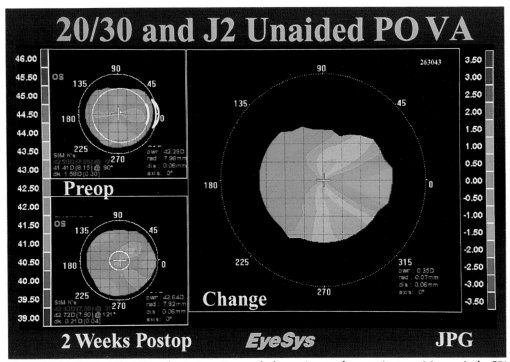

Figure 15-16. Preoperative, 2-week postoperative, and change images for a patient receiving a single CRI adjacent to a clear-corneal cataract incision. This patient sees 20/30 and J2 unaided.

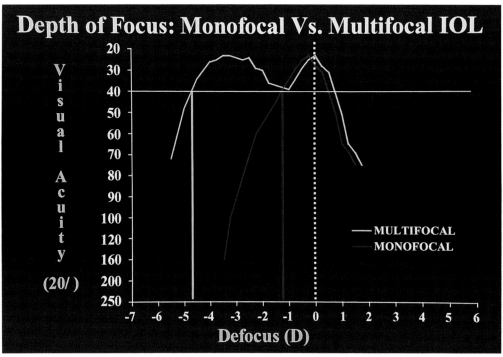

Figure 15-17. Schematic representation of defocus curves for monofocal and multifocal IOLs. The monofocal curve demonstrates approximately 1.25 D of 20/40 vision. The multifocal IOL provides for a dramatically increased depth of focus. Notice the characteristic two-peak curve afforded by the multifocal IOL.

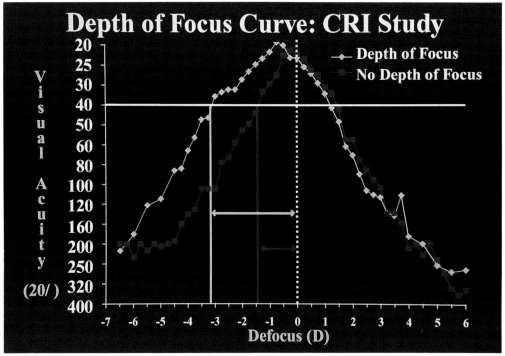

Figure 15-18. Depth of focus curves for patients in this study with 20/40 combined with J3 unaided vision and for those who do not have 20/40 combined with J3 vision. Notice the gradual broadening of the curve for patients having 20/40 combined with J3 vision.

CONCLUSION

The use of a single CRI in conjunction with the cataract incision, for the correction of moderate preexisting astigmatism, is effective in reducing cylinder while maintaining coupling. Increased depth of focus, or "omnimmetropia," has been observed in eyes receiving CRIs, a phenomenon which appears to be intimately related to corneal topography. The mechanism of action of the increased depth of focus involves broadening of the defocus curve, and is thus distinctly different from those afforded by various multifocal IOLs. However, corneal topography alone does not explain this effect in all cases, and we are continuing to investigate this phenomenon.

REFERENCES

1. Thornton SP. Theory behind corneal relaxing incisions/Thorton nomogram. In: Gills JP, Martin RG, Sanders DR, eds. *Sutureless Cataract Surgery.* Thorofare, NJ: SLACK, Inc; 1992:123-143.
2. Carlson NB, Kurtz D, Heath DA, et al. Negative relative accommodation/ positive relative accommodation (NRA/PRA). In: *Clinical Procedures for Ocular Examination.* Norwalk, CT: Appleton & Lange; 1990:133-134.
3. Holladay JT, Prager TC. Mean visual acuity. *Am J Ophthalmol.* 1991;111:372-374.

EVALUATING EXCIMER LASER PROCEDURES

Daniel S. Durrie, MD
Donald R. Sanders, MD, PhD
D. James Schumer, MD
Manus C. Kraff, MD
Robert T. Spector, MD
David Gubman, OD

Corneal topography has proven invaluable in evaluating the centration, surgical effect, and healing of excimer procedures.

CENTERING OF EXCIMER LASER PROCEDURES

Centration on Center of Pupil

Decentration of any refractive corneal procedure can result in blurred images, glare, ghost images, poor visual acuity, or poor contrast sensitivity.[1,2] Various methods of centering surgical corneal refractive procedures have been described.[3,4] Walsh and Guyton[2] and Uozato and Guyton[1] have pointed out that currently used centering surgical procedures emphasize centering about the visual axis of the eye, which in many cases is not defined properly. They and Maloney[5] believe that the optimum method for centering surgical (and excimer laser) refractive procedures utilizes the line of sight and the entrance pupil and not the visual axis.

Proper centering requires the patient to fixate on a point that is coaxial with the surgeon's sighting eye, and the cornea is marked at the point in line with the center of the patient's entrance pupil, ignoring the corneal light reflex. Besides the optical arguments for using the entrance pupil, the Stiles-Crawford effect demonstrates with normal pupils that light passing through the center of the pupil is more effective in stimulating the photoreceptors than light passing through the peripheral pupil because photoreceptors are aimed toward or oriented to the center of the pupil. Studies on eccentric pupils[6,7] have demonstrated that photoreceptors also actively orient themselves toward the center of an eccentric pupil.

These findings, therefore, suggest that the pupil and not the visual axis remains the proper optical reference for centering corneal refractive procedures.

Errors of from 0.5 to 0.8 mm were found using current methods of procedure centration. These errors arose from the use of the corneal light reflex as the sighting and marking point instead of the center of the pupil, or from inadvertent monocular sighting in techniques requiring binocular sighting.

Centration of Topographical Maps

How does the recommended centering of refractive procedures fit in with the centration of corneal topographic maps? With the EyeSys corneal topography unit, the patient fixates coaxial to the video camera image as recommended by Guyton and colleagues and Maloney. However, the center of the map is not coincident with the center of the pupil.

The center of the corneal topography map is referred to as the videokeratographic (VK) axis, or alternatively as the corneal vertex or vertex normal. Vertex normal can be more exactly defined as the line from the fixation point that intersects the corneal surface at right angles; the point of intersection on the cornea itself is called the corneal vertex. A light ray from the fixation point that travels down the vertex normal is reflected back on itself so the vertex normal must pass through the first Purkinje image of the fixation target. The corneal vertex does not usually coincide with the geometric center nor does it necessarily coincide with the visual axis but it does provide a reproducible point on the corneal surface.

In normal eyes the entrance pupil is not centered around the corneal vertex; the first Purkinje image of a fixation light usually lies nasal to the center of the entrance pupil.[8] In cases with distorted corneas or eccentric pupils there may be a great disparity between the center of the ring images and the center of the entrance pupil.

A major criticism of videokeratoscopes which center along the VK axis has been their failure in the past to provide information regarding the pupil center. Recently, however, new image enhancement and recognition software have been developed to detect and outline the patient's pupil and to mark the pupil center. This process was not trivial since corneoscopic ring images tend to mask the pupil margins. A very sophisticated computer algorithm was required to "subtract" the corneoscopic ring image from the photo and find the underlying pupil. With this new pupil recognition software, the corneal topography map can now be used to determine if corneal refractive procedures have been properly centered.

Figures 16-1A and B demonstrate corneal topographical maps in two cases with some disparity between the center of the ring images (VK axis) and the pupil center. The first two values in the cursor box in the lower right corner of the screen supply curvature information in radius of curvature (millimeters) and power in diopters, respectively, for the cornea at the location of the mouse cursor (large +). The third and fourth values from the top describe the position of the cursor relative to the center of the rings (VK axis). In these cases the mouse cursor is directly over the VK axis so that the first degrees and distance are equal to 0. These data are provided as direction in degrees and distance in millimeters from the center of the rings to the cursor position.

When the pupil is located during eye image processing, the position of the mouse cursor (in this case located at the VK axis) relative to the pupil center will also be provided as direction in degrees and distance in millimeters. Here we see in Figure 16-1A that the corneal vertex is 0.43 mm away from the center of the pupil in the direction of the 353° axis and in Figure 16-1B the corneal vertex is also 0.43 mm away from the center of the pupil but in the direction of the 329° axis. Figure 16-1B is a postoperative RK case. Note that in this case, pupil center is closer to the center of the flattened central zone indicating better centration than would be concluded if the VK axis rather than pupil center were used to determine centration.

Figure 16-2 demonstrates a case where the VK axis, pupil center, and center of the excimer laser ablation are all coincident.

Figure 16-3 demonstrates a slightly eccentric excimer laser ablation. The mouse cursor has been placed at the center

of the ablative zone where the corneal power is 34.75 D. The center of the ablative zone is 0.9 mm toward the 182° axis relative to the VK axis and 0.78 mm toward the 193° axis relative to the center of the pupil as documented by the printout in the cursor box in the lower right-hand corner of the figure.

Figure 16-4 demonstrates a symptomatic, markedly decentered excimer laser photorefractive keratectomy (PRK). The mouse cursor is centered in the ablative zone and demonstrates a corneal power of 42.96 D. The last two numbers in the cursor box indicate that the ablative zone is decentered 1.26 mm toward the 29° axis relative to the center of the pupil.

By looking at the corneal topography maps of their post-treatment excimer and other refractive surgery cases, surgeons can observe and hopefully correct any consistent problems in technique resulting in decentration. See Chapter 2 for a more complete discussion of the alignment of videokeratoscopes with regard to the major reference points and axes of the eye (line of sight, pupillary axis, visual axis, and VK axis).

EVALUATING EXCIMER PROCEDURES WITH CORNEAL TOPOGRAPHY

Topography can now assist in evaluating postoperative refractive surgery patients, including PRK cases. Following PRK, confirmation of a specific healing type can be confirmed through topography, which can help direct postoperative treatment options.

Using STARS™ Maps to Evaluate PRK

The STARS (*S*tandardized *T*opographic *A*nalysis of *R*efractive *S*urgery) display was designed specifically to assist in evaluating refractive surgery. The details were refined while following hundred of excimer laser patients in many different protocols at the Hunkeler Eye Clinic. These patients received PRK with the Summit Excimed, Summit Omnimed, or Chiron Vision/Technolas excimer lasers.

The format consists of five topographic maps on one screen (Figure 16-5). The preoperative, 1-month postoperative, and last exam are the three topographic maps on the top row, all on the same scale. The bottom two images are difference maps that vary according to the magnitude of change. The first difference map represents the change between preoperative and 1-month postoperative exams, referred to as the surgical effect, because it demonstrates the amount of corneal flattening that has occurred following PRK once the epithelium has remodeled. The second difference map represents the change between 1-month postoperative and the last exams, referred to as the healing effect,

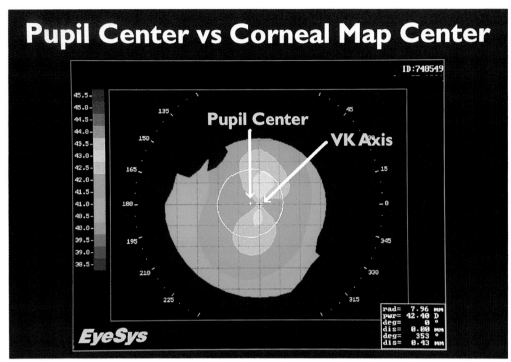

Figure 16-1A. Corneal topographical maps of the right eyes of two cases where the corneal vertex is nasal to the pupil center. Normal unoperated eye.

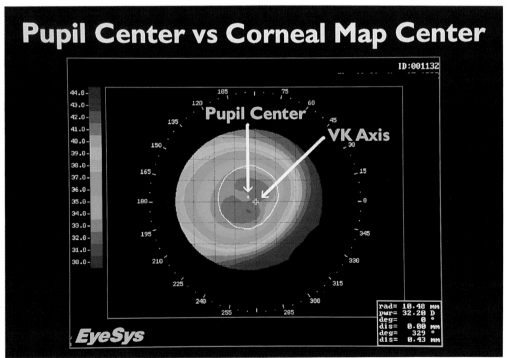

Figure 16-1B. Postoperative radial keratotomy case.

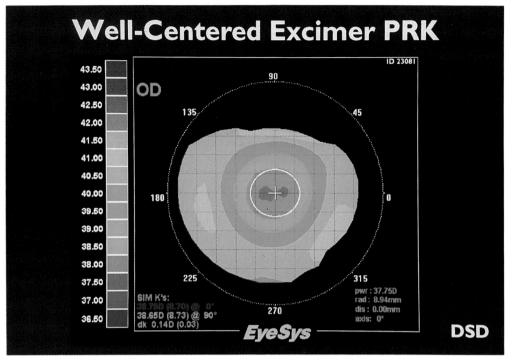

Figure 16-2. Post-treatment excimer laser PRK. The cursor numbers in the lower right indicates that the pupil center and corneal vertex are coincident. Observation of the topographical map indicates excellent centration of white pupil outline within the ablative zone.

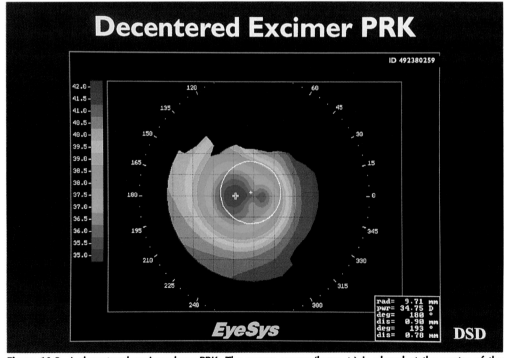

Figure 16-3. A decentered excimer laser PRK. The mouse cursor (large +) is placed at the center of the photoablative zone and the small + marks the pupil center. The first two degree and distance numbers at the lower right quantify the degree of decentration of ablation relative to the VK axis (small white circle). The second two numbers quantify the degree of decentration of the ablation relative to the pupil center.

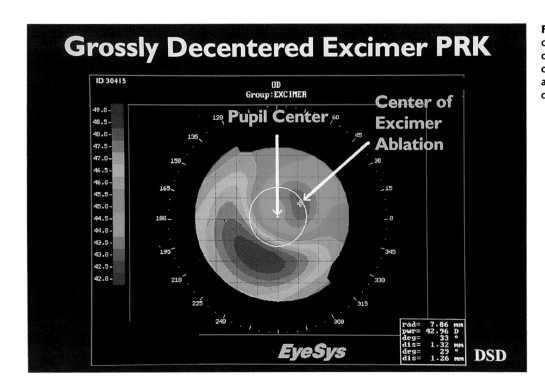

Grossly Decentered Excimer PRK

ID 30415

OD
Group:EXCIMER

Pupil Center

Center of Excimer Ablation

rad= 7.86 mm
pwr= 42.96 D
deg= 33 °
dis= 1.32 mm
deg= 29 °
dis= 1.26 mm

EyeSys DSD

Figure 16-4. A decentered excimer laser PRK. The mouse cursor (large +) is placed at the center of the photoablative zone and the small + marks the pupil center.

because the cornea typically steepens slightly beyond the 1-month visit following PRK.

This corneal steepening is associated with the development of a subepithelial haze and a regression of the refraction toward myopia. This regression is the reason the PRK algorithms slightly overcorrect myopia, so that most patients are slightly hyperopic at 1 month. As the subepithelial haze develops, corneal steepening ensues, and the refraction regresses back to the intended correction.

Healing Patterns

After following hundreds of post-PRK patients, three separate healing patterns became evident. The most typical healing pattern, Type I, is seen in approximately 85% of patients following treatment with the Summit Excimed laser (Figure 16-5A). The patient is slightly hyperopic at 1 month postoperatively, and there is a developing subepithelial haze noted on biomicroscopy. Between the 1-month and 6-month visits the hyperopia and haze resolve as the cornea steepens slightly. Note how the slit lamp images correlate with the topography (Figure 16-5B).

A Type II healing pattern is seen in approximately 10% of patients. With this healing pattern, no or very little subepithelial haze develops, the cornea does not significantly steepen, and therefore the patient remains slightly hyperopic (Figures 16-6A and 16-6B).

Techniques have been developed to correct a Type II healing pattern. One technique used is an epithelial debride-

ment. Allowing the patient to "heal" the epithelium without a topical steroid allows for haze formation and corneal steepening even after 12 months post-PRK. Figure 16-7 shows the topographic effect after an epithelial debridement. Note the corneal steepening on the difference map.

A Type III healing pattern is seen in approximately 5% of patients. This group has a significant increase in subepithelial haze formation, the cornea steepens beyond the typical amount, and the patient regresses back toward myopia (Figures 16-8A and 16-8B).

Techniques have also been developed to correct a Type III healing pattern. As soon as this pattern can be identified, an increase of topical steroids is used. In addition, a topical NSAID is used. Together, this regimen has not only stopped the Type III healing pattern, but in some cases has reversed the regression. Figure 16-9 shows the topographic maps after the topical treatment in a Type III healer. The treatment decreased the subepithelial haze and reduced the myopia.

Figure 16-10 shows another Type III healer who was treated with steroids at 6 months postoperatively. Before the steroid treatment, the patient had 2.5 D of residual myopia. An additional 1.28 D of flattening was achieved in 2 weeks of treatment. Although some of the effect of the steroid treatment regressed after the steroids were withdrawn, the patient still had residual effect at 1 year postoperatively, reducing the spherical equivalent by 1 D over the presteroid level.

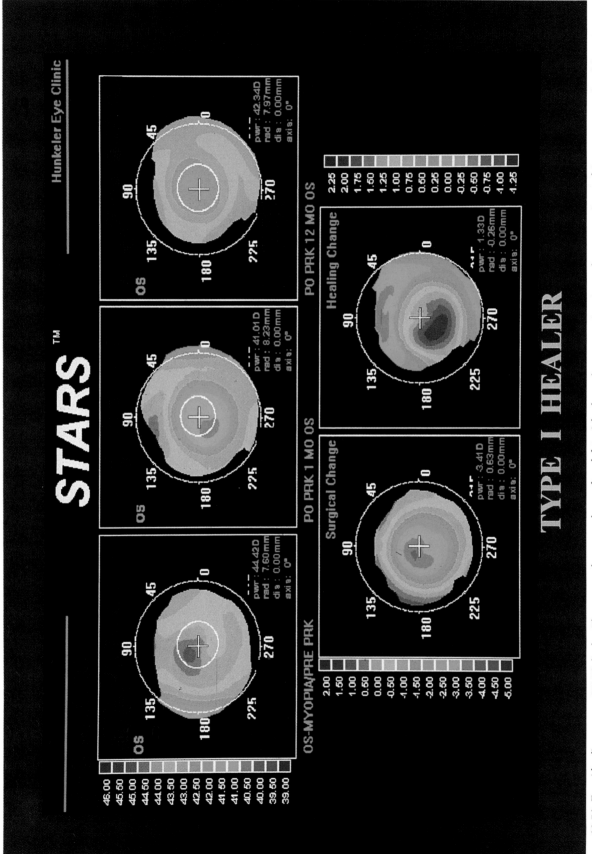

Figure 16-5A. Type I healing pattern, STARS display. The topography across the top from left to right shows the preoperative, 1-month postoperative, and 1-year postoperative visits, respectively. The bottom left topography is a difference map depicting the surgical change between preoperative and 1 month postoperative. The bottom right topography is a difference map demonstrating the typical healing effect or corneal steepening that occurs following photorefractive keratectomy.

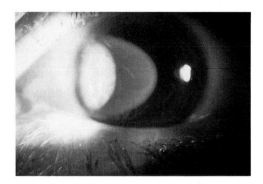
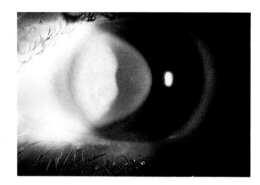
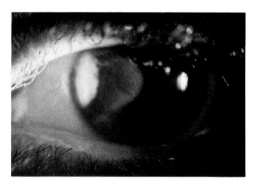

Figure 16-5B. Clinical biomicroscopy photos. Upper left, postoperatively. Upper right, 1-month postopreratively. Lower center, 1 year postoperatively. The 1-month postoperative photo shows the typical formation of slight haze with its resolution by 1 year.

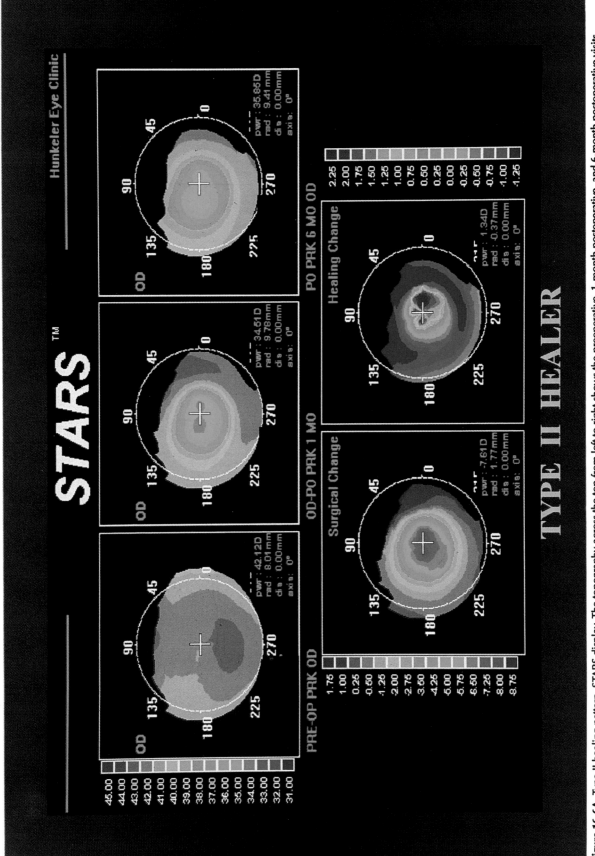

Figure 16-6A. Type II healing pattern, STARS display. The topography across the top from left to right shows the preoperative, 1-month postoperative, and 6-month postoperative visits, respectively. The bottom left topography is a difference map depicting the surgical change between preoperative and 1 month postoperative. The bottom right topography ia a difference map demonstrating the inadequate healing effect that occurs in a Type II healing pattern, although in this case slight central steepening is seen.

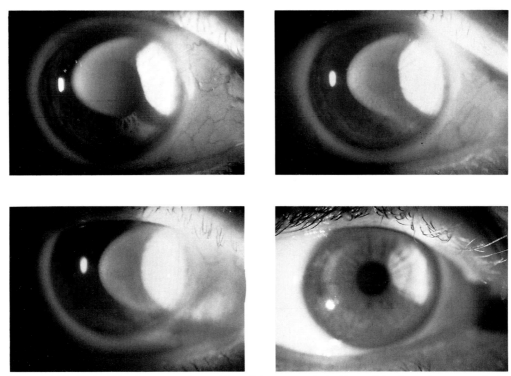

Figure 16-6B. Clinical biomicroscopy photos. Upper left, preoperatively. Upper right, 1 month postoperatively. Lower left, 6 months postoperatively. Lower right, post-debridement. The post-epithelial debridement photo demonstrates the haze formation and corneal steepening that occur following this procedure.

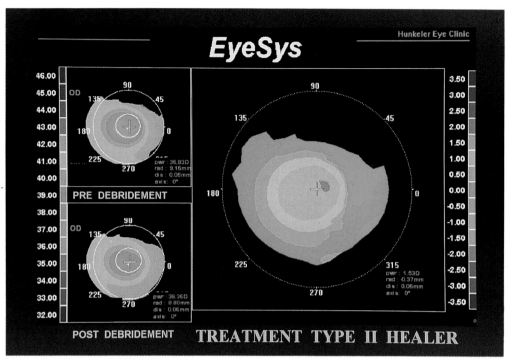

Figure 16-7. Topographic difference map demonstrating the treatment for a Type II healer. This patient underwent an epithelial debridement 12 months following photorefractive keratectomy. The cornea was allowed to heal without any topical steroids. Note the central corneal steepening that occurred following this procedure. This patient's hyperopia resolved.

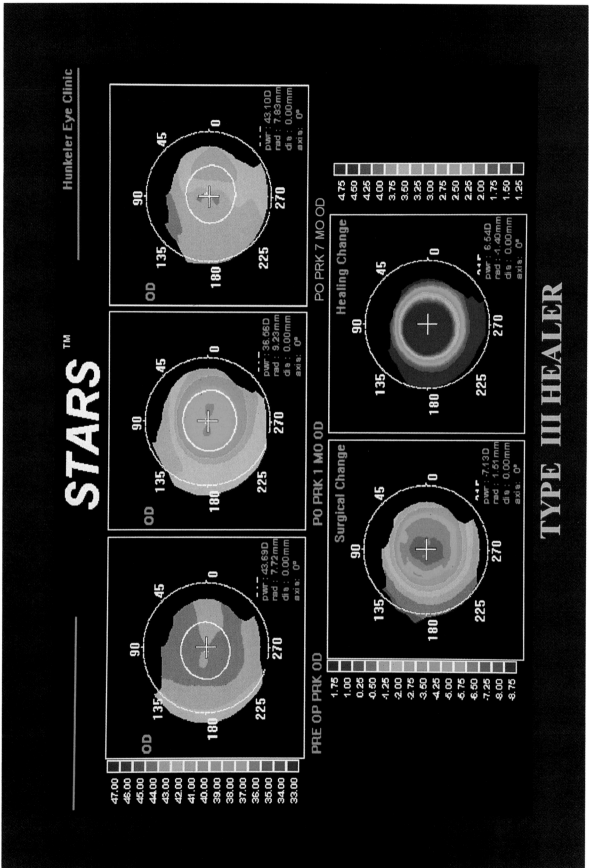

Figure 16-8A. Type III healing pattern, STARS display. The topography across the top from left to right shows the preoperative, 1-month postoperative, and 7-month postoperative visits, respectively. The bottom left topography is a difference map depicting the surgical change between preoperative and 1-month postoperative visits. The bottom right topography is a difference map demonstrating the atypical healing effect from a Type III healer. Notice the amount of corneal steepening that occurs with this healing type.

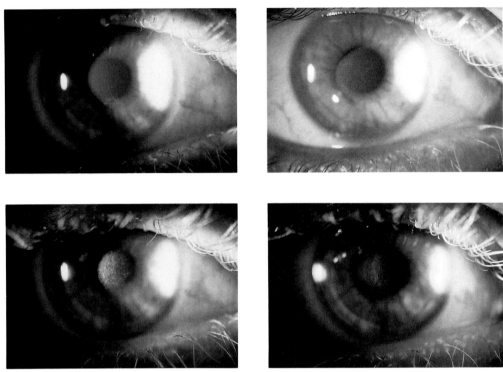

Figure 16-8B. Clinical biomicroscopy photos. Upper left, preoperatively. Upper right, 1 month postoperatively. Lower left, 2 months postoperatively. Lower right, post-treatment with topical steroids and NSAIDS. The 1-month postoperative photo shows the atypical formation of haze. The haze progresses with a continued regression of effect at the 7-month visit. At the 8-month visit (lower right), the haze and corneal steepening respond to topical treatment.

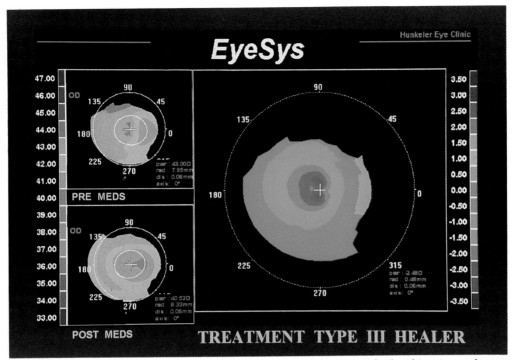

Figure 16-9. Topography difference map demonstrating the treatment for a Type III healer. This patient underwent topical treatment with both FML forte and Voltaren® QID. Note the central corneal flattening that occurred following this topical treatment alone. The patient's myopia improved.

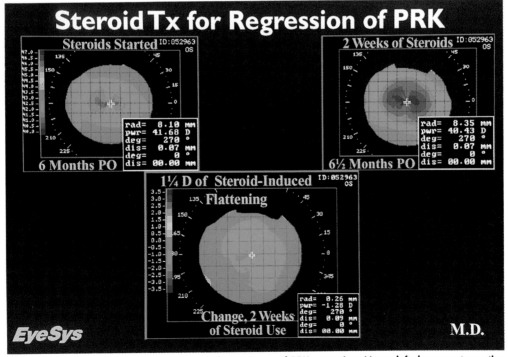

Figure 16-10. Case receiving topical steroids for treatment of PRK regression. Upper left shows postoperative topographical appearance at the visit at which steroid treatment was started, upper right shows appearance 2 weeks later, and bottom shows difference map, demonstrating additional flattening induced by the treatment. *Courtesy of Dr. Michael Deitz.*

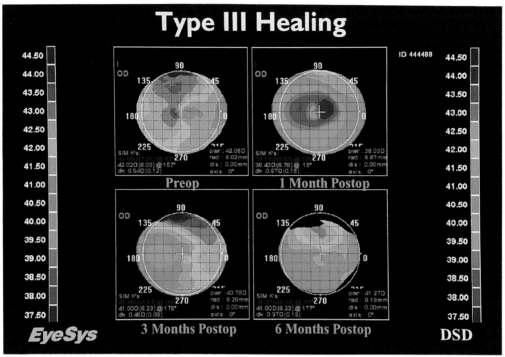

Figure 16-11A. Case receiving excimer retreatment for PRK regression. Upper left shows preoperative, upper right shows 1-month postoperative, lower left shows 3-month postoperative, and lower right shows 6-month postoperative topographical appearance. The 6-month topographical map demonstrates an almost complete loss of correction.

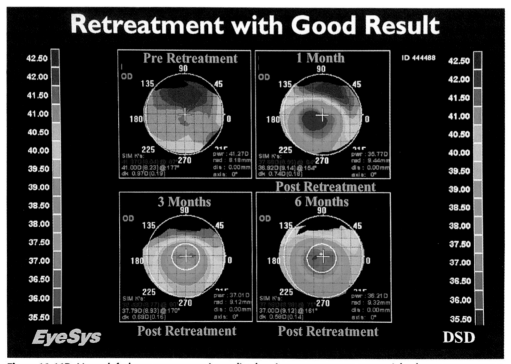

Figure 16-11B. Upper left shows appearance immediately prior to retreatment, upper right shows appearance 1 month post-retreatment, and lower left and right show 3- and 6-month post-retreatment appearance, respectively. The topography following retreatment demonstrates a more normal healing pattern.

Regression of effect can also be addressed by retreatment. Figure 16-11A shows another case with Type III healing who had significant corneal haze and almost total loss of correction by 6 months post-treatment. This case was retreated with the subepithelial fibrosis removed and experienced a much decreased haze response, which resulted in an excellent visual and refractive response (Figure 16-11B). The topography demonstrates a more normal healing pattern following the second treatment.

Multi-Zone Ablations for High Myopia

Attempting to correct high myopia with deeper ablations tends to result in more severe regression. As the cornea re-epithelializes, the steep edge of a deep ablation tends to be filled in, resulting in a reduction of effect. One way to avoid this process is to use a multi-zone ablation. With this technique, progressively smaller apertures are used to create greater effect centrally. Figures 16-12 and 16-13 demonstrate the preoperative and change image topography of cases receiving multi-zone ablations. The early postoperative change image in both these cases demonstrates about 15 D of central flattening and about 9 D of flattening peripherally. The different ablation zones can easily be seen on the change images.

Central Islands

An interesting phenomenon seen in some PRK cases was discovered through corneal topography. In some cases, the excimer did not ablate the center of the cornea as much as the immediate periphery, causing a central island which is steeper than the surrounding region. Figure 16-14A shows a case with a 2.5 D difference in flattening produced by the ablation between the center and the surrounding region. Figure 16-14B shows that over time this central island resolved, becoming flatter over time, until by 3 to 4 months it had virtually disappeared. Figure 16-15A shows another central island with a 2 D difference in effect between the center and the surrounding region. This central island started out small and progressed with time (Figure 16-15B).

PRK for Undercorrected RK

We have had some experience treating undercorrected radial keratotomy (RK) cases with the excimer. In the first case (Figures 16-16), the post-RK pre-PRK topography (Figure 16-16, left) demonstrates that the cornea is flatter centrally with some residual astigmatism. The 1-month

post-PRK appearance demonstrates a profound central flattening with a large flat zone. In another case (Figure 16-17), topography reveals little evidence of effect from RK (Figure 16-17, left) and again an excellent effect from the PRK (Figure 16-17, right).

Evaluating PARK for Correction of Astigmatism

Treatment of corneal astigmatism requires selective flattening of the steeper meridian, and, depending on the refractive error, concomitant treatment of myopia. The VisX 20/20 laser provides two methods of treating astigmatism with photoastigmatic refractive keratectomy (PARK)—the sequential method, with which the astigmatism is treated first and then the myopia, and the elliptical method, with which the astigmatism and sphere are treated simultaneously. The elliptical method produces a smoother ablation with no transition zones, but is not as effective in patients who require a larger cylinder correction than myopic correction.

Figure 16-18 demonstrates the topography of a 29-year-old male with myopic astigmatism. Preoperatively, the refraction was -4.00 +2.00 x 70 with 20/25^{+2} best-corrected vision. The patient was treated with an elliptical program with a setting of -2.67 -1.84 x 160. Postoperatively the refraction was -0.25 +0.25 x 80 with 20/20 best-corrected vision. Note the vertical pattern of flattening in the change graph, corresponding to the area of steepness postoperatively.

Figure 16-19 shows topography of a 40-year-old male 1-year status post penetrating corneal laceration, resulting in repair of the laceration followed by a pars plana lensectomy and vitrectomy. The patient was intolerant to aphakic contact lenses with refraction of +8.50 +6.00 x 90 with 20/100 best-corrected vision. A hard contact lens over the refraction yielded a best-corrected vision of 20/60. The treatment plan was to treat the entire corneal astigmatism with the sequential program, followed by implantation of a posterior chamber intraocular lens at a future date. The software parameters with a sequential ablation program were plano -5.58 x 180. Six months following the excimer treatment, the patient's refraction was +13.00 +1.00 x 165 with 20/20 best-corrected vision. After implantation of a posterior chamber IOL onto the remaining posterior capsule, the refraction was -0.25 +2.25 x 180 with 20/25 uncorrected acuity and 20/20 best-corrected vision. The topographical change image (right) demonstrates the induced flattening following the same pattern where the preoperative topography indicated steepness.

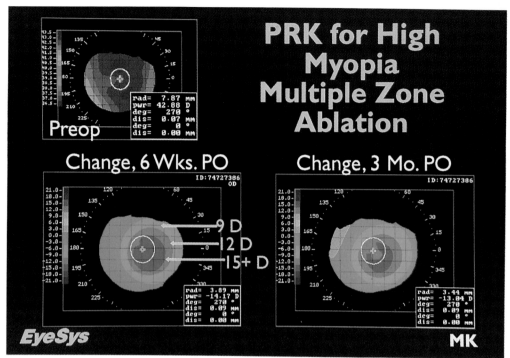

Figure 16-12. High myopia case receiving multiple zone ablation. Upper left shows preoperative appearance, lower left shows induced corneal changes at 6 weeks postoperatively, and right shows induced changes at 3 months.

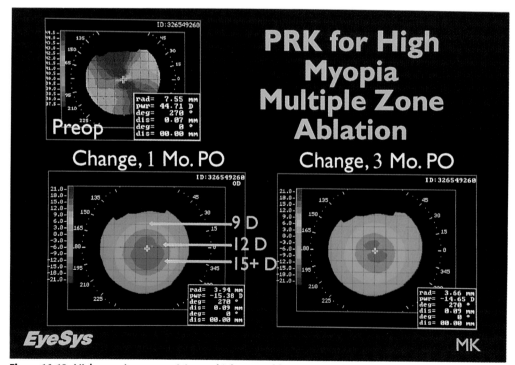

Figure 16-13. High myopia case receiving multiple zone ablation. Upper left shows preoperative appearance, lower left shows induced corneal changes at 1 month postoperatively, and right shows induced changes at 3 months.

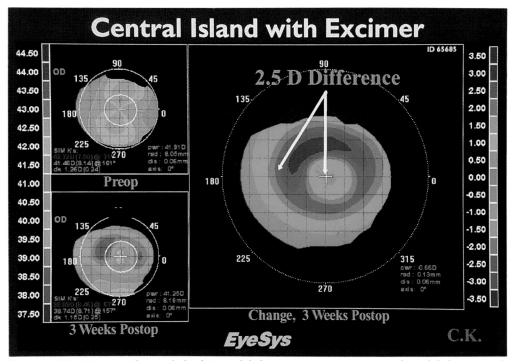

Figure 16-14A. PRK case with central island. Upper left shows preoperative appearance, lower left shows 1-week postoperative appearance, and right shows induced corneal changes. There is a 2.5 D difference in flattening induced by the ablation between the center and the surrounding region.

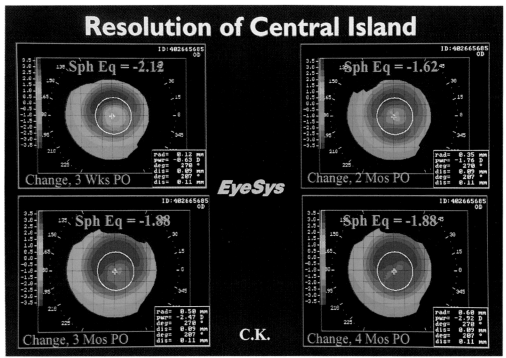

Figure 16-14B. Over time the central island has resolved.

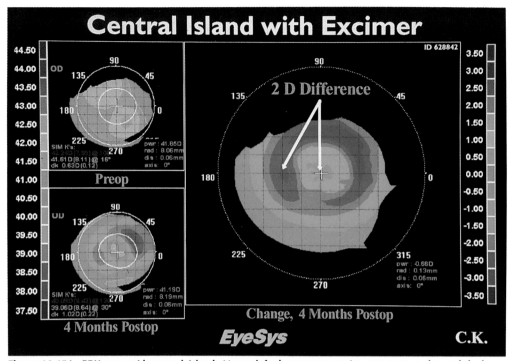

Figure 16-15A. PRK case with central island. Upper left shows preoperative appearance, lower left shows 1-month postoperative appearance, and right shows induced corneal changes. There is a 2 D difference in flattening induced by the ablation between the center and the surrounding region.

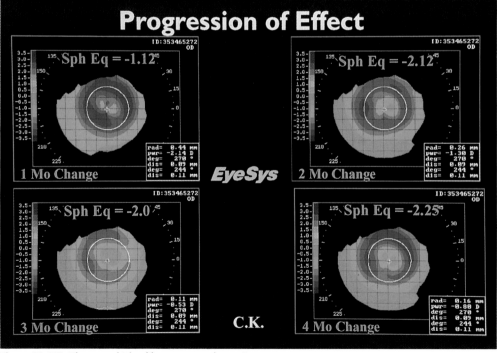

Figure 16-15B. The central island has progressed over time.

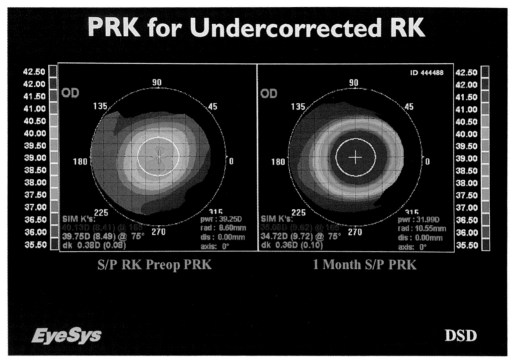

Figure 16-16. Corneal topography of case receiving PRK for undercorrected RK. Left, status post-RK prior to PRK. Right, status post-PRK.

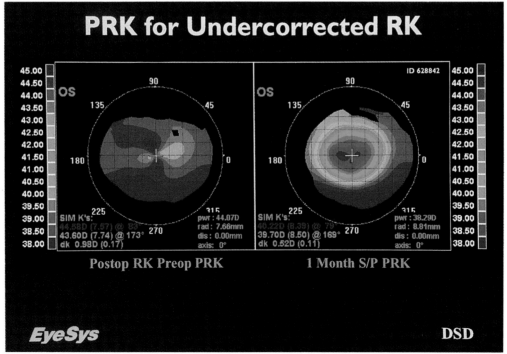

Figure 16-17. Corneal topography of case receiving PRK for undercorrected RK. Left, status post-RK prior to PRK. Right, status post-PRK.

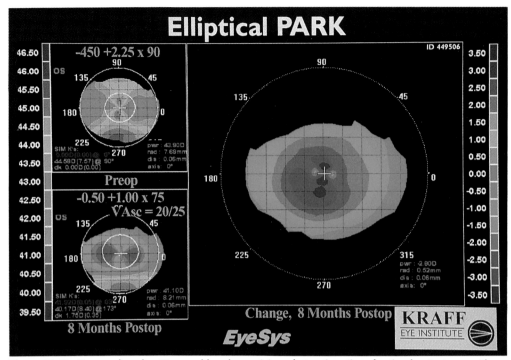

Figure 16-18. Topography of a 29-year-old male receiving photoastigmatic refractive keratectomy with an elliptical ablation for myopic astigmatism. Upper left shows pre-ablation, lower left shows post-ablation, right shows induced changes.

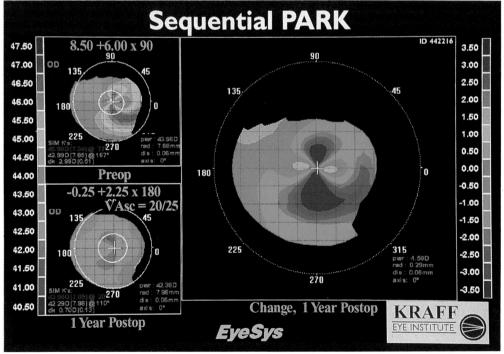

Figure 16-19. Topography of a 40-year-old male status post repair of corneal laceration, pars plana lensectomy, and vitrectomy. Upper left shows pre-ablation, lower left shows post-ablation, and right shows induced changes.

SUMMARY

Corneal topography has become an indispensable part of pre-treatment and post-treatment evaluation of the excimer patient. While it closely parallels refractive change, it provides much more clinically relevant information. Corneal topography has greatly enhanced our understanding of healing patterns, treatment induced anomalies such as central islands, and the effect on astigmatism.

REFERENCES

1. Uozato H, Guyton DL. Centering corneal surgical procedures. *Am J Ophthalmol.* 1987;103:264-275.
2. Walsh PM, Guyton DL. Comparison of two methods of marking the visual axis on the cornea during radial keratotomy. *Am J Ophthalmol.* 1984;97:660.
3. Steinberg EB, Waring GO III. Comparison of two methods of marking the visual axis on the cornea during radial keratotomy. *Am J Ophthalmol.* 1983;96:605.
4. Thornton SP. Surgical armamentarium. In: Sanders DR, Hofmann RF, Salz JJ, eds. *Refract Corneal Surgery.* Thorofare, NJ: SLACK Inc; 1986:134.
5. Maloney RK. Corneal topography and optical zone location in photorefractive keratectomy. *Refract Corneal Surgery.* 1990;6:363-371.
6. Enoch JM, Laties AM. An analysis of retinal receptor orientation. II. Prediction for psychophysical tests. *Invest Ophthalmol.* 1971;10:959.
7. Bonds AB, MacLeod DIA. A displaced Stiles-Crawford effect associated with an eccentric pupil. *Invest Ophthalmol Vis Sci.* 1978;17:754.
8. Uozato H, Makino H, Saishin M, Nakao S. Measurement of the visual axis using a laser beam. In: Breinin GM, Siegal IM, eds. *Advances in*

CORNEAL TOPOGRAPHY IN LAMELLAR REFRACTIVE SURGERY

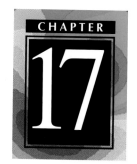

Stephen A. Updegraff, MD

Luis A. Ruiz, MD

Stephen G. Slade, MD

Lamellar refractive keratoplasty developed from the concepts and work of Jose Barraquer, working in his clinic in Bogota, Colombia.[1-4] The original myopic keratomileusis technique was a very involved process. However, the encouraging results for high myopia, the potential for a corneal procedure to correct aphakia, and the surprisingly clear appearance of the cornea following surgery led many surgeons to become interested in lamellar refractive surgery.[5-7] Early on, the results of these procedures were evaluated based on Snellen visual acuity, and problems with surface irregularities could only be elucidated by examining the keratoscope mires and with hard contact lens over refraction. Video corneal topography provides a new outlook on lamellar refractive techniques that has increased our understanding of the optics of these procedures.

MYOPIC KERATOMILEUSIS—THEORY AND TECHNIQUE

Lamellar refractive surgery corrects myopia by altering the anterior curvature of the cornea. This flattening at the crucial tear film-air interface is achieved by removing stroma from within the cornea and leaving Bowman's membrane and the epithelium virtually intact. As the correction is based upon refractive changes at the surface of the cornea, a technology to evaluate the change, quality, and stability of the topography is essential. Classic myopic keratomileusis has evolved dramatically over the past years. Barraquer himself advanced the art rapidly. He extensively modified the contact lens lathe to include micrometer gauges and freezing circuits to more accurately shape the tissue and introduced a motorized microkeratome to remove the corneal disc.[4] The microkeratome is based upon the principle of a carpenter's plane. All microkeratomes, except for the Draeger keratome which has a circular blade, have in common an oscillating blade and a suction device that holds the eye in position and elevates the intraocular pressure. The keratome applanates the cornea against the undersurface of the keratome so that a lamellar disc of tissue is removed (Figure 17-1).[8] The original Barraquer keratome had a set of suction rings to fixate the globe that would each permit a different diameter of cornea to be exposed to the keratome. The thickness of the cut was determined by a set of removable plates which changed the gap between the blade and the base of the keratome.[9]

The resected corneal tissue, after being dyed in kiton green for better visualization, was placed upon the head of the lathe and frozen into position while a frozen cutting tool was used to carve the cornea, either for hyperopia or myopia (Figure 17-2). The tissue thickness, radius, cut, and diameter were programmed into the lathe by aid of a computer. The limiting factor on the amount of correction was the central corneal thickness remaining after the lathing. Six to 15 D of myopia were able to be corrected. Higher degrees of myopia could be corrected theoretically if a thicker donor cornea were used, or the size of the optical zone decreased.[9]

The main difficulty with myopic keratomileusis was the learning curve of the keratectomy and the complexity of the cryolathe. A keratome driven across the eye by hand is very dependent upon the speed of the passage to determine the thickness of the cut.[4] Any irregularity in this cut will be exposed as irregular astigmatism in the patient.[10] The cryolathe itself was also a difficult instrument to master and maintain. Although several investigators initially reported good outcomes,[7,8] the complexity of the technique and low margin for surgeon error prevented widespread use.

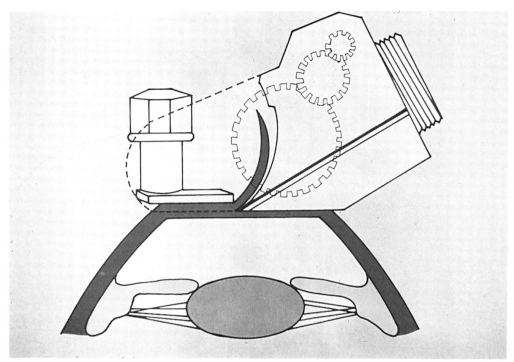

Figure 17-1. The keratome creates a lamellar dissection by applanating the cornea, and incises the underlying stroma like a carpenter's plane.

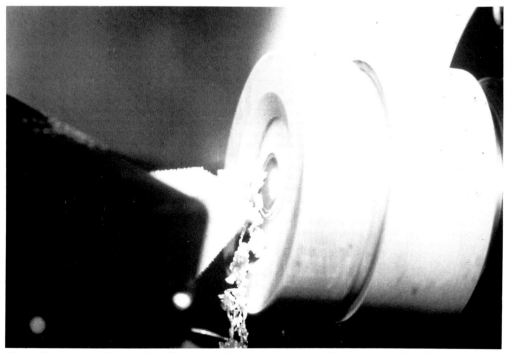

Figure 17-2. Cryolathing of a lamellar corneal disc. A myopic correction is obtained by thinning the disc centrally.

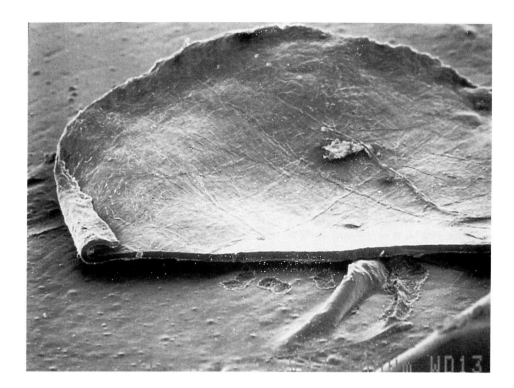

Figure 17-3. Scanning electron microscopy of a disc following ALK showing the lamellar orientation of the resected stroma.

AUTOMATED LAMELLAR KERATOPLASTY OR IN SITU KERATOMILEUSIS FOR MYOPIA: THEORY AND TECHNIQUE

Many attempts were made to make lamellar keratoplasty available to more ophthalmologists by either eliminating the need for a keratectomy or the use of the cryolathe. Epikeratoplasty, which eliminated the need for the surgeon to own a cryolathe or operate a keratome, came closest in theory, but in the end did not enjoy widespread acceptance.[11-13] The Barraquer, Krumeich, Swinger (BKS) keratomileusis technique was another attempt to eliminate the cryolathe by using the microkeratome to perform the refractive cut. The BKS system did not gain widespread acceptance due to the complexity as well as the inherent inaccuracy of a manual keratectomy.[14] However, the concepts behind the BKS device led researchers to investigate the tissue damage present in corneal tissue after freezing and to demonstrate the clinical advantage of rapid healing present when corneal tissue is not heavily processed.[15-18] These findings, combined with the dioptric limitation of shaping the lamellar disc with classic myopic keratomileusis, led to the reintroduction of keratomileusis in situ.

Keratomileusis in situ, where a second shaping resection is made upon the bed after a primary cap is resected, was developed in Bogota by Dr. Luis A. Ruiz. Early on, Dr. Barraquer abandoned this technique due to the inaccuracy of the critical second refractive keratectomy and focused his attention on refining the process of shaping the lamellar disc.[9]

The refractive change in classical keratomileusis is done upon the resected cap of tissue by the cryolathe, while in keratomileusis in situ this is performed upon the bed by the microkeratome. Keratomileusis in situ involves cutting a single lamellar disc of tissue as a cap, or a hinged flap, and a second disc on the bed to thin out the central cornea. The first disc is then replaced and drapes into the resected bed, altering the anterior curvature of the cornea. The second disc removed is a lamellar section as evidenced by scanning electron microscopy (Figure 17-3). The draping effect gives a larger effective optical zone than the diameter of the resected portion.

The accuracy of the keratome is critical to in situ myopic keratomileusis where the thickness of the second resection is directly responsible for the power correction. The speed and consistency of the pass is critical in determining the thickness of the resection.[4] Recognizing that improvement in the outcome for in situ myopic keratomileusis could only come from the development of a predictable second pass, Dr. Ruiz designed a keratome that aided the surgeon in making the crucial second refractive cut.

This keratome, the one most commonly used today, was developed in the late 1980s (Figure 17-4). Dr. Ruiz's automated geared microkeratome controls the speed of the pass across the cornea so that a more consistent cut is possible. This advance in equipment has greatly popularized the technique. In addition, improvements to the suction ring increased the ease of the procedure. An adjustable suction

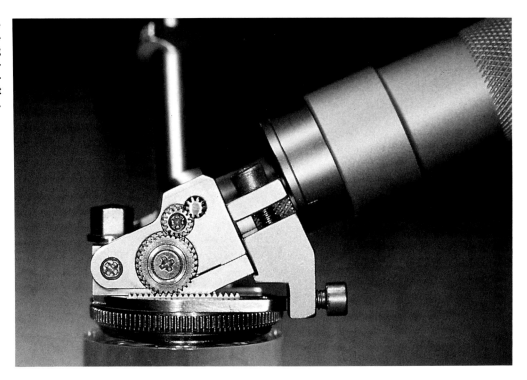

ring is now able to create any specific diameter so that different rings are no longer needed. Keratectomies with this new device display a fine smoothness (Figure 17-5). Early results with this technique were very promising. Initially, the first disc or corneal cap was sutured back into position, but it was later found that sutures were not necessary. Various theories as to why the cap sticks into position have been proposed, including:

1. Surface tension
2. The inherent stickiness of the collagen and ground substance of the cornea
3. The partial relative vacuum of the endothelial cell pump.

Without sutures, there is less induced astigmatism and the recovery time improves. Cases may be done safely with topical anesthesia with this quick, simplified technique. The patients have a more rapid recovery in vision and a more comfortable postoperative course because the corneal tissue is not devitalized or frozen. A further advance is the flap technique: not completely removing the covering cap, but simply leaving a hinge or a flap so that after the second cut is made, the flap is laid back into position (Figure 17-6). If a large hinge is made, sub-clinical topographical changes can be seen which have been of no refractive significance to date for ALK-M (Figures 17-7A and B). Due to the flattening near the hinge, reduced correction in ALK-Hyperopia has been observed when the hinge is too large.

A main goal of ALK remains improved refractive accuracy, which depends upon the thickness and diameter of the resected disc. Ruiz's automated keratome, along with its improved calibration and standardized blades, appears to be moving in this direction. Disadvantages with ALK include potential irregular astigmatism and loss of caps. Reported irregular astigmatism rates have been lower with the ALK technique (2%)[19] than with classic myopic keratomileusis (8% to 20%).[6,7] The danger of losing the cap has been lessened by using the flap technique. ALK has reduced the complexity of lamellar refractive surgery, improved recovery times, and offers a wide range of potential correction. As currently done, ALK seems to be a safe, effective, and reasonably accurate technique for myopia from 4 to 25 D.

As Lee Nordan, MD, reported in his series of classic myopic keratomileusis,[7] ALK also appears to be "astigmatism neutral," affecting only the spherical component (Figures 17-8A and B). Dr. Nordan also noted that incisional keratotomy is a very useful tool in conjunction with lamellar surgery in that it exhibits a potentiating effect by altering both the anterior and posterior corneal curvature. Incisional keratotomy is routinely used to correct residual myopia (Figures 17-9A and B) and astigmatism following ALK. As ALK technique improves, the upper limit for performing radial keratotomy (RK) as a primary procedure of choice decreases, so that even if incisional keratotomy enhancement is necessary, a much larger optical zone is used than that required to correct the preoperative myopia. In this way, a minimally invasive approach is achieved with potentially fewer side effects and improved stability.

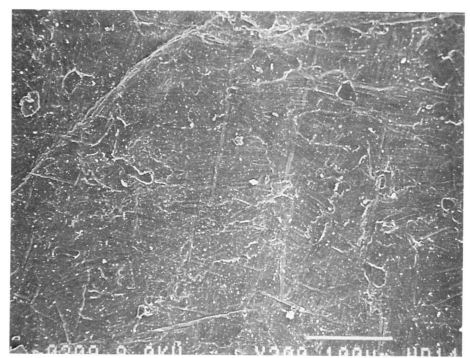

Figure 17-5. Scanning electron microscopy of the stromal surface following the first pass of the automated microkeratome displaying a smooth lamellar bed (200X).

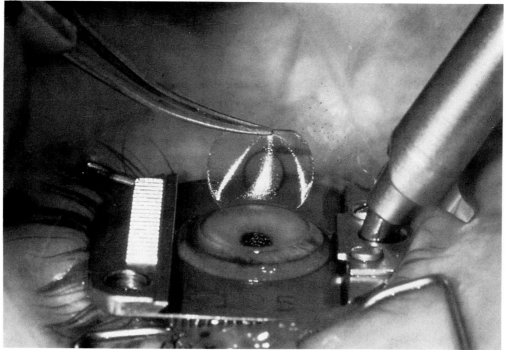

Figure 17-6. After the first lamellar pass, a 160 μm hinged flap is made.

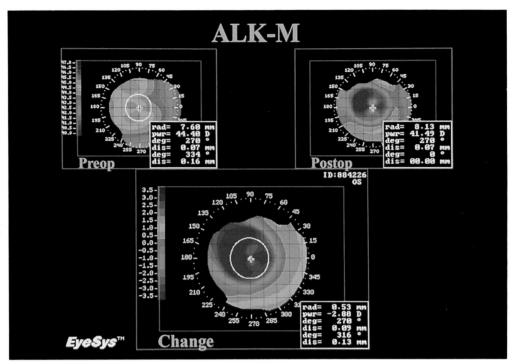

Figure 17-7A. Significant central flattening following standard ALK.

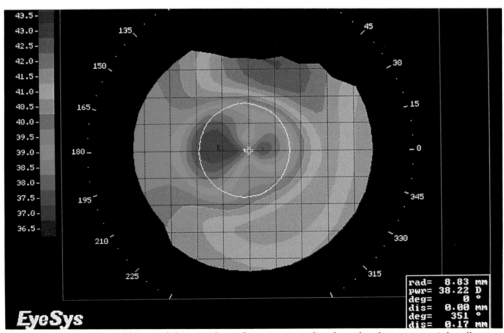

Figure 17-7B. A large nasal hinge exhibits significant flattening extending from the clear zone peripherally.

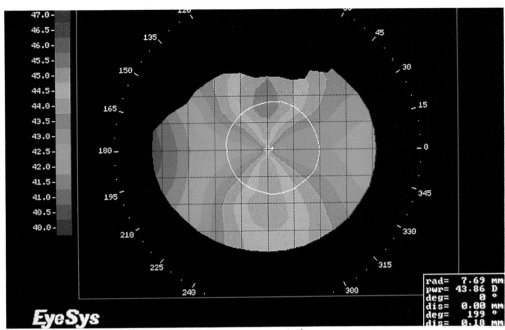

Figure 17-8A. Manifest refraction -9.00 + 4.00 x 90 preoperatively.

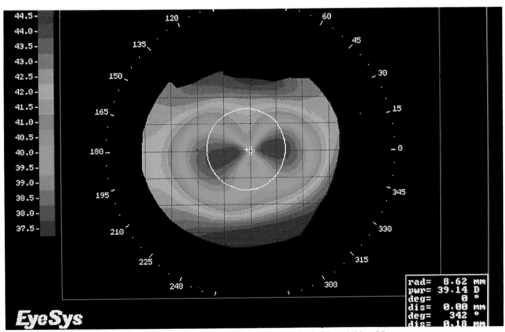

Figure 17-8B. Postoperative manifest refraction following ALK-M is -2.50 +4.00 x 90.

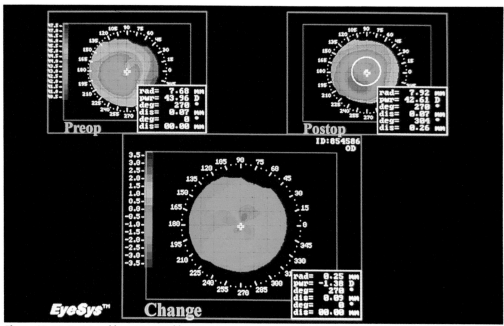

Figure 17-9A. Incisional keratotomy of four incisions at a 5-mm optical zone to correct -1.5D of residual myopia following ALK for myopia.

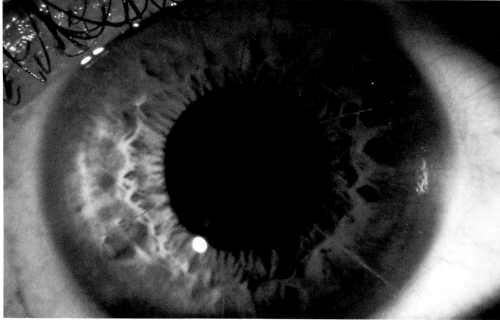

Figure 17-9B. Clinical slit lamp photograph.

ALK may be combined with previous corneal surgery, such as penetrating keratoplasty, to visually rehabilitate the patient. We have used ALK to treat undercorrected or regressed epikeratoplasty, which appears to be a more predictable and safer procedure than frontal ablation with the excimer laser (Figures 17-10A and B).[20,21]

Although complications of ALK are rare, they can often be elucidated by corneal topography analysis. One problem is central islands and regression of a myopic correction. The diameter of the resected bed is critical to the refractive effect. We postulate that for a given plate depth of resection, if the diameter is significantly increased, the overlying cap will conform to the large diameter lamellar resected bed, and thus the corneal cap surface assumes the same preoperative radius of curvature or one that is smaller. Topographically an ALK central island or central steepening is observed, which results in undercorrection or no change from the preoperative refraction (Figure 17-11). The desired central flattening in ALK is dependent upon the formation of the initial nonlamellar edge or peripheral knee of the resected bed which for most refractive resections is 4.2 mm. This finding stresses the importance of maintaining and checking suction, avoiding a false meniscus, and proper applanation diameter prior to making the critical myopic refractive resection.

With all corneal refractive procedures, centration of the keratectomy is crucial to the outcome as well. Although some surgeons break suction prior to proceeding with the refractive cut, the suction ring typically assumes the position of the first depression of the ring in the sclera, and if it is decentered the second pass will be off center as well. Although patients may have good visual acuity despite decentration, it is likely that under scotopic conditions, glare and decreased contrast sensitivity will increase (Figures 17-12 through 17-14).

While most complications with ALK can be avoided, perhaps the most vexing problem is the proliferation of epithelial inclusions in the interface. This complication can be severe enough to induce topographical irregularities, as well as stromal melting of the overlying corneal cap (Figure 17-15). Thus, we recommend the debridement of the interface and reattaching the cap.

Significant central flattening may be achieved with the removal of the corneal cap only, without a second resection (Figures 17-16A and B). Despite the early comparison to PRK with the phrase "mechanical excimer" or superficial lamellar keratectomy, more evaluation of this technique has yet to be done.

Severe persistent anterior stromal haze unresponsive to steroid therapy has been observed, particularly in young patients (Figure 17-17). We reserve this technique for therapeutic removal of anterior stromal opacities, especially in older patients, who do not seem to scar as much. Although rare, in the face of a lost myopic cap we evaluate the refractive outcome and wound healing prior to performing homoplastic lamellar keratoplasty.

AUTOMATED LAMELLAR KERATOPLASTY OR IN SITU KERATOMILEUSIS FOR HYPEROPIA: THEORY AND TECHNIQUE

Lamellar surgical techniques for hyperopia in the past have included reshaping of a corneal cap so it is thinner in the periphery and steeper centrally (classical freeze hyperopic keratomileusis), insertion of alloplastic or homoplastic material in the lamellar interface (keratophakia), or a deep lamellar keratectomy of a specific diameter creating a presumably controlled posterior bulging of the cornea, creating central steepening (original Ruiz technique).

ALK-H improves on the technique by using an adjustable suction ring, automated keratome, and no suturing of the cap. The present Ruiz technique is currently under investigation in the United States. It appears to be most predictable for low to moderate hyperopia (1 to 4 D) although up to 9 D of hyperopia can potentially be corrected. Like ALK-M, ALK-H is astigmatism neutral (Figure 17-18). Since one pass is needed for this procedure and the optical zone diameters are theoretically smaller than for myopic lamellar surgery, centration of the procedure is of utmost importance (Figure 17-19). Decentration of ALK-H is difficult to correct.

The same technique for cap placement in ALK-M is used for ALK-H. However, due to the thickness of the cap, even with a flap, loss of the cap is more likely to occur with ALK-H. In this situation, we recommend lamellar homoplastic keratoplasty as the procedure of choice due to the possibility of progressive iatrogenic corneal ectasia and scarring.

ALK-H is presently the procedure of choice for stable RK patients with overcorrection (Figures 17-20A and B). Due to cases of progressive corneal steepening following ALK-H in patients who had the initial incisional keratotomy 3 months prior, this procedure is reserved for those patients 1 year after their last incisional keratotomy.

Another type of corneal steepening procedure is keratophakia, which was first described by Barraquer in his first publication in the US literature.[22] Because of the development of the cryolathe and carving of the cap, this procedure was supplanted. The automated keratome designed by Dr. Ruiz permits a return to exploring this technique to correct aphakia where intraocular lens implantation would be contraindicated or surgically impractical. Our early experience with homoplastic keratophakia is encouraging, significant steepening is evidenced by topography, and the interfaces have remained clear (Figures 17-21A and B).

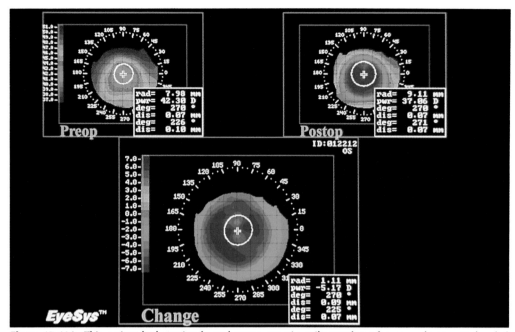

Figure 17-10A. This patient had previously undergone myopic epikeratoplasty for an undercorrected radial keratotomy several years earlier. The epikeratoplasty initially obtained complete correction but regressed to -5.00 D over several years and remained stable for 2 years. The patient underwent ALK-M and obtained a full correction, which has been stable with 1-year follow-up.

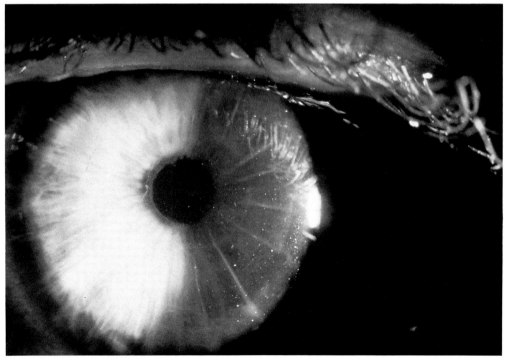

Figure 17-10B. Clinical slit lamp photograph.

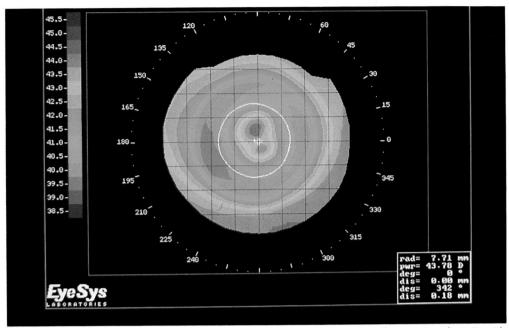

Figure 17-11. A central island following ALK-M revealing central steepening of approximately 4 D with surrounding flattening. This central island resulted in a marked undercorrection.

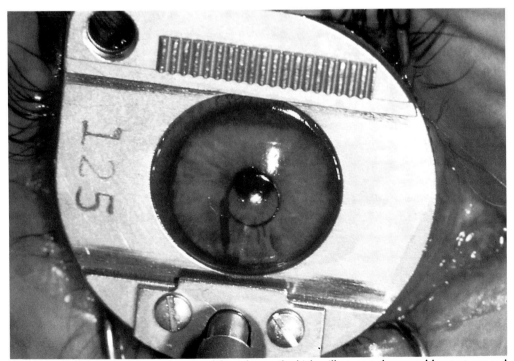

Figure 17-12. The suction ring is decentered from the pupil which will cause a decentered keratectomy and subsequent decentration of the second pass.

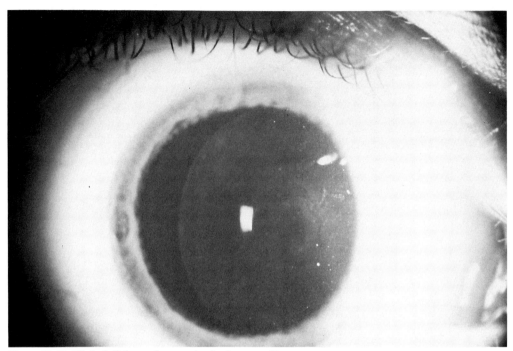

Figure 17-13. Clinical slit lamp photograph of a decentered keratectomy.

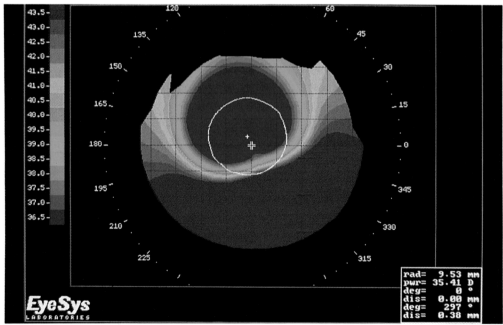

Figure 17-14. Decentered optical zone following ALK.

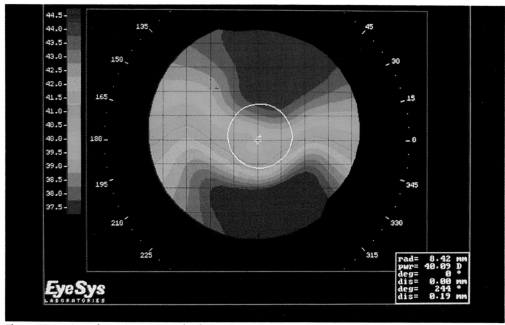

Figure 17-15. Irregular astigmatism and inferior steepening secondary to growth of nests of epithelium in the interface.

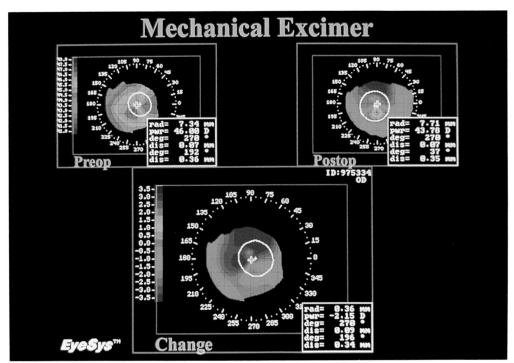

Figure 17-16A. A single pass keratectomy with removal of the cap can yield significant central flattening.

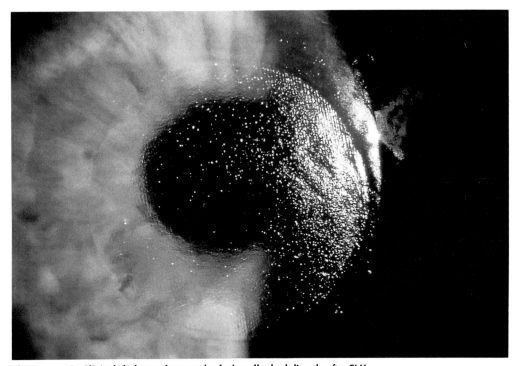

Figure 17-16B. Clinical slit lamp photograph of a lamellar bed directly after SLK.

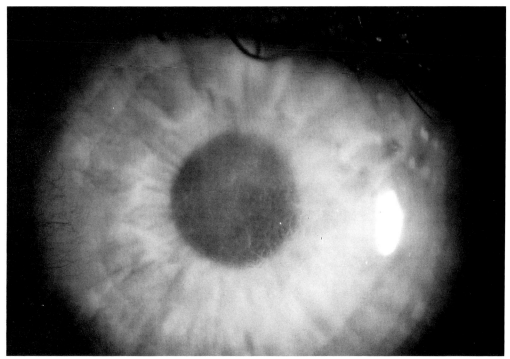

Figure 17-17. 4+ anterior stromal haze 3 months following SLK.

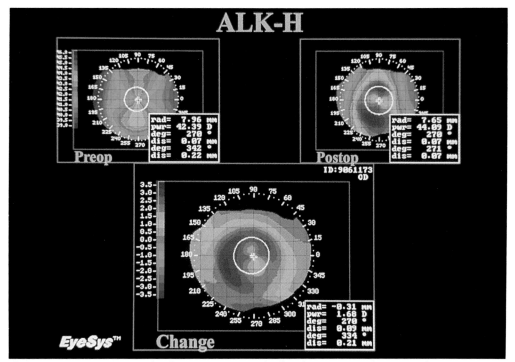

Figure 17-18. ALK-H is considered astigmatism neutral. The change map indicates significant steepening; however, the preoperative astigmatism of 2 D at 90° is still evident postoperatively.

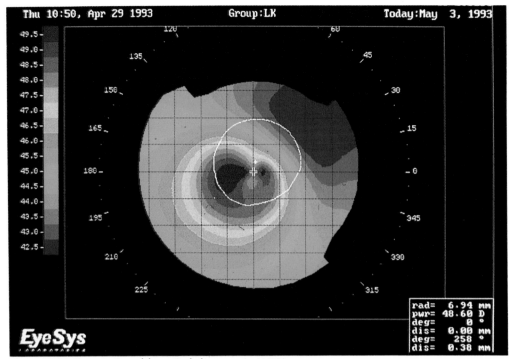

Figure 17-19. Decentration of the optical clear zone in ALK-H.

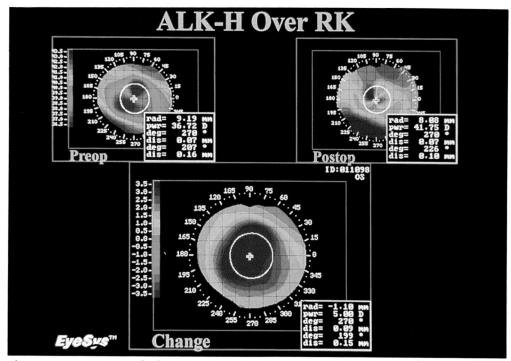

Figure 17-20A. Preoperatively this RK patient's refraction was +1.50. The change map indicates 5 D of keratometric steepening following ALK-H. The patient's postoperative refraction was +0.25 D, which has remained stable for 2 years.

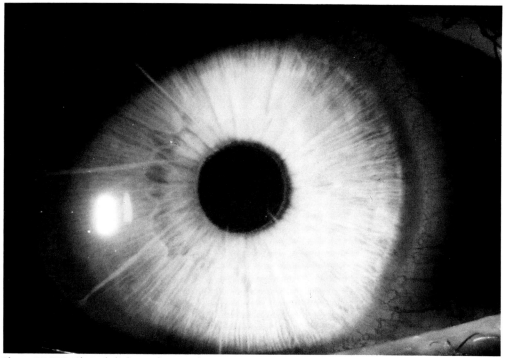

Figure 17-20B. Clinical slit lamp photograph.

IN SITU PHOTOREFRACTIVE KERATOMILEUSIS

ALK has proven very useful for high myopia, while still being limited by a lack of absolute accuracy, which has led investigators to explore ways other than the microkeratome to make the second critical refractive cut. We have begun using the excimer laser to make the second cut of in situ myopic keratomileusis. Peyman et al were the first to investigate the application of a laser to remove stromal tissue under a lamellar flap to obtain a refractive change.[23] Ioannes Pallikaris, using an excimer ablation, provided the most extensive histopathologic evaluation of in situ photorefractive keratomileusis under a corneal flap on rabbit eyes.[24] Lucio Buratto later reported good results in a large series of human eyes, placing an excimer ablation on the undersurface of the 300 μm disc of tissue removed with the microkeratome, or on the bed after a free cap had been removed.[25] The next large series of excimer MKM to the cap to be done was the Summit FDA protocol,[26] started in New Orleans by Stephen Brint and Stephen Slade in the summer of 1991. The current technique, ALK-E, in which the excimer ablation is placed under a lamellar flap to the bed, was then first performed by Stephen Slade in Houston under the Summit FDA protocol. Dr. Ruiz of Bogota has refined these techniques and has developed a new approach for hyperopic and presbyopic ablations to the bed as well as for combined astigmatic ablations (Figures 17-22A and B). Recently, we have prospectively evaluated the excimer laser technique to a 300 μm cap versus ablation to a lamellar bed beneath a 160 μm corneal flap in Bogota, Colombia.[27] At 6 months the bed technique revealed the most accuracy.

Corneal topography analysis of cap ablations reveals that significant parallax error can induce tilting of the cap during ablation with the Summit excimer laser, resulting in an ovoid ablation (Figure 17-23).

Ablation to the bed, which typically is 7 mm in diameter with the Chiron Keracor 116 Excimer Laser, creates a lenticular surface of the bed with the overlying cap mimicking this contour. The central island scenario in standard ALK is the result of a cap contouring to a lamellar bed rather than a lenticular one. Hence, the phenomenon of a central island has not yet been observed with ALK-E for myopia (Figure 17-24).

Corneal topography shows that decentered ablations to the bed can occur, even with a centered keratectomy (Figure 17-25). A mildly decentered keratectomy is less problematic because the ablation can be centered over the pupil, unlike standard ALK, where the suction ring commits the surgeon to a decentered second pass.

The excimer laser offers the potential accuracy to precisely remove corneal tissue. When combined with lamellar surgery, the refractive outcome is not as dependent on wound healing or changes in the optics of the corneal epithelium[28] and offers quicker visual recovery and less pain. As is true with all lamellar surgery, the procedure is astigmatism neutral only if a spherical ablation is performed. However a prime advantage is that the excimer laser is also able to correct astigmatism during the same surgery for the spherical component, unlike standard ALK.

ALK-E patients, due to the virtually intact epithelium and Bowman's membrane, have less postoperative discomfort than standard PRK patients. First day uncorrected vision is often 20/40 or better. Large zones of central flattening are evident on corneal topography. The vision generally stabilizes earlier than with either PRK or RK, as wound healing does not play as large a role. The standard PRK haze is not noted with this technique. The combination of these techniques may be quite fortuitous.

FUTURE TRENDS

Optimism over the future of lamellar refractive surgery is increasing rapidly. These procedures allow patients to be treated with a non-freeze, non-sutured, minimally invasive operation under topical anesthesia. There is a rapid return to vision and excellent patient comfort. Irregular astigmatism rates are encouragingly low. Lamellar refractive techniques are very much in development, as are keratomes, blades, and our knowledge of how best to use the excimer. Different spot sizes, optical zones, multi-zone treatments, ablation parameters, and our understanding of the fluidics of the corneal stroma[29] will all continue to evolve.

Fortunately, the early pioneers in this arena had the vision and persistence to strive for large predictable corrections of ametropia without performing intraocular surgery. The potential risks of intraocular surgery outweigh those of lamellar surgery.[30] However, in order for lamellar techniques to be the first choice for large refractive errors, the accuracy and optical performance of that obtained by intraocular lens implantation must be achieved.[31] Our ability to evaluate our surgery with corneal topography to assess the optical effect and quality of the corneal surface does and will continue to greatly benefit our patients.[32-34]

The combination of the excimer laser to do the refractive cuts and improved automated microkeratomes to do the keratectomies may prove to be a more predictable procedure than PRK or standard ALK alone. Perhaps the main advantage of lamellar refractive surgery is the ability to avoid wound healing responses to provide an "intrastromal ablation" when the dream of true intrastromal ablation remains distant.

We anticipate many improvements in lamellar refractive

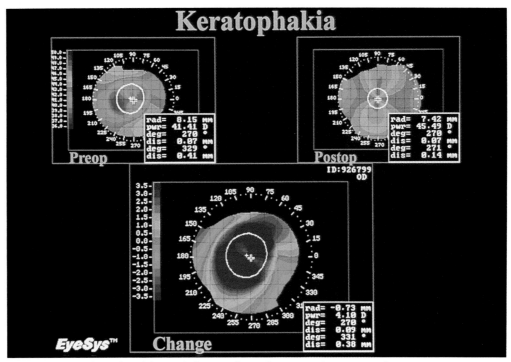

Figure 17-21A. Early work with keratophakia reveals significant central steepening of 4 D.

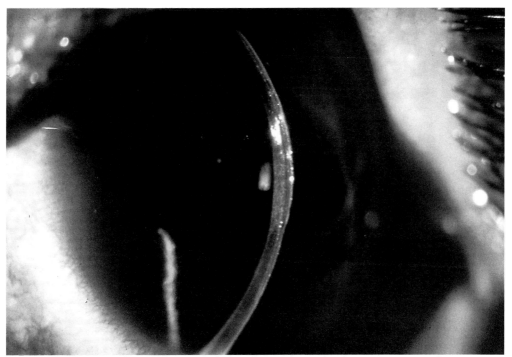

Figure 17-21B. Slit lamp photography reveals the lamellar interface and a clear cornea at 6 months.

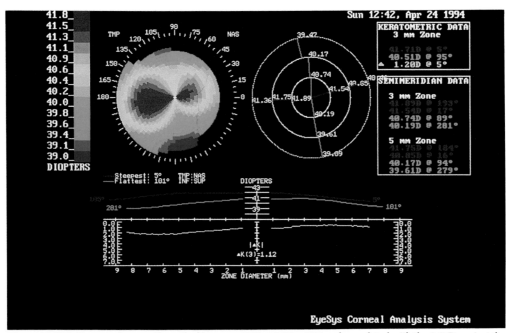

Figure 17-22A. Preoperative manifest refraction was -7.00 +1.50 x 180 and correlated with the 1.2 D against the rule asigmatism apparent with corneal topography analysis.

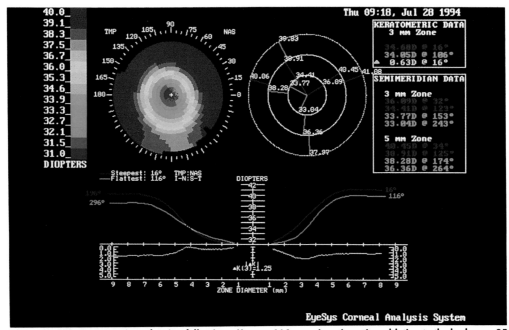

Figure 17-22B. Postoperative refraction following a Keracor 116 myopic astigmatism ablation to the bed was -.25 sphere with a well-centered ablation.

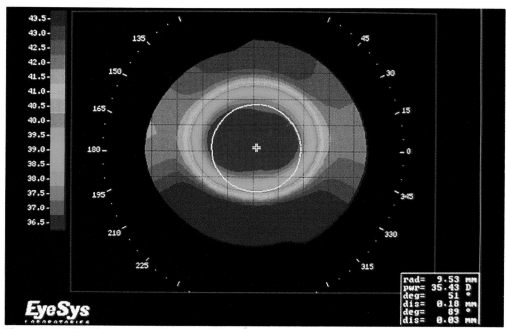

Figure 17-23. Significant central flattening following Summit excimer laser ablation to the cap; however, a markedly ovoid ablation is apparent due to tilting of the cap from parallax error of the operating microscope.

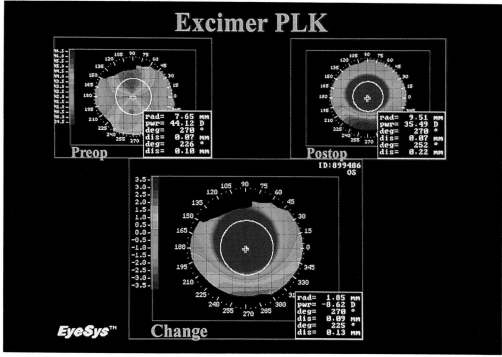

Figure 17-24. Significant central flattening following a well-centered ALK-E.

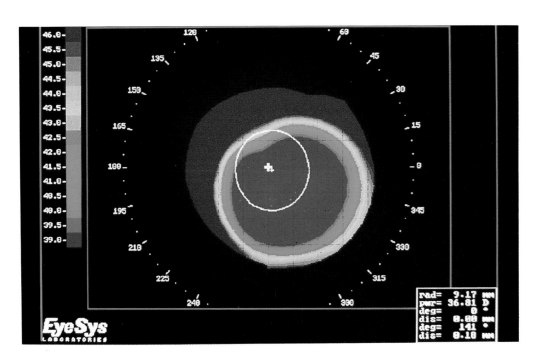

Figure 17-25. A decentered excimer laser ablation to the bed.

surgery which we will be able to evaluate and appreciate with video computerized topography.

REFERENCES

1. Barraquer JI. Queratoplastia refractiva. *Estudios Inform Oftal Inst Barraquer.* 1949;10:2-21.
2. Barraquer JI. Results of hypermetropic keratomileusis. In: Binder PS, ed. *Refractive Corneal Surgery: The Correction of Aphakia, Hyperopia and Myopia.*
3. Barraquer JI. Results of myopic keratomileusis. *J Refract Surg.* 1987;3:98-101. 1983;23:25-44.
4. Barraquer JI. Keratomileusis for myopia and aphakia. *Ophth.* 1981;88:701-708.
5. Troutman RC, Swinger CA. Refractive keratoplasty: keratophakia and keratomileusis. *Trans Am Ophthalmol Soc.* 1978;76:329-39.
6. Swinger CA, Barker BA. Prospective evaluation of myopic keratomileusis. *Ophthalmol.* 1984;91:785-792.
7. Nordan LT, Fallor MK. Myopic keratomileusis: 74 consecutive non-amblyopic cases with one year of follow-up. *J Refract Surg.* 1986;2:124-128.
8. Hofmann RF, Bechara SJ. An independent evaluation of second generation suction microkeratomes. *Refract Corneal Surg.* 1992;8:348-354.
9. Barraquer JI. Keratomileusis. *Int Surg.* 1967;48:103-117.
10. Maguire LJ, Klyce SD, et al. Visual distortion after myopic keratomileusis: computer analysis of keratoscopy photography. *Ophth Surg.* 1987;18:352-356.
11. Kaufman HE. The correction of aphakia. *Am J Oph.* 1980;89:1-10.
12. Werblin TP, Klyce SD. Epikeratophakia: the surgical correction of aphakia. I. Lathing of corneal tissue. *Curr Eye Res.* 1981;1:591-597.
13. Goosey JD, Prager TC, Goosey CB, et al. Stability of refraction during two years after myopic epikeratoplasty. *Refract Corneal Surg.* 1990;6:4-8.
14. Swinger CA, Krumeich J, Cassiday D. Planar lamellar refractive keratoplasty. *J Refract Surg.* 1986;2:17-24.
15. Binder PS. What we have learned about corneal wound healing from refractive surgery: Barraquer lecture. *Refract Corneal Surg.* 1989;5:98-120.
16. Binder PS, Zavala EY, Baumgartner SD, et al. Combined morphological effects of cryolathing and lyophilization on epikeratoplasty lenticles. *Arch Ophthalmol.* 1986;104:671-679.
17. Zavala EY, Krumeich J, Binder PS. Laboratory evaluation of freeze vs nonfreeze lamellar refractive keratoplasty. *Arch Ophthalmol.* 1987;105:1125-1128.
18. Buratto L, Ferrari M. Retrospective comparison of freeze and non-freeze myopic epikeratophakia. *Refract Corneal Surg.* 1989;5:94-97.
19. Slade SG, the ALK Study Group. *Keratomileusis in-situ: a prospective evaluation.* American Academy of Ophthalmology poster presentation, 1993.
20. Updegraff SA, McDonald MB, Slade SG. *ALK versus PRK for the treatment of undercorrection or myopic regression following epikeratoplasty.* International Society for Refractive Keratoplasty presentation, October 1993.
21. Colin J, Sanguilo R, Malet F, Volant A. Photorefractive keratectomy following undercorrected myopic epikeratoplasties. *J Fr Ophth.* 1992;15(6-7):384-388.
22. Barraquer JI. Modification of refraction by means of intracorneal inclusions. *Int Ophthalmol Clin.* 1966;6:53-78.
23. Peyman GA, Badaro RM, Khoobehi B. Corneal ablation in rabbits using an infrared (2.9-μm) erbium:YAG Laser. *Ophthalmol.* 1989;96:1160-1169.
24. Pallikaris IG, Papatzanaki ME, Stathi EZ, et al. Laser in situ keratomileusis. *Lasers Surg Med.* 1990;10:463-468.
25. Buratto L, Ferrari M, Rama P. Excimer laser intrastromal keratomileusis. *Amer J Ophthalmol.* 1992;113:291-295.
26. Slade SG, Brint SJ, et al. Phase I myopic keratomileusis with the Summit Excimer Laser. In press.
27. Ruiz L, Slade SG, Updegraff SA. A prospective single-center clinical trial to evaluate ALK and ALK combined with PRK using the excimer laser versus PRK alone for the surgical correction of moderate to high myopia. Bogota, Colombia. In press.
28. Simon G, Ren Q, Kervick G, Parel J. Optics of the corneal epithelium. *Refract Corneal Surg.* 1993;9:42-50.
29. Dougherty P, Wellish K, Maloney R. Excimer laser ablation rate and corneal hydration. 1994;118:169-176.
30. Javitt JC. Clear lens extraction for high myopia. *Arch Ophth.* 1994;112:321-323.
31. Holladay JT, Prager TC, Ruiz RS, et al. Improving the predictability of intraocular lens power calculations. *Arch Ophthal.* 1986;104:539-41.
32. Maguire LJ. Topographical principles in keratorefractive surgery. *Int Ophthalm Clin.* 1991;31:1-6.
33. Camp JJ, Maguire LJ, Cameron BM, et al. A computer model for the evaluation of the effect of corneal topography on optical performance. *Am J Ophthalmol.* 1990;109:379-386.
34. Florakis GJ, Jewelewicz DA, Michelsen HE, Trokel SL. Evaluation of night vision disturbances. *Ref Corneal Surg.* 1994;10(3):333-338.

CORNEAL TOPOGRAPHY IN THE EVALUATION OF THE CORNEAL TRANSPLANT PATIENT

Roger Steinert, MD
Johnny L. Gayton, MD
Robert G. Martin, MD

Corneal topography is valuable in evaluating the corneal curvature changes induced by corneal transplantation (Figure 18-1). However, as the rate of corneal transplants remaining clear in the long term has improved, increasing attention has been directed at control of postoperative astigmatism. An anatomically clear graft with poor optical function is a functional failure. Over the past decade many surgeons changed suturing techniques to improve their results with postoperative astigmatism, including different styles of single and double running sutures and different suture materials. In the mid 1980s, surgeons began using combined interrupted and running sutures.

SELECTIVE SUTURE REMOVAL

Selective suture removal of tight interrupted sutures in the steep meridian helped to reduce suture-in astigmatism. With the advent of computer-assisted topographic analysis as a clinical tool, discrimination of the precise etiology of the astigmatism improved further. The most immediately obvious application was to identify the exact location of the tight interrupted suture(s) causing the astigmatism (Figures 18-2A and B) and to evaluate the immediate effects on the cornea of the suture removal (Figures 18-3A through 18-4B). Not only can one evaluate the effects of removing interrupted sutures, but also the combined effects of removing running and interrupted sutures (Figure 18-5).

These illustrations demonstrate how keratometry may be misleading since clearly the corneal power changes are neither orthogonal nor symmetrical across a given meridian (ie, 0° to 180° axis or 90° to 270° axis).

SUTURE ROTATION

Van Meter et al[1] introduced a further refinement in postoperative suture adjustment by utilizing a 24 bite running suture as the sole closure. Tension on the suture is then adjusted postoperatively, guided by the computer-assisted topographic analysis. In a prospective randomized study, we have shown both more rapid recovery and less final astigmatism with the 24 bite running suture adjustment technique compared to a technique utilizing eight interrupted sutures combined with a 16 bite running suture.[2] Figures 18-6 to 18-9 represent detailed case reports documenting the value of this technique and powerfully demonstrate the use of corneal topography in postoperative suture adjustment.

RELAXING INCISIONS

Obviously none of the dramatic effects outlined in the cases above are useful once all the sutures have been removed. At this point, corneal relaxing incisions (CRIs) provide a useful alternative. Frequently, these cases present with asymmetric, non-orthogonal astigmatism, requiring asymmetric surgery. Only corneal topography could provide the detailed information about the corneal distortion that is needed to formulate surgical plans in these cases. Figure 18-10 demonstrates topography of a 52-year-old male with 12 D of astigmatism 10 years following penetrating keratoplasty. Contact lens fitting was unsuccessful due to lens decentration. Relaxing incisions in the graft-host junction were placed along the 30° and 190° semi-meridians. Three months postoperatively the keratometric cylinder was reduced to 3.6 D.

Figure 18-1. Penetrating kerato-plasty for keratoglobus 1 day preoperatively (upper left) and 1 day postoperatively (lower left). Note the marked conver-sion of central steepness to rela-tive central flatness. Right, subtraction, or change, map shows the dramatic postopera-tive flattening in excess of 20 D. *Courtesy of Douglas Koch, MD.*

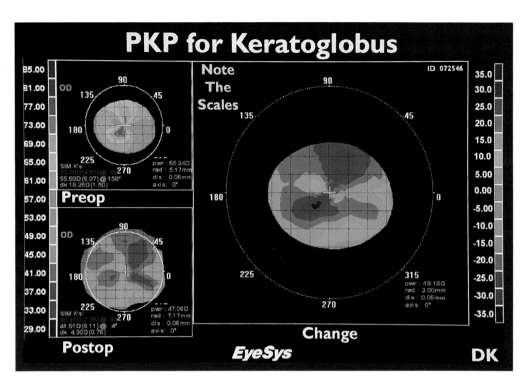

The topography of a 77-year-old woman who received penetrating keratoplasty for bullous keratopathy is shown in Figure 18-11. Nine months later she received a single 2-mm arcuate relaxing incision to correct superotemporal steepness. Preoperatively, her refraction was -3.50 +7.25 x 39, with 20/40 corrected acuity and 20/150 uncorrected acuity. Three weeks following the procedure, as shown in the topography, her refraction was -2.00 +3.00 x 79, with 20/50 corrected acuity and 20/80 uncorrected acuity. The change image (right) illustrates the flattening induced at the incision site and the steepening induced 90° away.

Figure 18-12 shows the topography of a 72-year-old woman who had extracapsular cataract extraction and pene-trating keratoplasty for decompensated bullous keratopathy. Ten months later she received a single 3-mm arcuate relaxing incision to correct 8 D of refractive cylinder. The topographic change image demonstrates the tremendous effect of the relaxing incision. In addition to flattening in the incision meridian, over 7 D of steepening occurred 90° away, as shown in the change map. Five months postoperatively the refraction was +1.00 +0.50 x 33.

Figures 18-13A and B show topography of a 75-year-old female 4 years post penetrating keratoplasty and 12 years post cataract and IOL surgery OD. Preoperatively, the refraction was -4.50 +6.25 x 25 with best-corrected visual acuity of 20/70. Because topography revealed asymmetry in astigmatism, two 50° arcuate incisions were placed across the 35° semi-meridian superiorly and one 50° arcuate incision

was placed across the 215° semi-meridian inferiorly. The arcuate incisions were kept within the graft button.

Figure 18-13A compares the preoperative and 2-week postoperative topographical appearance. The change graph demonstrates the marked flattening in the incision meridian with steepening 90° away. At 3 months postoperatively (Figure 18-13B), the coupling has regressed, leaving only the flattening in the incision meridian. Although there is residual keratometric cylinder, refraction is -0.75 -0.50 x 85 and the best-corrected visual acuity has improved to 20/25.

Figure 18-14 displays the topography of a 34-year-old female who received penetrating keratoplasty in both eyes in 1988 for keratoconus. CRIs were performed on the right eye. Preoperatively the refraction was -1.75 +2.25 x 125 with 3 D of keratometric cylinder. Corneal topography determined placement of the incisions. Two incisions were made at the graft/host interface at 0.6 mm depth, each 40° of arc. Postoperatively the refraction was -1.00 sph, and keratometry was 41.87/42 x 84. Topography demonstrated flattening in the incision meridian and steepening 90° away. The postoper-ative image indicates a breakup of the astigmatism pattern with a nearly spherical central cornea.

After the successful result in the right eye, CRIs were performed on the left eye (Figure 18-15). These incisions were also placed at the graft/host interface at 0.6 mm depth. A longer arcuate incision was placed nasally because of asymmetry of astigmatism as determined by topography. The surgery resulted in an overcorrection, which progressed later

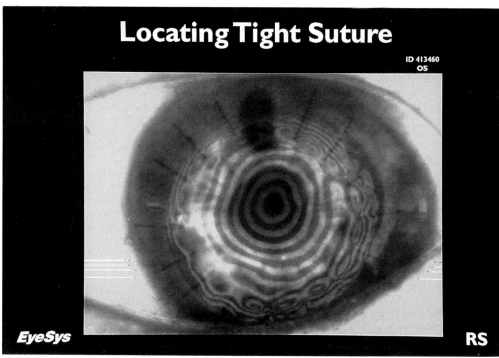

Figure 18-2A. Localization of tight interrupted suture. Placido image—location of tight suture not obvious.

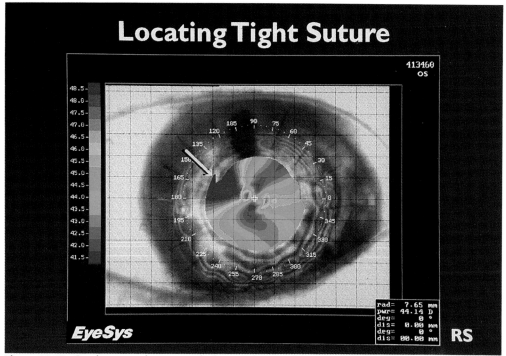

Figure 18-2B. Overlay corneal map—marked area of steepening (arrow) localizes the suture(s) that needs removal.

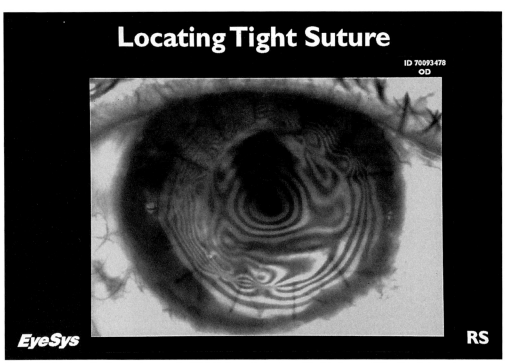

Figure 18-3A. Localization and removal of tight interrupted suture. Placido image difficult to interpret.

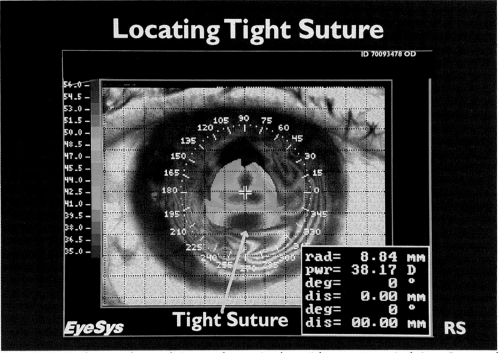

Figure 18-3B. Overlay corneal map. Inferior area of steepening due to tight suture (arrow) is obvious. *Courtesy of Douglas Koch, MD.*

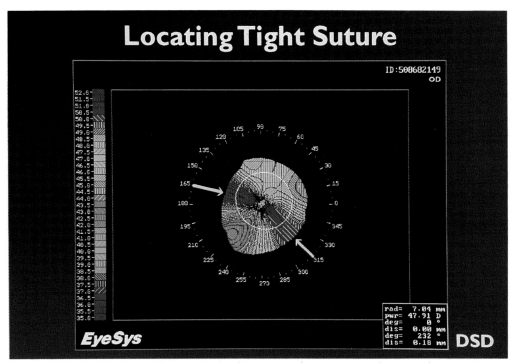

Figure 18-4A. Localization and removal of tight interrupted suture. Corneal topography reveals steep hemi-meridians at 165° and 315° (arrows, 150° apart) corresponding to areas with tight sutures.

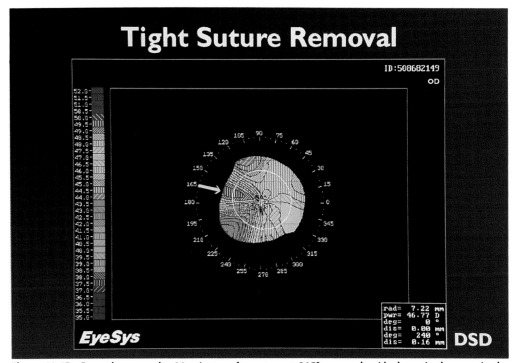

Figure 18-4B. Corneal topography 30 minutes after suture at 315° removed, with dramatic decrease in the astigmatism. The examiner advised the patient to wait until the next visit to consider suture removal at 165° (arrow). *Courtesy of Daniel Durrie, MD.*

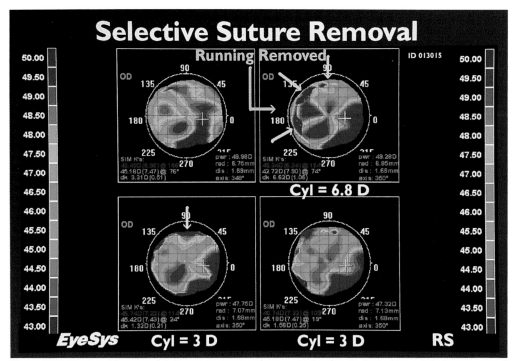

Figure 18-5. Topographic map of right cornea 4 years after penetrating keratoplasty. Upper left, best-corrected vision was 20/70. Note irregular astigmatism. Upper right, following removal of the running suture, the corneal topography is more regular. Interrupted sutures remain at the 8:00, 10:00, and 12:00 positions (arrows). Lower left, following removal of the 8:00 and 10:00 sutures, astigmatism has been reduced from 6.83 to 3.00 D, although some irregularity is present. The 12:00 suture is still in place (arrow). Lower right, following removal of the 12:00 suture, astigmatism is still 3.00 D, but the cornea is more regular. Best-corrected vision is 20/30. Note the persistent steep zone inferonasally.

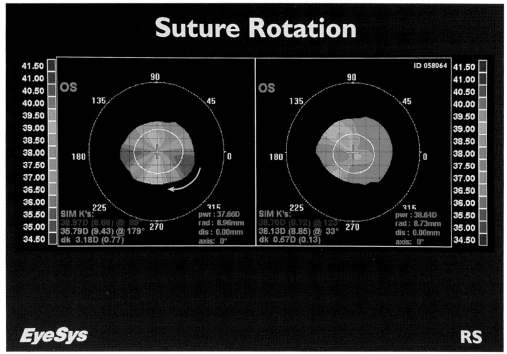

Figure 18-6. The patient is a 27-year-old female with keratoconus who underwent penetrating keratoplasty in the left eye utilizing the 24-bite 10-0 nylon running suture technique. The first topographic image, 1 month postoperatively (left), shows fairly regular astigmatism. Both keratometrically and refractively, she has 4 D of astigmatism with the steep orientation vertically. The suture was adjusted by moving suture material from the flattest hemi-meridian as indicated by the peripheral blue coloration at 4:00, or the hemi-meridian centered at 330.° Suture material was moved from this flat hemi-meridian inferiorly toward the 6:00 position at 270° (arrow). Repeat topography approximately 35 minutes later (right) shows marked improvement in overall sphericity with reduction in cylinder. There is still some component of irregular astigmatism. At this point the wound is left to settle down and re-evaluation will be performed in 1 month. The patient notes qualitatively marked improvement in uncorrected vision.

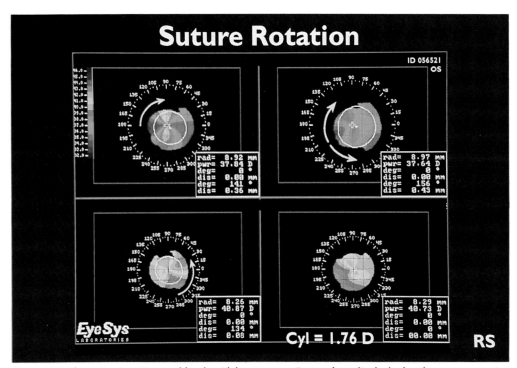

Figure 18-7. The patient is a 30-year-old male with keratoconus. Five weeks earlier he had undergone penetrating keratoplasty in his left eye. The baseline topography (upper left) shows steepening vertically and flattening horizontally, with more prominent steepening at the 90° hemi-meridian. The tension on the running suture was adjusted by tightening suture loops from 180° (9:00) and moving the suture material toward 90° (12:00, arrow). Upper right, re-evaluation 1 hour later shows dramatic reduction in total astigmatism but a shift toward some irregular astigmatism with maximal steepening at the 125° hemi-meridian and maximal flattening at 195°. This astigmatism was then adjusted on a second immediate revision by tightening suture loops centered at 195° and moving tension both toward 140° and toward 270° as indicated by the topographic analysis (suture shifted from 8:00 toward 10:30 and toward 6:00, arrows). Lower left, re-evaluation 30 minutes later shows further reduction in net astigmatism but marked asymmetry with a maximally steep hemi-meridian at 30° and a maximally flat meridian at 290°. Accordingly a third revision was performed, tightening loops at 290° and moving them toward 30° (5:00 toward 2:00, arrows) Lower right, the final keratograph 30 minutes later shows a return to relatively regular astigmatism with a net keratometric astigmatism of 1.76 D. This series of adjustments and consecutive topographic analyses were performed to demonstrate the power of the computer-assisted corneal topography to follow and direct the suture adjustment. Our more typical procedure is to begin suture adjustment 1 month postoperatively, as soon as the surface is smooth enough to permit it, but rarely do we perform more than one adjustment at a given session. Some realignment of the suture occurs in the weeks following the adjustment, and we will typically allow 2 to 4 weeks to pass before bringing the patient back for re-analysis with refraction, repeat topographic analysis, and further adjustment if needed.

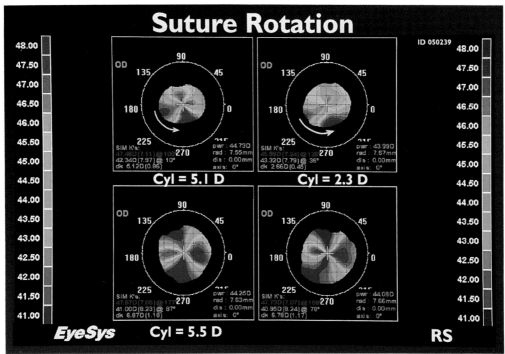

Figure 18-8A. This 21-year-old female underwent penetrating keratoplasty due to central corneal scarring from a pseudomonas ulcer acquired during extended wear soft contact lens use. Suturing utilized the 24-bite 10-0 nylon running suture technique. Upper left, 1 month postoperatively the topography exhibited 5 D of central astigmatism with mild asymmetry of the hemi-meridians but good orthogonality. Guided by the topography, suture material was tightened in the flattest hemi-meridian at 195° and passed to the steepest hemi-meridian centered at 285° (8:00 to 5:00, arrow). Upper right, by the third postoperative month repeat topography showed less central astigmatism by conventional keratometry (5 D had been reduced to 2.3 D), but the residual astigmatism was asymmetric, limiting best spectacle correction to 20/40. A second suture manipulation was therefore performed, shifting more suture material from the flattest hemi-meridian centered at 200° to the steepest hemi-meridian centered at 290° (arrow). Lower left, 90 minutes later repeat topography showed marked improvement in the regularity of the astigmatism with return of orthogonality but with a net increase in conventional keratometric cylinder (2.3 D increased to 5.5 D). Lower right, by the fifth postoperative month, no spontaneous improvement in the residual astigmatism had occurred.

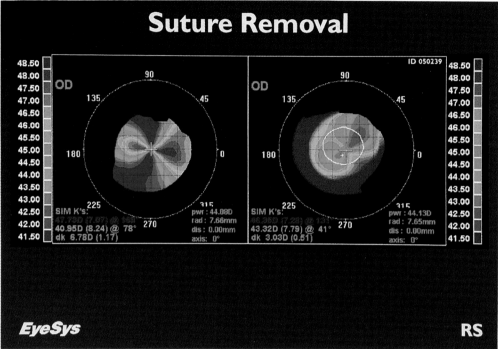

Figure 18-8B. After a graft rejection episode successfully reversed with intense topical steroids, the suture spontaneously loosened and was removed. The wound appeared anatomically stable. Topographic analysis (right) 1 year postoperatively showed mildly asymmetric astigmatism with conventional keratometric cylinder of 3 D. Compare this image to topography with suture-in 8 months earlier (left). This case dramatically illustrates the power of suture adjustment on astigmatism, both regular and irregular. Also clearly illustrated by the suture-out topography 1 year postoperatively is the appearance of an entirely different topographic pattern, which is consistent with the literature suggesting that, based on historical controls, there is no evidence yet that suture manipulation affects the ultimate astigmatism after full suture removal. Until a suture manipulation technique does demonstrate such an effect, the working hypothesis is that postoperative suture manipulation has the goal of improving suture-in astigmatism. Depending upon the patient's age and underlying pathology, as well as the surgeon's own technique, nylon sutures are typically retained between 1 and 5 years. Restoration of good acuity during this period is therefore an important goal.

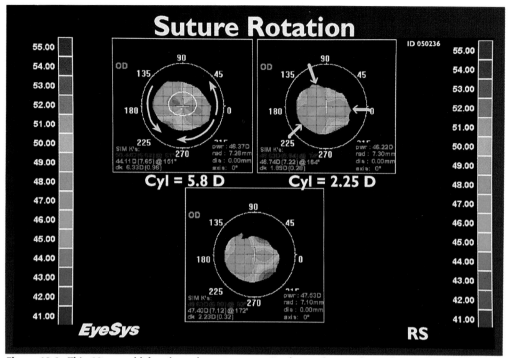

Figure 18-9. This 83-year-old female underwent penetrating keratoplasty in her right eye for pseudophakic bullous keratopathy. The 24-bite running 10-0 nylon suture technique was used. Early postoperative filamentary keratitis gradually cleared and topographic analysis became possible 10 weeks postoperatively. Upper left, initial astigmatism disclosed regular astigmatism with 5.8 D of keratometric cylinder. Suture tension was adjusted moving suture material from the flat hemi-meridian at 345° both toward 60 and 240° and from the opposite flat hemi-meridan at 150° toward the steep hemi-meridian at 240° (arrows). Upper right, 5 months postoperatively a marked reduction in total astigmatism had occurred, but with development of an interesting pattern of three flat hemi-meridians (arrows). Nevertheless, refractive astigmatism dropped from 5.5 D prior to the manipulation to 2.25 D. No further suture manipulations were undertaken. The irregular astigmatic component diminished by 7 months postoperatively (bottom).

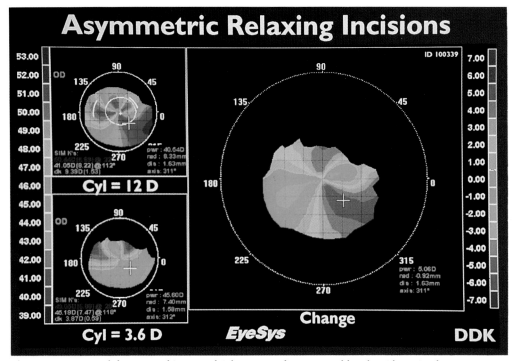

Figure 18-10. Upper left, topographic map of right cornea of a 52-year-old male with 12 D of astigmatism 10 years following penetrating keratoplasty. Contact lens fitting was unsuccessful due to lens decentration. Sixty degree relaxing incisions in the graft-host junction along the 30° and 190° semi-meridians were placed (curved lines). Lower left, 3-month postoperative appearance. Keratometric cylinder is now 3.6 D axis 32°. Right, difference map shows that the greatest change consisted of steepening of the flat zones approximately 90° from the sites of the incisions. *Courtesy of Dr. Douglas Koch.*

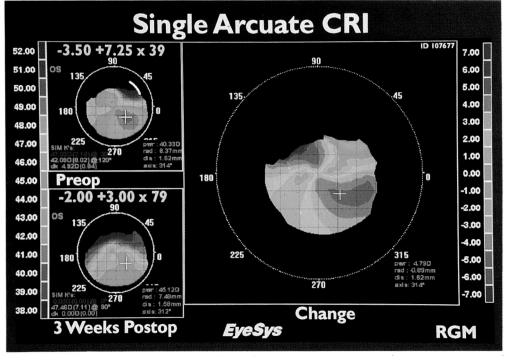

Figure 18-11. Topography of a post penetrating keratoplasty case receiving a 2-mm relaxing incision at area of greatest steepness. The change image (right) indicates flattening at the incision site with almost 5 D of steepening 90° away.

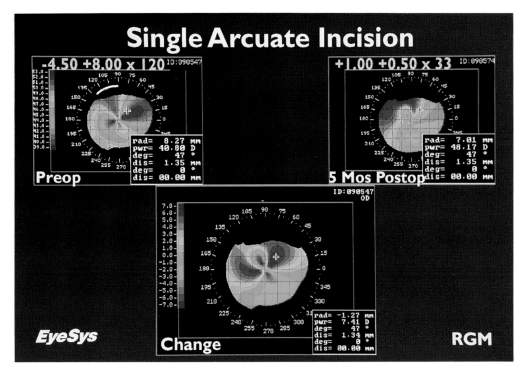

Figure 18-12. Topography of a case status post penetrating keratoplasty and cataract extraction, receiving a single 3-mm superior relaxing incision. The change image (bottom) indicates flattening in the incision meridian with over 7 D of steepening 90° away. The postoperative image (right) demonstrates residual corneal distortion, but the central cornea is more regular than preoperatively.

postoperatively. At 3 months, a pair of CRIs was performed at the graft/host interface to counteract the overcorrection. Because of the strong response to the first pair of CRIs, this pair was initially made at 0.4 mm depth. These incisions mildly reduced the overcorrection, but the effect regressed. After this regression, the topography appears virtually unchanged. The incisions were deepened to 0.5 mm depth and then again to 0.6 mm depth. Following the second redeepening, the keratometry was 39.75/43 x 89. Topography indicated a more spherical central cornea, although peripheral superonasal steepness persists.

EVALUATING OTHER REFRACTIVE SURGERIES POST PENETRATING KERATOPLASTY

In addition to high postoperative astigmatism, post penetrating keratoplasty cases frequently present with significant myopia. Radial keratotomy (RK) can be performed in the donor button, either alone or in combination with astigmatic keratotomy.

Figure 18-16 shows topography of a 64-year-old woman who had penetrating keratoplasty in 1992. One year later she received four-incision RK at a 4.75-mm optical zone and a single CRI to correct 4.25 D of myopia and 3.5 D of astigmatism. Four months postoperatively the refraction was -3.25 + 1.00 x 45, with 20/30 corrected acuity. Five months postoperatively the RK was enhanced by reducing the optical

zone to 4.25 mm. One week following the enhancement the refraction was -1.25 + 1.00 x 15, with 20/30⁻ best-corrected, as well as uncorrected, visual acuity. The lower right image on the topography demonstrates the flattening achieved by the enhancement.

Figure 18-17 shows topography of an 80-year-old man aphakic in the left eye who received penetrating keratoplasty for Fuch's dystrophy and secondary IOL implantation, and then four pairs of relaxing incisions 1 year later. Four years later he received four-incision RK and two 2.4-mm arcuate CRIs at the areas of greatest steepness, as demonstrated by topography. Preoperatively the refraction was -13.25 + 12.00 x 52. One week postoperatively the refraction was -5.25 + 5.75 x 65. The change image demonstrates almost 7 D of flattening in the 45° meridian.

Figure 18-18 shows the topography of a 72-year-old male who underwent penetrating keratoplasty in the left eye for Fuch's dystrophy. Three years after all sutures had been removed, the patient presented with significant myopia and astigmatism. Refraction was -12.75 + 5.50 x 64. Keratometry found 4 D of cylinder at 63.° Corneal topography revealed asymmetric steepness superiorly which extended into the visual axis. Accordingly, eight radial incisions at the 3-mm optical zone were performed in addition to a superiorly placed relaxing incision at the graft/host interface, 60° of arc.

The topographic change image demonstrates the effect of the combined surgeries. There is marked flattening in the

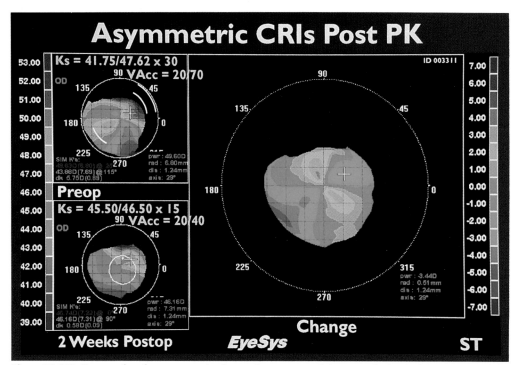

Figure 18-13A. Topography of post penetrating keratoplasty case receiving two relaxing incisions superonasally and one inferotemporally within the donor button. Two-week postoperative topography. The change image (right) indicates flattening in the incision meridian with coupling, that is, steepening 90° away.

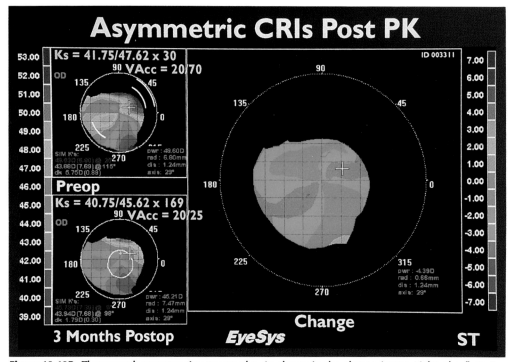

Figure 18-13B. Three-month postoperative topography. As shown in the change image (right), the flattening persists, but the coupling has regressed. *Courtesy of Spencer P. Thornton, MD, FACS.*

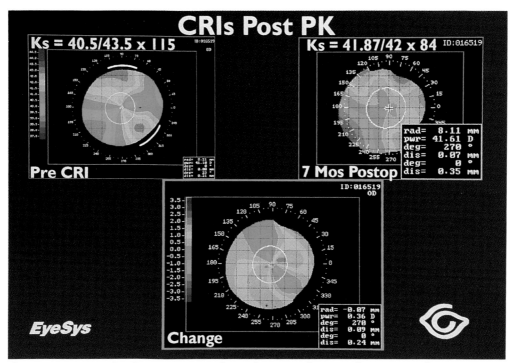

Figure 18-14. Topography of a post penetrating keratoplasty case who received two arcuate relaxing incisions at the graft/host interface for non-orthogonal astigmatism, placed at the areas of greatest corneal steepness as determined by preoperative corneal topography. The change image (bottom) demonstrates a coupling effect has occurred, with flattening at the incision sites and steepening 90° away. The postoperative image (right) shows the astigmatism pattern effectively broken up.

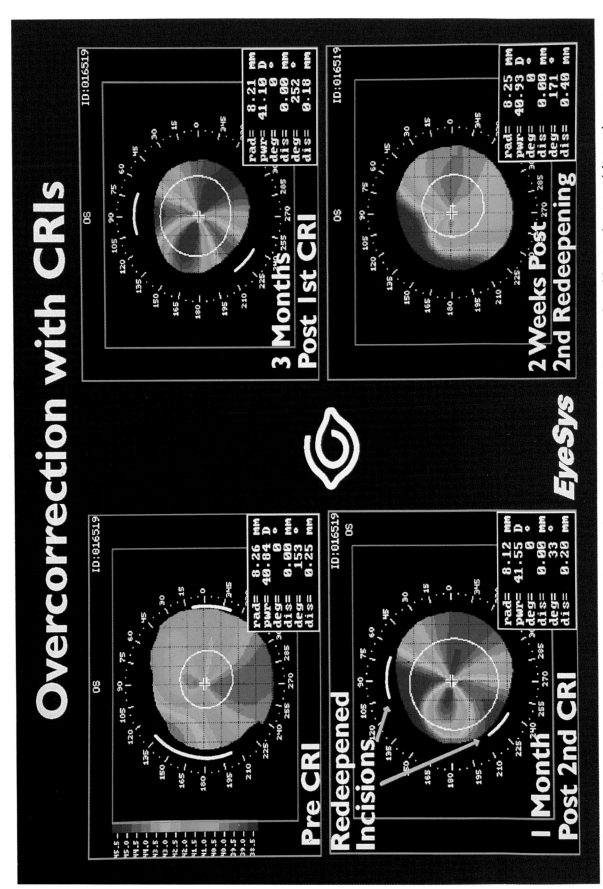

Figure 18-15. Fellow eye of patient shown in Figure 18-14. A pair of arcuate relaxing incisions made at a depth of 0.6 mm at the graft/host interface (upper left) caused severe overcorrection (upper right). Guided by the topography, an additional pair of CRIs were placed at the graft/host interface at a depth of 0.4 mm to counteract the overcorrection. The lower left image illustrates the corneal appearance following the second pair of CRIs after regression of effect had occurred. The lower right image shows the appearance after these CRIs were redeepened twice to a total depth of 0.6 mm. While there remains corneal distortion, the topography indicates a tremendous reduction of the astigmatism.

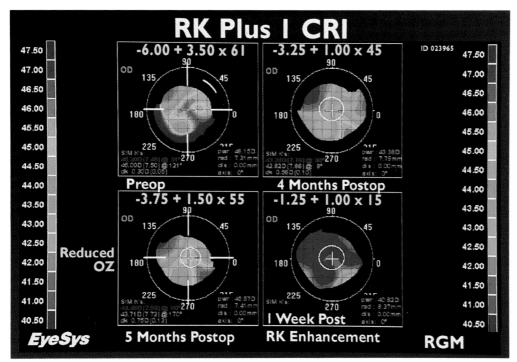

Figure 18-16. Topography of post penetrating case receiving four-incision RK at the 4.75-mm optical zone and a single CRI. Upper left shows the preoperative appearance and upper right shows the 4-month postoperative appearance, demonstrating flattening induced by the incisions. Bottom left shows the 5-month postoperative appearance. At this visit, the RK optical zone was reduced to 4.25 mm. Bottom right shows the corneal appearance 1 week following the enhancement. The cornea has been markedly flattened by the enhancement.

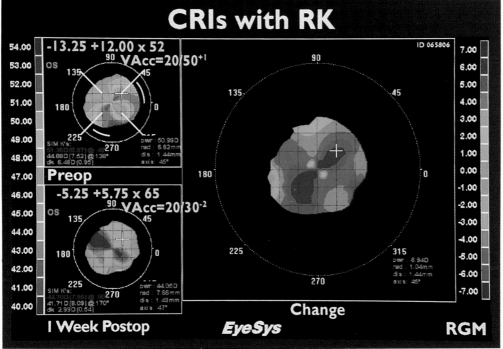

Figure 18-17. Topography of case post penetrating keratoplasty and secondary IOL implantation, and post previous astigmatic keratotomy, receiving four-incision RK and two 2.4-mm relaxing incisions. Upper left shows preoperative corneal appearance, lower left shows 3-month postoperative appearance, and right shows surgically induced changes. Topography indicates marked flattening and astigmatism reduction.

Figure 18-18. Corneal topography of a post penetrating keratoplasty case who received eight-incision RK and a superior corneal relaxing incision at the graft/host interface. There is no coupling effect seen in the change image (right) due to the presence of radials. Although there is residual steepness seen in the postoperative image (lower left), the pupillary area (white circle) is more spherical postoperatively.

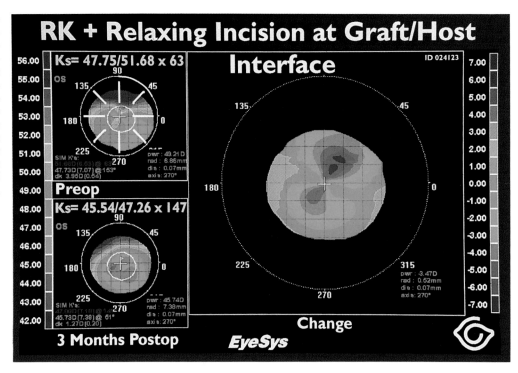

meridian of the CRI, but due to the radials there is no coupling effect, that is, no steepening 90° away. Although the postoperative image still demonstrates superior steepening, the steep region is more peripheral. Keratometry found only 1.72 D of cylinder. Final refraction is -3.00 + 0.75 x 115.

Figure 18-19 demonstrates astigmatism management using wedge resection. A 37-year-old female status post penetrating keratoplasty for keratoconus had progressively poor contact lens tolerance due to difficulty of fit and topical allergies. The pretreatment topography shows baseline astigmatism of over 9 D. Because of the excessive flattening inferotemporally, the wound was broken down in that area and resutured. At 6 months post resuturing, with 3 sutures still in place, partial return of the temporal flattening is seen, shifted superiorly. Dramatic further flattening had occurred with severely asymmetric astigmatism. The patient could not be refracted better than 20/100 and the remaining three

sutures were removed. With all sutures removed, the wound appeared normal to clinical exam. Nevertheless the best refracted acuity was 20/200 with a refraction of 7.75 -5.00 x 170.

Accordingly a wedge resection was performed. At 2 months post wedge resection, after removal of the three tightest sutures, topography demonstrates less astigmatism, although steep in the area of the wedge resection. Asymmetry was still a factor. All sutures were removed at the time because the wound appeared well scarred 2 months postoperatively. The patient returned post suture removal. Even though the wound appeared secure, and over 1 mm of corneal tissue had been resected from the wound by the wedge resection, the overall topographic pattern and values bear a striking resemblance to the topography seen prior to the wedge resection (upper right), indicating that perhaps the sutures had been removed prematurely.

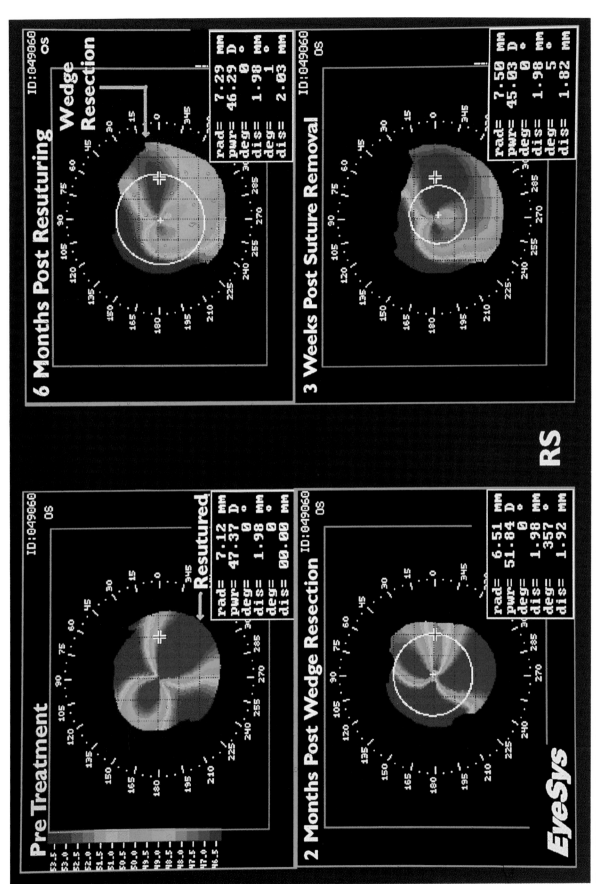

Figure 18-19. Resuturing of graft followed by wedge resection. Upper left, appearance prior to resuturing inferotemporally. Upper right, 6 months following resuturing. A wedge resection was performed temporally. Lower left, 2 months post wedge resection. All sutures were removed after this image was taken. Lower right, 3 weeks after sutures were removed, flattening has recurred in the location of the wedge resection.

SUMMARY

As the above described examples amply demonstrate, corneal topography has virtually transformed the post surgical management of refractive error in the corneal transplant case.

REFERENCES

1. Van Meter WS, Gussler JR, Soloman KD, Wood TO. Postkeratoplasty astigmatism control: single continuous suture adjustments versus selective interrupted suture removal. *Ophthalmology.* 1991;98:177-183.
2. Filatov V, Steinert RF, Talamo J. Postkeratoplasty astigmatism with single running suture or interrupted sutures. *Am J Ophthalmol.* 1993;115(6):715-21.

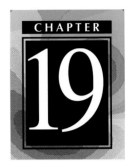

THE HOLLADAY DIAGNOSTIC SUMMARY

Jack T. Holladay, MD, FACS

The Holladay Diagnostic Summary (HDS) is intended to provide the clinician with a single report that contains all of the information about:
1. The true refractive power of the cornea at every point
2. The shape of the cornea compared to normal at every point
3. The optical quality of the cornea at every point
4. Fifteen specific corneal parameters, such as effective refractive power used in intraocular lens calculations, to quantitatively describe the cornea.

MAPS IN GENERAL

The "key" giving the value for the color "green" and the color "step" size is in the upper left or upper right corner of each map. The black mark at the center of all maps is the center of the rings. It is often referred to as vertex normal since the reflected image must be perpendicular at this point. The small white circle, usually near the black mark, is the pupil center. The medium white circle has an average diameter of 3 mm and the large white circle has an average diameter of 6 mm. The actual shape of the white perimeters is identical to the shape of the patient's actual detected pupil at the time of the photograph, ie, if the pupil is tear shaped because of a peaked pupil, all three white perimeters will be tear shaped. The 3- and 6-mm pupil perimeters are present on every map because they are helpful in explaining visual changes that may be a function of pupil size. The white reference grid is in 1-mm increments. The black numbers around the large black circle are the axis of the semi-meridian.

POWER MAPS

The "true" refractive power of the cornea at any point must be relative to the fovea along the visual axis. Power maps in the past have not used true refractive power, but instead "surface normal power." Surface normal power gives the power at any point on the cornea, assuming every ray is perpendicular to the cornea. For very small pupils (< 1 mm diameter), this approximation is true for distant objects, since the rays within this 1-mm region are almost perpendicular to the cornea. As we move beyond 1 mm from the visual axis along the cornea, we find significant errors in the "true" refractive power are made. At 5 mm the error in refractive power is approximately 6.5 D.

To determine the actual refractive power at any point on the cornea, one must apply Snell's law of refraction.[1] If the cornea were completely spherical, like a steel calibration ball, the radius of curvature would be the same at every point, but the refractive power increases as we move toward the periphery of the cornea. If a person's cornea were 7.7 mm radius at all points (average human central corneal radius), the refractive power would be 43.83 D at the center, but at 2 mm from the center the power is 44.68 D, at 3 mm 45.84 D, at 4 mm 47.64 D, and at 5 mm the refractive power would be 50.40 D. The "true" refractive power map of a spherical surface should not be a single color over the whole surface, but should show a gradual increase in power toward the periphery. This characteristic of a spherical surface gradually increasing toward the periphery is known as spherical aberration. This is why single lenses that require a clear image are aspheric, such as the indirect ophthalmoscopic viewing lens. One should always ask for a map of a spherical calibration ball to determine the accuracy of the instrument and to verify that the map demonstrates a progressive increase in power toward the periphery of approximately 6.5 D by 5 mm (Figure 19-1).

The normal human cornea is not spherical, but is aspherical to reduce spherical aberration. The normal corneal radius of curvature flattens toward the periphery by approximately 7% by 5 mm, correcting about one half of the eye's total spherical aberration. The normal cornea would therefore increase in power by approximately one half of the powers mentioned above, from 43.83 D at the center to 46.95 D at 5 mm from the center, an increase of 3.12 D. The remaining spherical aberration of the eye is corrected by the crystalline lens that is also aspheric and has a higher index of refraction in the center than at the periphery. The normal eye has very little remaining spherical aberration. If there is any remaining spherical aberration, it would result in a myopic shift in the refraction as the pupil dilates, commonly referred to as "night myopia." Approximately 10% of the population experience night myopia due to residual spherical aberration.[2] In those individuals with night myopia, the induced myopia rarely exceeds 0.50 D.

Refractive Map Standard Scale

The refractive power map on the standard scale is the map on the upper left of the HDS. The range is the same as a standard manual keratometer from 37 to 51 D, in 1 D increments. Green, the central color, is always 44 D and is the

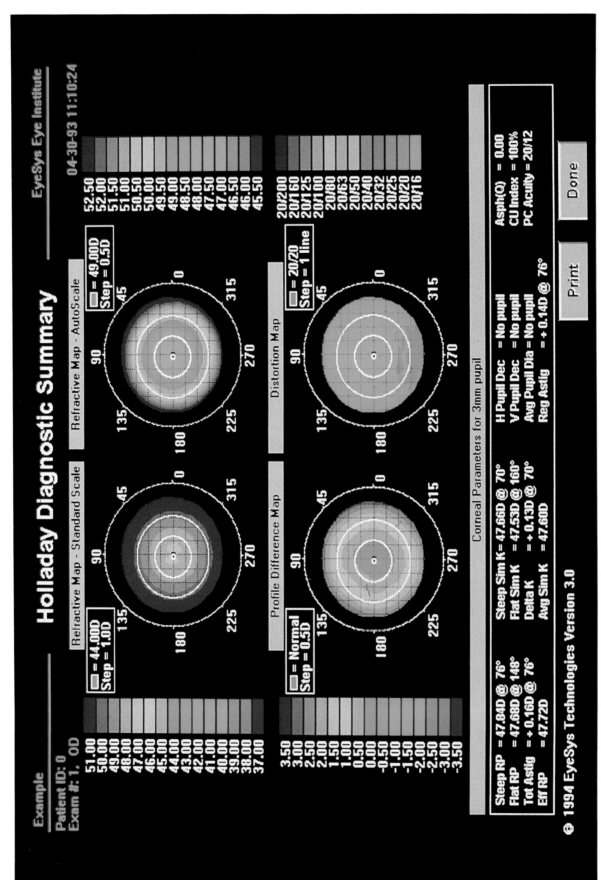

Figure 19-1. Holladay Diagnostic Summary of 47.5 D steel calibration ball.

average central corneal power of the human. Because this scale is always the same, a quick glance reveals whether the central cornea is very steep (toward red) or very flat (toward blue). The normal cornea will increase by approximately 3 D at the periphery, and should therefore change by three colors toward the red along any semi-meridian.

Refractive Map Auto Scale

The refractive power map on the auto scale is the map on the upper right of the HDS. This map displays the same data as the standard scale, but chooses the range of powers and step size to utilize the 15 colors for the best visual display. The exact value for green and the step size are shown in the key at the top of the map. The step size can be 0.25, 0.50, 1.00, or 2.00 D, whichever value best displays the data.

Profile Difference Map

The profile difference map is on the lower left of the HDS. This map compares the shape of the patient's actual cornea to the "normal" aspheric cornea. The normal aspheric cornea has an asphericity (Q) of -0.26, which means that it becomes flatter than a sphere as we move toward the periphery, sometimes referred to as a "prolate" surface since the central curvature is the steepest.[3] Using the patient's central corneal power and an asphericity of -0.26, the theoretical refractive power at every point is calculated. The actual refractive power of the patient at every point is then compared to the ideal aspheric cornea. The difference at every point is then plotted in diopters on the map. At any point, if the patient's cornea is steeper than the normal aspheric cornea, then the difference is plus and is toward the red. If the patient is flatter than the normal aspheric cornea, then the difference is negative and is toward the blue. The scale is always in step sizes of 0.50 D and the range is from -3.50 to +3.50 D. Green indicates that there is no difference between the patient's cornea and normal.

It is of interest to note that the profile difference map correlates well with the appearance of the red reflex with the retinoscope or the direct ophthalmoscope when held at approximately 66 cm (26 inches) from the eye along the visual axis. This correlation occurs because the shadows seen in the retinoscopic reflex, such as with keratoconus, are due to irregular astigmatism that cannot be completely neutralized with a spherocylindric refraction. Patterns seen with the retinoscope such as scissoring, radial astigmatism, and spherical aberration will appear the same on the profile difference map. This map is especially helpful in the diagnosis of corneal diseases in which the cornea changes its overall shape, such as with keratoconus, keratoglobus, and pellucid marginal degeneration.

Distortion Map

The distortion map shows the optical quality of the cornea at every point. The distortion is mapped using traditional Snellen lines of visual acuity ranging from blue (20/16) to red (20/200). Green is 20/20. The map assumes the best spherocylindric correction is in place, grades the optical distortion in Snellen equivalents, then plots the appropriate color at every point. This map is very helpful in correlating visual performance and optical irregularities in the cornea. For example, in anterior membrane dystrophy, the refractive power maps and the profile map may be completely normal, but the distortion map usually shows many areas of optical irregularity documenting the reason for poor vision. Serial maps at different times of the day or over several days can document the fluctuation in optical quality of the cornea, and consequently, the fluctuation in vision. It should be noted that optical distortions of the cornea outside the 3-mm pupil zone should have very little effect on visual performance, except when the pupil is dilated.

CORNEAL PARAMETERS FOR 3-MM PUPIL

There are four columns of corneal parameters at the bottom of the HDS. These values are helpful when quantitative parameters are necessary to describe the cornea, such as with intraocular lens calculations and keratorefractive procedures. A description of each of these parameters and its usefulness to the clinician is given.

Column 1: Refractive Power Measurements

The steep refractive power (steep RP) is the strongest refractive power in any single meridian of the cornea. The refractive power is given in diopters followed by the axis of the meridian. The system uses all points within the 3-mm pupil zone to find the meridian with the strongest refractive power, not just the values along the 3-mm perimeter. The flat refractive power (flat RP) is the weakest refractive power in any single meridian of the cornea. Note that these two meridians are not necessarily 90° apart. If they are not 90° apart, then there is oblique irregular astigmatism present. This occurrence cannot be fully corrected with spherocylindric lenses. The difference between the steep RP and the flat RP is the total astigmatism, given in plus cylinder and therefore referenced at the steep RP. The effective refractive power (Eff RP) is the refractive power of the corneal surface within the 3-mm pupil zone. This value is commonly known as the spheroequivalent power of the cornea within the 3-mm pupil zone. This value should be used for the power of the cornea in intraocular lens calculations as well as keratorefractive procedures. It is especially helpful in corneas with irregular astigmatism, such as keratoconus, penetrating keratoplasties, and corneas that have undergone keratorefractive procedures. The most common example today is in patients who have had radial keratotomy (RK) and have now developed a cataract.

Column 2: Simulated Keratometry Measurements

The simulated keratometry measurements are primarily for historical reference and comparison with the standard manual keratometer. The standard keratometer measures two points, approximately 3.2 mm apart, to determine the power of the cornea in that meridian. The instrument is then rotated 90° and the procedure repeated. In short, the keratometer measures four points to determine the flattest and steepest meridians of the cornea. In a normal cornea four sample points are usually enough to yield accurate values of the central corneal power. In irregular corneas (RK, PKP, PRK, and corneal scars), the four samples are usually not sufficient to provide an accurate estimate of the central corneal refractive power, especially true of RK corneas with small optical zones (3.0 mm or less), where the four points measured by the standard keratometer are at a transition zone of the cornea that requires many more than four points to describe the changes in refractive power accurately. The greater the differences in the refractive power measurements in column 1 and the simulated keratometry in column 2, the greater the degree of irregular astigmatism, and the greater the need to use the refractive power measurements (Eff RP) for any quantitative calculations.

The steep simulated K-reading (Steep Sim K) is the steepest meridian of the cornea using only the points along the 3-mm pupillary perimeter, not the entire zone. The flat simulated K-reading (Flat Sim K) is the flattest meridian of the cornea using only the points along the 3-mm pupillary perimeter. As with the standard keratometer, these two meridians are forced to be 90° apart. Delta K is the difference between the Steep Sim K and the Flat Sim K given in diopters at the axis of the Steep Sim K. The Avg Sim K is the average of all of the simulated K's within the 3-mm pupil zone. The discrepancy between the Eff RP and the Avg Sim K is another measure of the degree of irregular astigmatism. Although the Eff RP should always give a more reliable value for the corneal power than the Avg Sim K, the discrepancy indicates that one should expect a higher degree of variability in the results of an intraocular lens calculation than with a normal cornea.

Column 3: Pupil Parameters and Regular Astigmatism

The system detects the perimeter of the pupil at the time of the photograph, then calculates the centroid of the pupil. A

very small white perimeter (0.2-mm diameter) is shown, the same shape as the original pupil, at the centroid of the pupil. A medium white perimeter is shown with an area equal to that of a circle with a 3-mm diameter, and a large white perimeter with an area equal to that of a circle with a 6-mm diameter. The exact shape of these larger perimeters is also the same as the original pupil perimeter at the time of the photograph. Note: if no pupil is detected by the system, a small (0.2-mm diameter), medium (3-mm diameter), and large (6-mm diameter) circle are shown and centered at the nominal decentration of 0.2 mm out (temporal) from the center of the map. "No pupil" will be reported when this situation occurs. When a pupil is detected, the relationship of the centroid of the pupil to the center of the map (black mark) is then determined. The horizontal pupil decentration (H Pupil Dec) is the horizontal distance in mm from the center of the map to the centroid of the pupil, where "out" (temporal) means the pupil is out with respect to the center of the map and "in" (nasal) means the pupil is in with respect to the center of the map. This value is commonly referred to clinically as angle kappa, and is nominally approximately 0.2 mm out in the human.

The vertical pupil decentration (V Pupil Dec) is the vertical distance in mm from the center of the map to the centroid of the pupil, where "up" (superior) means the pupil is up with respect to the center of the map and "down" (inferior) means the pupil is down with respect to the center of the map. The nominal value for the human is almost zero.

The Average Pupil Diameter (Avg Pupil Dia) is the average diameter of the pupil at the time of the photograph. Since the photograph is taken under bright light conditions, without dilation, the pupil diameter is usually less than 3.0 mm.

Regular Astigmatism (Reg Astig) is the amount and axis of astigmatism that can be neutralized with a spherocylindric correction. This cylinder and axis are very helpful in refracting patients with irregular corneas. The program finds the best fit power and axis of the cylinder that best corrects the irregularity. The Reg Astig often provides a good starting point for refraction, and sometimes eliminates the need for refinements with time consuming crossed-cylinder refraction techniques, particularly in patients where the endpoint is ambiguous. The Reg Astig will always be less than or equal to the Tot Astig, because the Tot Astig also includes irregular astigmatism, not just regular astigmatism. The disparity in the two values is therefore a measure of the degree of irregular astigmatism.

Column 4: Miscellaneous Measurements

As mentioned previously, most investigators use the Asphericity (Q) in the conic equation to describe the corneal aspbericity.[3] The normal value for asphericity (Q) is -0.26, indicating that the normal human cornea flattens by about 7% in its radius of curvature compared to a sphere at a distance of 5 mm from the center. The asphericity for a sphere would be 0.00 and, if the patient's cornea flattens more than the normal asphericity, then the magnitude of the asphericity would exceed -0.26. For example, an asphericity of -0.50 almost completely eliminates any contribution of spherical aberration from the cornea.

The Corneal Uniformity Index (CU Index) is a measure of the uniformity of the distortion of the cornea within the 3-mm pupil expressed as a percentage. A CU Index of 100% indicates that the optical quality of the cornea is almost perfectly uniform over the 3-mm pupil, which does not indicate that the cornea has good optical quality, simply that it is uniform. It could be uniformly bad or good. A CU Index of 0% indicates that the optical quality of the cornea is very non-uniform over the 3-mm pupil. For example, a patient with diffuse microcystic edema from elevated intraocular pressure would be expected to have reduced vision, but from a uniform poor optical quality of the cornea. In contrast, a person with localized areas of bullous keratopathy would be expected to have reduced vision, but from a non-uniform poor optical quality of the cornea. The CU Index is therefore useful in the differential diagnosis of corneal pathology where generalized or localized characteristic patterns are present. Normal values usually exceed 80%.

The Predicted Corneal Acuity (PC Acuity) provides a single value in units of Snellen Acuity of the optical quality of the cornea within the 3-mm zone. The PC Acuity estimates the predicted acuity if the cornea is the limiting factor in the visual system. The PC acuity can be very helpful in differentiating corneal from lenticular disease. For example, in a patient with a best-corrected visual acuity of 20/60 who has anterior membrane dystrophy and a nuclear sclerotic cataract, it is often difficult to determine whether the cornea or the cataract is the major factor in the reduced vision. If the PC Acuity is 20/25, then clearly the cornea is not significantly reducing the vision, and cataract extraction is indicated and expected to improve the vision. If the PC Acuity were 20/60, however, then removal of the cataract would not be expected to significantly improve the vision.

Together, the CU Index and the PC Acuity are very helpful in characterizing corneal abnormalities and monitoring changes over time. These values should correlate visually with the appearance of the central 3-mm zone on the distortion map, but the program takes into account other parameters, such as the Stiles-Crawford effect, which makes visual estimation only approximate.

CLINICAL EXAMPLES

Steel Calibration Ball

The calibration ball is chosen as the first example (Figure 19-2), because it best illustrates many of the topics we have discussed as well as tests the accuracy of the system on a known surface.

Refractive Map Standard Scale: The central 3 mm is blue-green, indicating that the refractive power of the central cornea is slightly less than average. The central area is circular and the rings are concentric, indicating a spherical surface. The refractive power increases toward the periphery by 5 color steps, or 5 D, which is approximately 4.7 mm from the center as determined on the 1 mm white grid. There is no pupil on the calibration ball, so the program creates 0.1-, 3.0-, and 6.0-mm circles located 0.2 mm OUT (temporal) to the center on the map.

Refractive Map Auto Scale: This map shows the same data as above, but with more detail because the color scale has been chosen to best utilize the 15 colors. The program chose green to be 43.50 D and a color step size of 0.50 D. The change in power toward the periphery can be seen in greater detail.

Profile Difference Map: This surface is not like the normal aspheric cornea, but increases in power toward the periphery to +2.50 D more than the normal. This map indicates that the 42.50 D calibration ball has much more power in the periphery than the normal cornea. The term for this change is called spherical aberration, and simply indicates that this surface is more like a sphere than the normal aspheric cornea. A patient with this map may be expected to experience night myopia, due to this significant spherical aberration.

Distortion Map: The optical quality of this surface is almost perfect because it is almost completely blue (20/16). This map therefore represents the ideal optical quality of the cornea.

Corneal Parameters for 3-mm Pupil: The steel calibration ball can be used to test the accuracy of the system. The Effective Refractive Power (Eff RP) is 42.53 D with a total astigmatism (Tot Astig) of 0.10 D at 72.° The exact values should be 42.50 D and 0.00 D of total astigmatism. We can see from the Profile Difference Map that the differences have occurred because the ball was not perfectly centered when the photograph was taken; the ball was slightly decentered approximately 0.2 mm toward 72.° The Simulated Keratometry is very similar, but notice that the axis of the Delta K (40°) and Tot Astig are not the same, and the Average Simulated K (Avg Sim K = 42.44) and Eff RP are different. The axis is different because the astigmatism is so small that

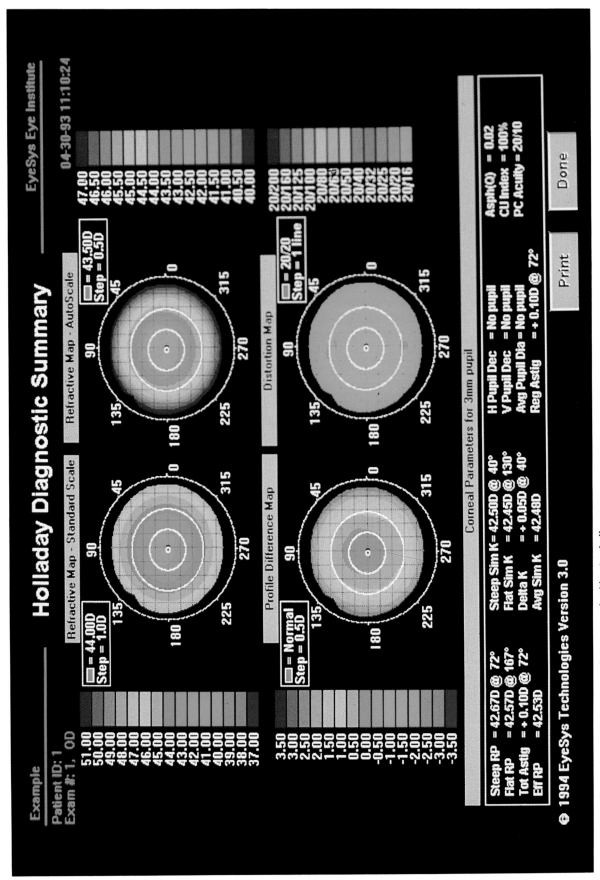

Figure 19-2. Holladay Diagnostic Summary of 42.5 D steel calibration ball.

with only four samples the keratometric values are 32° off. The 0.05 D of greater power with the Effective Refractive Power is real and is due to the correct use of Snell's law for the Eff RP.

"No pupil" was detected on the ball, so the 0.2-, 3.0-, and 6.0-mm diameter circles are displayed on the maps and centered at 0.2 mm OUT (temporally). The Reg Astig is virtually the same as the Total Astigmatism, indicating that there is no irregular astigmatism from the steel ball. The Asphericity (Q) is 0.00, indicating this surface is a sphere. The CU Index is 100%, indicating the surface is perfectly uniform, and the PC Acuity is 20/16, indicating that the surface has a perfect optical quality within the 3-mm pupillary zone.

Regular Astigmatic Cornea

Figure 19-3 shows an exam from the left eye of a 30-year-old female with no ocular pathology. Her best-corrected visual acuity is 20/16 with -3.00 + 3.25 X 90° in her left eye. She has never worn contact lenses and has no history of corneal problems.

Refractive Map Standard Scale: The horizontal meridian is green, indicating normal corneal power, but the vertical meridian is steeper than normal, indicating there is with-the-rule astigmatism. The pattern is very symmetrical and is often referred to as a "symmetrical bowtie."

Refractive Map Auto Scale: The auto scale has increased the color of green to 45.50 D and changed the color step size to 0.50 D to show more detail. The bowtie is still very symmetrical, indicating regular astigmatism.

Profile Difference Map: The inferior semi-meridian follows the exact asphericity of the normal cornea and is within + 0.50 D to the left (nasal). The right side (temporal) of the cornea appears to gradually increase in power by approximately + 1.50 D by 5 mm. The superior semi-meridian appears to be increasing like the temporal cornea, but the upper lid has blocked our view beyond 3.2 mm. These individual variations among the four quadrants are not unusual beyond the 3.0-mm pupil zone. Within the 6-mm pupil zone there is only 0.50 D of variation, indicating that these variations should have very little effect on the quality of vision even when the pupil is moderately dilated.

Distortion Map: The optical quality of the cornea is excellent, with no distortions within the 3-mm pupil and only a few small irregularities in the horizontal meridian within the 6-mm zone. The distortion seen on the right side (temporally) at 3:00 should have no effect on the vision, because it is almost 4.5 mm from the pupil center.

Corneal Parameters for 3-mm Pupil: The Steep RP is 46.26 D at 91° and the Flat RP is 42.97 diopters at 1,° with a

Tot Astig of + 3.31 D at 91.° Notice that the two principal meridians are 90° apart, indicating regular astigmatism. Remember, the Steep RP and Flat RP are not forced to be perpendicular. The Eff RP is 44.67 D, which is the effective refractive power of the cornea within the 3-mm zone. Notice that this value is not exactly equal to the average (44.62 D) of the Steep RP and the Flat RP. This difference of 0.05 D is very slight because the cornea is normal. If the cornea is abnormal, the difference can be much greater. The Simulated Keratometry values in column 2 are quite similar to the Refractive Powers, because this is a normal cornea. Notice, however, that the axis of the Delta K is 84,° 7° away from the actual axis of corneal astigmatism. This error occurs because the simulated K values only look along the 3-mm perimeter, as does the standard keratometer.

In column 3 we see that the pupil is 0.06 mm IN and 0.07 mm DOWN, with respect to the center of the map, and the pupil has an average diameter of 2.57 mm at the time of the exam. The Reg Astig is + 3.28 D at 91,° which agrees almost exactly with the refraction, indicating that all of the patient's astigmatism is corneal and there is no significant lenticular component. The Asph (Q) is -0.04, which should be expected from the appearance of the Profile Difference Map, because of the increase in power as we moved toward the periphery in three of the four quadrants. The patient is nearer the asphericity of a steel ball (Q = 0.00) than the normal corneal asphericity (Q = -0.26). The CU Index is 100%, which can be seen from the distortion map where the central 3 mm is completely uniform with no distortions. The PC Acuity is 20/10, indicating that the central 3 mm of the cornea has a perfect optical quality.

Keratoconus Cornea

Figure 19-4 shows a 26-year-old male with progressively decreased best-corrected visual acuity with spectacles over the past 8 years in his left eye. His current spectacle prescription is -8.25 + 4.25 X 40 with a visual acuity of 20/80. He has never worn contact lenses.

Refractive Map Standard Scale: The map is very irregular with an extremely steep area that exceeds 51 D in the lower right quadrant (inferotemporally). There is a significant variation in refractive power within the 3-mm pupil zone (blue to red), indicating that this localized steep area should affect the vision.

Refractive Map Auto Scale: On the auto scale map, the program has chosen the green color to be 48 D to better utilize the 15 colors, while the step size remains at 1 D. The peak of the cone can be more accurately located on the new scale between the 3-mm and 6-mm pupil zone at 5:00. The more sensitive scale confirms the significant variation in

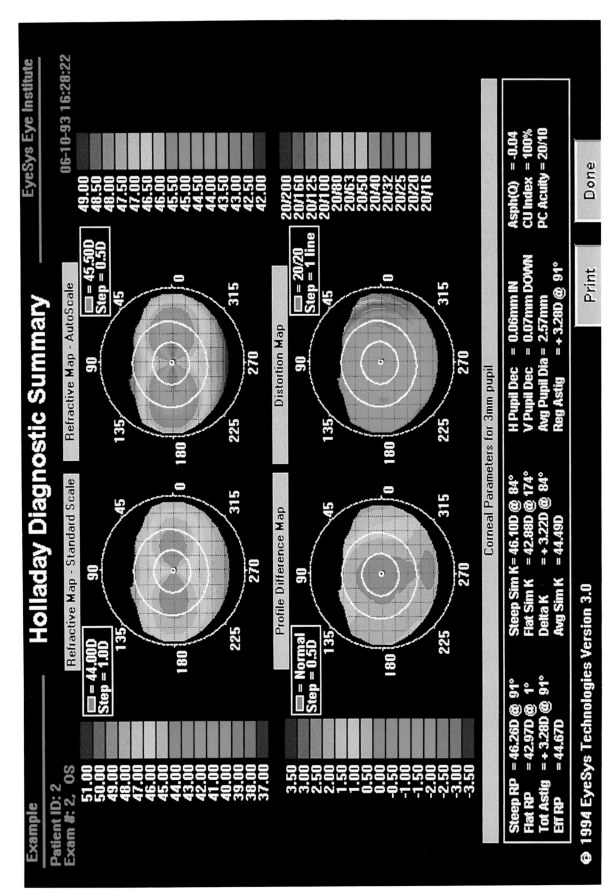

Figure 19-3. Holladay Diagnostic Summary of a regular astigmatic cornea.

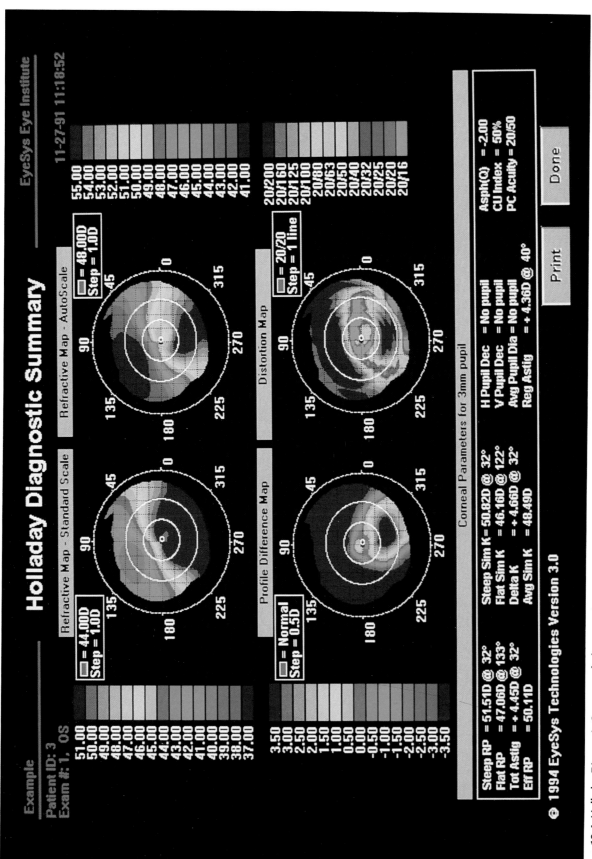

Figure 19-4. Holladay Diagnostic Summary of a keratoconic cornea.

refractive power within the 3-mm pupil zone.

Profile Difference Map: This map delineates the cone most accurately, and as previously mentioned appears very similar to the red reflex seen with retinoscopy near neutralization. The exact peak of the cone can easily be seen. Note that a 7.5-mm corneal trephine would completely encompass the cone. The "sea" of dark blue in the other three quadrants simply means that these regions are far too flat for a nominal central corneal refractive power of 50.11 D (Eff RP).

Distortion Map: The distortion map may at first seem somewhat surprising, because there are many areas of distortion in addition to the area of the cone. It must be remembered that the program and the patient will try to find the best spherocylindrical correction for the 3-mm pupil zone. Within the 3-mm zone we see distortions that range from 20/16 to 20/200, once again, indicating a significant detrimental effect on vision. The area on the cone is very distorted with the entire area appearing red. The distorted areas on the superior cornea are a result of the power being so much lower than the central area, by almost 9 D. This area would be 9 D out of focus when the central 3 mm is in focus, resulting in poor overall optical quality.

Corneal Parameters for 3-mm Pupil: The Steep RP is 51.51 D at 32° and the Flat RP is 47.06 D at 133,° with a Tot Astig of +4.45 D at 32.° Notice that the steep and flat meridians are 101° apart, not 90,° indicating the presence of irregular astigmatism of oblique axes. This finding is not unusual for keratoconus, corneal scars, and other corneal pathology that create a radial asymmetry of the cornea. The Eff RP is 50.11 D, which is 6 D steeper than normal. It would be suspected that a large degree of the patient's myopia is due to the excess corneal power and not due to increased axial length of the eye. The simulated keratometry is up to 1 D different from the refractive power measurements, due to the limitation of four samples along the 3-mm pupil perimeter. In this patient the error in standard keratometry is relatively small, but in other patients the difference can be much greater, depending on the exact characteristics of the cornea.

There was "no pupil" detected in this patient, so the default 0.2-, 3-, and 6-mm diameter circles are shown. The Reg Astig is +4.36 D at 40,° which is less than the Tot Astig, and at a different axis. This difference indicates there is irregular astigmatism present, and the best spherocylindric correction for this surface is not at the axis of the steepest meridian (Steep RP), but 8° away at 40.° Placing the nearest available cylinder of +4.25 D at 40° in the trial frame, then performing a spherical refraction, is much simpler than dealing with crossed-cylinders and less frustrating to the patient, since the endpoints are never clear. The Reg Astig is very close to the actual refraction, so we know there is very

little lenticular astigmatism. The Asph(Q) is -2.00, which indicates that the cornea flattens much too rapidly in the periphery, relative to the central zone, which should be expected from our discussion of the Profile Difference Map.

The CU Index is 50%, revealing a very non-uniform cornea, with a PC Acuity of 20/50, which correlates very well with the patient's actual vision of 20/60 in this eye. These parameters indicate a severe, non-uniformly distorted cornea within the central 3-mm zone that can account for the poor vision of 20/60.

8-mm PKP with Two Sutures Remaining

Figure 19-5 shows a 72-year-old male 1 year post penetrating keratoplasty in his right eye for pseudophakic bullous keratopathy. The patient has two remaining sutures at 4:00 and 11:00, and his refraction is +1.00 + 1.00 X 150° with which he sees 20/40. There is a history of cystoid macular edema with a retinal acuity of 20/30 using the PAM (potential acuity meter). His best-corrected vision with a trial hard contact lens is also 20/40.

Refractive Map Standard Scale: The central color is mostly light blue indicating that the central refractive power of the cornea is approximately 2 D flatter than normal or about 42 D. The large dark blue area to the right of the 6-mm zone is an artifact from a missing ring that should have been edited out on the ring eye picture. We will therefore ignore this region on all of the maps.

Refractive Map Auto Scale: The auto scale has chosen 42 D for green. The 3-mm and 6-mm central pupil zones are very consistent in power showing at most 1 D of variation near 4:00 between the 3-mm and 6-mm rings.

Profile Difference Map: The profile difference is zero everywhere except for the right (nasal) 3:00 region between the 3-mm and 6-mm rings, where it is approximately 1 D steeper than the normal aspheric cornea. Notice, the entire 3-mm zone is almost perfect.

Distortion Map: The central 3-mm pupil zone indicates excellent optical quality (almost completely blue), with yellow distortions appearing at 4:00 and 11:00, corresponding to the location of the remaining sutures. The red ring corresponds to the graft-host junction that is 8.0 mm in diameter. Although these sutures are causing distortion outside the 3-mm pupil zone, they are also holding the cornea in an almost spherical shape. The patient may experience some decreased vision when the pupil dilates at night due to the sutures, but removing them may induce a significant amount of astigmatism. The amount of astigmatism induced by their removal can only be judged clinically at the slit lamp by the tension of the suture and by estimating the amount of compressed tissue. In this patient the sutures were very tight

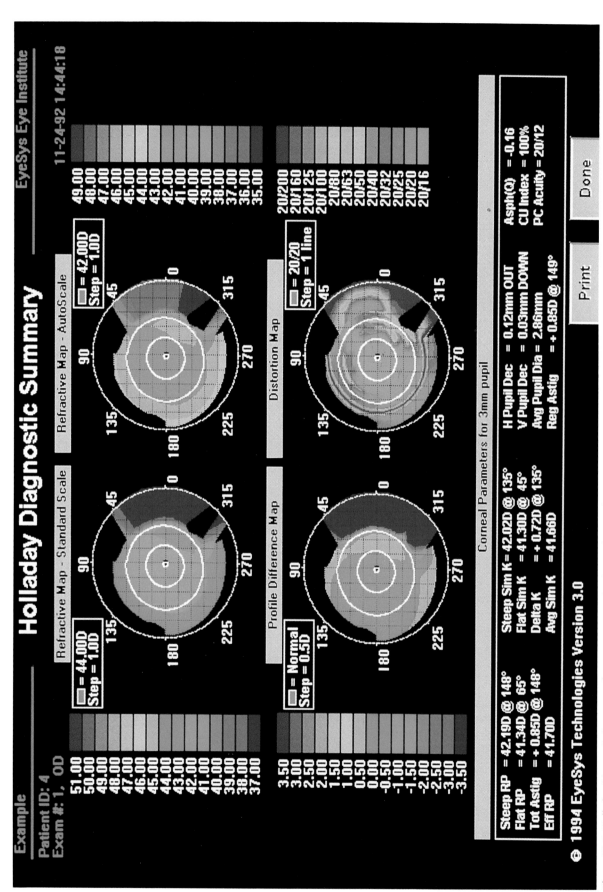

Figure 19-5. Holladay Diagnostic Summary of an 8-mm penetrating keratoplasty with sutures remaining at 4:00 and 11:00.

and therefore were not removed.

Corneal Parameters for 3-mm Pupil: The Steep RP is 42.19 D and the Flat RP is 41.34 D at 65,° with a Tot Astig of +0.85 D at 148.° Notice that these two meridians are not perpendicular, but are only 83° apart, indicating a small degree of irregular astigmatism of oblique axes. This would not be expected to affect the vision, however, because the magnitude of the Tot Astig is only 0.85 D and is virtually the same as the Reg Astig of +0.85 D at 149.° The magnitude of the Simulated K's is very close to the values of the refractive power, but the axes are from 13° to 20° different due to the few sample points with the standard keratometer. The Eff RP is 41.70 D.

The H Pupil Dec is 0.12 mm OUT (temporal) and V Pupil Dec is 0.03 DOWN (inferior), with an Avg Pupil Dia of 2.86 mm at the time of the exam. The pupil shows no irregularities and the location is normal. The Asph(Q) is -0.16, which is almost exactly the average human value, which we expected from the completely central green color of the Profile Difference Map. The CU Index is 100% and the PC Acuity is 20/16 as we suspected from the Distortion Map that revealed a completely uniform blue color within the 3-mm pupillary zone. The patient's vision, however, was only 20/40 with refraction much less than the PC Acuity. This finding indicates that the cornea is not the limiting factor in the patient's vision; it is the macula. This is also confirmed by the PAM and a trial hard contact lens. The trial hard contact lens is usually more reliable in these patients with a history of cystoid macular edema, because the PAM sometimes overestimates the potential retinal acuity.

Radial Keratotomy Cornea

Figure 19-6 is of a 26-year-old female, 1 day after an eight-incision, 3-mm optical zone RK in the left eye. The vision was corrected to 20/20 with a correction of -2.50 +4.00 X 98°. Although corneal topography was not done preoperatively, it was noted that the preoperative K-readings were much steeper than normal, 49.25 D at 5° X 49.75 D at 95° with a preoperative refraction of -4.50 sphere. It was determined in retrospect that the patient may have been a forme fruste of keratoconus that was undetected and resulted in an abnormal response to the RK and consequently a large degree of induced astigmatism.

Refractive Map Standard Scale: This map reveals over 4 D of symmetrical with-the-rule astigmatism, with the vertical meridian being much steeper than normal.

Refractive Map Auto Scale: The auto scale increases the green to 46.50 D and reduces the step size to 0.50 D revealing a mild asymmetry in the bowtie.

Profile Difference Map: The curvatures in all directions

outside the central 2 mm are progressively steeper than normal, indicating the peripheral cornea is much steeper than average for the central power, which is to be expected in keratorefractive procedures for myopia, since the optical zone becomes flatter with respect to the periphery. The center is always chosen as the reference, since this area is most important to vision. The irregular contour of the green area indicates that the cornea is not a normal shape.

Distortion Map: The central 3-mm pupil zone is mostly blue with a few areas of green, indicating that the patient's vision with a 3-mm or smaller pupil should be very good. The eight radial yellow distortions correspond to the eight RK incisions. These distortions are dramatically enhanced because it is only 1 day following the surgery. There could be a great deal of variation if serial photographs were taken, since the incisions have not been fully epithelialized and the tear film is highly variable.

Corneal Parameters for 3-mm pupil: The Steep RP is 47.75 D at 97° and the Flat RP is 43.37 D at 11,° with a Tot Astig of +4.38 D at 97.° The Eff RP is 45.60 D, much steeper than the average corneal power following RK (37-40). However, compared to the preoperative K's, the EFF RP is approximately 4 D less, which corresponds to the change in the spheroequivalent of the refraction. The Simulated Keratometry measurements were from 4° to 8° off in the axes, but very close to the refractive power values. In these types of cases the standard keratometry can be quite variable, and differ by several diopters. The Reg Astig is +4.37 at 98° which is very close to the magnitude and axis of the postoperative refractive cylinder, indicating that the astigmatism is all corneal.

The Asph(Q) is +0.20, indicating that within the 3-mm zone, the cornea steepens more rapidly than the normal cornea. Remember that it is only 1 day after the surgery and there is probably some corneal edema still present. The CU Index is 90% and the PC Acuity is 20/20, indicating that the central 3-mm zone is of good optical quality with very little distortion. Notice the values are not 100% and 20/16 like our perfect steel ball in Figure 19-2 or the patient with regular astigmatism in Figure 19-3. This patient's cornea is less than perfect, but the cornea is still able to achieve 20/20 vision. It may, however, be the limiting factor in the visual acuity.

Excimer PRK Cornea

Figure 19-7 shows a 24-year-old female who had an excimer laser PRK with a 4.5-mm optical zone in her right eye 6 months ago. She is correctable to 20/16 with a -0.25 + 0.75 X 100. She did mention that she had noticed some glare or "ghosting" around headlights at night, but said that it did not cause much of a problem.

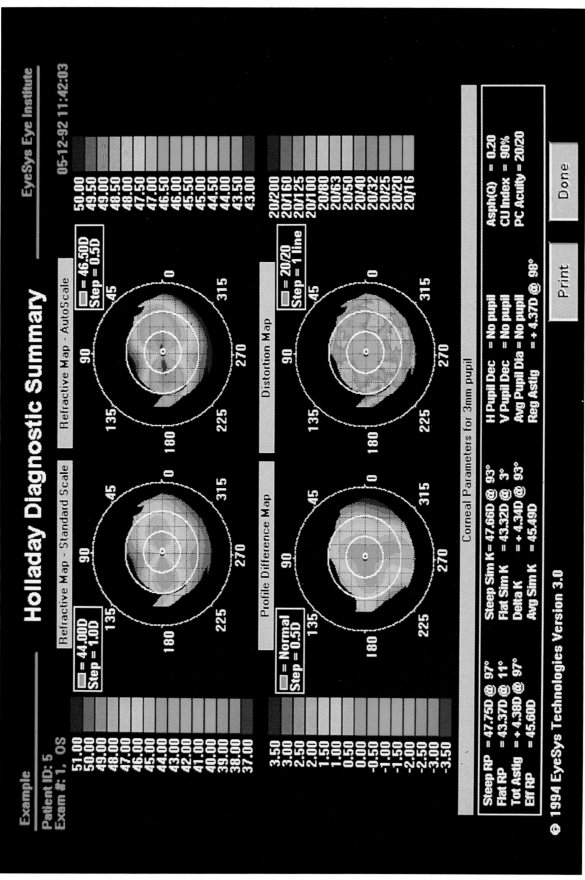

Figure 19-6. Holladay Diagnostic Summary of a cornea 1 day post eight-incision RK.

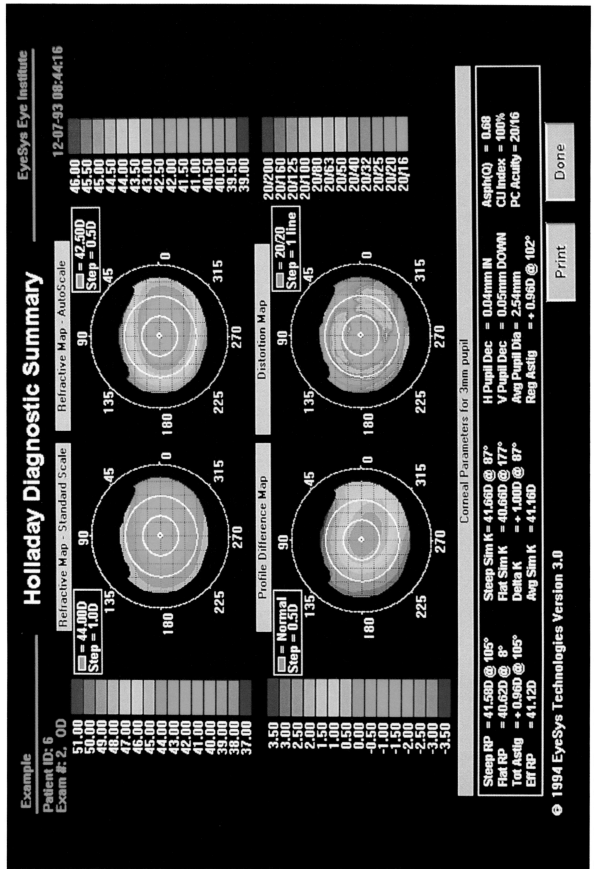

Figure 19-7. Holladay Diagnostic Summary of a cornea 6 months post-PRK.

Refractive Map Standard Scale: The central zone is uniformly light blue, indicating the central cornea is 3 D flatter than normal, with almost no astigmatism present.

Refractive Map Auto Scale: The auto scale has chosen green as 42.50 D and a step size of 0.5 D. On this scale we see that there is a "sea" of light blue that is horizontally oval and not concentric with the pupil, but slightly displaced to the right (nasally).

Profile Difference Map: The central green area is also oval, due to elongation at 4:00. The central green area is also not concentric with the pupil. The cornea progressively increases in power peripherally, by four colors, demonstrating that this cornea is much steeper in the periphery than normal for this central power.

Distortion Map: The central 3-mm pupillary zone is very good with a few areas of green. The arcs of yellow between the 3-mm and 6-mm pupillary zone correspond to the edge of the ablated 4.6-mm optical zone. Once again we see that this optical zone is not concentric with respect to the pupil.

Corneal Parameters for 3-mm Pupil: The Steep RP is 41.58 D at 105° and the Flat RP is 40.62 D at 8,° with a Tot Astig of +0.96 D at 18°. The Eff RP is 41.12 D, approximately 3 D flatter than normal. The Reg Astig is +0.96 D at 102°, which is almost identical to the Tot Astig, indicating there is no irregular astigmatism. The Simulated Keratometry varies from 11° to 18° from the Refractive Power axes, but is very close to the powers. The difference is small because the 4.5-mm zone of the ablation is outside the 3.2-mm perimeter sampled by the standard keratometer. The pupil is almost concentric with the map, having a H Pupil Dec of 0.04 mm IN (nasal) and V Pupil Dec of 0.05 mm DOWN (inferior), and an Avg Pupil Dia of 2.54 mm at the time of the photograph. The Asph(Q) is +0.68, indicating the central 3-mm zone of the cornea is steepening more than a spherical ball. This asphericity would be expected following PRK because the paracentral region is far too steep for the central power. The CU Index is 100% and the PC Acuity is 20/16, indicating a uniform central 3-mm zone with excellent optical quality, but not quite perfect.

The ghosting of headlights at night is most likely due to the edge of the 4.5-mm optical zone that can be seen on the Distortion Map. The fact that the optical zone is slightly decentered to the right (nasally) may also be a complicating factor.

REFERENCES

1. Michaels DD. *Visual Optics and Refraction A Clinical Approach.* 3rd ed. St. Louis, MO: CV Mosby; 1985.
2. Holladay JT, Lynn M, Waring GO, et al. The relationship of visual acuity, refractive error and pupil size following radial keratotomy. *Archives of Ophthalmology.* 1991;109:70-76.
3. Atchison DA. Optical design of introcular lenses. I. On-axis performance. *Optometry and Vision Science.* 1989;66(8):492-506.

Index

alignment, videokeratograph, 17-23, 18-20
  corneal apex, relationship to, 21-22
  error, measurement of, 20
  refractive surgery, relation to, 22-23
  repeatability, 21
astigmatism
  asymmetrical, 26-28
  keratotomy, 26-33
    cataract surgery, 215-222
      after, 199-202
      screening, 215
      topographical results, 215-221
    corneal topography, 199-202
    penetrating keratoplasty, after, 202
  symmetrical, 26

cataract surgery
  with astigmatic keratotomy, 215-222
    screening, 215
    topographical results, 215-221
  corneal topography, 172-192
    combined procedures, evaluating, 179-183
    incision size/sutureless surgery, effect of, 173-175
    sutures, effect of, 172-173
    wound
      construction/location—clear-corneal incisions, effect of, 175-179
      management techniques, evaluating, 179
central islands, excimer laser procedures, 255
clinical applications, 157-323
computerized videokeratography, 9
  applications of, 10-13
  Placido-based device, 9
contact lens fitting display, EyeMap EH-270, 41
cornea
  analysis system, EyeSys 2000, 55-75
  multifocal, 225-239
  relaxing incisions, 225-239
  topography
    engineering, history of, 90-95
    in evaluation of corneal transplant patient, 288-306
    excimer procedures, 242-260

healing patterns, 245-255
EyeMap EH-270, 37-52
  telocentric method, 47
image accuracy, 13
keratometric measurement, astigmatism, 26-33
lamellar refractive surgery, 263-284
  automated lamellar keratoplasty, or in situ keratomileusis for hyperopia, 271-279
  in situ photorefractive keratomileusis, 280
normal, 10-13
overview, 3-15
pathology
  characterization of, 159-169
  detection of, 159-169
qualitative measurement of, 6-13
in refractive surgical procedures, 195-212
  astigmatic keratotomy, 199-202
    post cataract surgery, 199-202
    post penetrating keratoplasty, 202
  epikeratophakia, 203-208
  hexagonal keratotomy, 208
  radial keratotomy, 195-199
  refractive surgery enhancements, 202-203
transplant patient, evaluation of corneal topography, 288-306
  refractive surgeries, post penetrating keratoplasty, evaluation of, 299-305
  relaxing incisions, 288-299
  suture
    removal, selective, 288
    rotation, 288
curvature, cornea, normal, 4-6

dioptric plot
  comparative, EyeMap EH-270, 41
  EyeMap EH-270, 38
  with side-by-side image plot, EyeMap EH-270, 40

epikeratophakia, corneal topography, 203-208
excimer laser procedures, 241-261
  centering of, 241-242
  central islands, 255

corneal topography, 242-260
  healing patterns, 245-255
multi-zone ablations for high myopia, 255
PARK, for correction of astigmatism, 255-260
topography maps, centration of, 241-242
EyeMap EH-270
  case examples, 46
  clinical applications, 46-47
  comparative dioptric plot, 41
  contact lens fitting display, 41
  corneal topography, telocentric method, 47
  difference plot, 41
  dioptric plot, 38
    with side-by-side image plot, 40
  measurement, 46-51
  meridional contour, 41
  method of analysis, 47-48
  three-dimensional display, 40-41
  video displays, 38-45
EyeSys 2000 corneal analysis system, 55-75, 63, 74
  absolute scale, high resolution, 58
  accuracy, 62-63
  affordability, 63-69
  artifact detection/correction, 63
  autocorrection, 63
  auto-focus, 63
  backup, database, 69
  calibration, automatic, 63
  color map, tangential, 58-62
  contact fitting software, 69
  conversion capabilities, export/import, 69
  corneal coverage, 55
  customizable displays/reports, 62
  difference maps, 62
  fitting protocol, 69
  fluorescein, simulated, 69
  focus verification, 62
  hardware, high performance, 55
  Holladay Diagnostic Summary, 56
  lens
    categories, 69
    fitting, trial, 69
  Microsoft Windows-based software, 63
  multi-map comparison tools, 62
  normalized scale, adjustable, 58
  ordering, 69
  overview, 55
  patient
    database software, 63
    identification photo, 63

    photo identification, 69
    selection, 69
  peripheral corneal topographer technology, 63
  preoperative/postoperative examinations, 56
  print, exam protocols with, 63
  refractive nomogram software, 69-74
  reproducibility, 62-63
  ring edge detection, 62
  save, exam protocols with, 63
  simplicity of use, 63
  software, high performance, 56-62
  STARS display, 56
  surgical change/healing change maps, 56
  three-camera technology with profile view, 55
  Tyler's Quarterly database, 69
  upgradability, 63-69

HDS. See Holladay Diagnostic Summary
hexagonal keratotomy, corneal topography, 208
Holladay Diagnostic Summary, 309-323
  astigmatic cornea, regular, 315
  auto scale, refractive map, 320, 323
  clinical examples, 313-323
  corneal parameters for 3-mm pupil, 311-313,
    313-315, 318-320, 323
  distortion map, 311, 313, 318, 320, 323
  excimer PRK cornea, 320-323
  EyeSys 2000 corneal analysis system, 56
  keratoconus cornea, 315-320
  keratometry measurements, simulated, 312
  measurements, miscellaneous, 312-313
  power maps, 309-311
  profile difference map, 311, 313, 318, 320, 323
  pupil parameters and regular astigmatism, 312
  radial keratotomy cornea, 320
  refractive map
    auto scale, 311, 313, 315-318, 318
    standard scale, 309-311, 313, 315, 318
  refractive power measurements, 311-312
  standard scale, refractive map, 320
  steel calibration ball, 313-315
hyperopia, keratomileusis, 271-279

image accuracy, corneal topography, 13
incision, corneal relaxing, 225-239
keratometry
  limitations of, 4-6
  measurement, corneal topography,

astigmatism, 26-33
  misleading, 28-32
keratomileusis, 280
  for hyperopia, 271-279
  for myopia, 265-271
keratoplasty, automated lamellar, 265-271

lamellar refractive surgery, corneal topography, 263-284
  automated lamellar keratoplasty
    or in situ keratomileusis for hyperopia, 271-279
    or in situ keratomileusis for myopia, 265-271
  myopic keratomileusis, 263-264
  photorefractive keratomileusis, in situ, 280

maps, 242-245. See also individual maps
  topographical, evaluation of, 3-4
MasterVue topography systems, 77-87
  alignment, 77
  clinical outcomes module, 83
  contact lens fitting module, 81-83
  corneal power maps, 78
  data conversion, 78
  displays, 81
  exam
    collecting, 78
    full, 78
    managing, 81
    viewing, 78
  focusing, 77
  future developments, 83-87
  imaging with, 77-78
  keratometric view, 78
  networking, 81
  numerical view, 78
  optional modules, 81-83
  output, 81
  overview, 87
  photokeratoscope view, 81
  profile view, 81
  QuickVue, 78
  RK nomogram module, 83
meridional contour, EyeMap EH-270, 41
multifocal cornea, 225-239
multi-zone ablations for high myopia,
    excimer laser procedures, 255
myopia, keratomileusis, 265-271

omnimmetropia, 225-239
ORBSCAN system
  alignment, 98
  corneal topography, 95-101
    engineering, history of, 90-95
  non-Placido topography, 101-102
  pachymetric maps, 98-101
  pachymetry, 90-103
  topographic map, 98-101

pachymetry, ORBSCAN system, 90-103
PAR corneal topography system, 105-120
  astigmatism, 111-112
  clinical applications, 110-119
  cornea, normal, 110-111
  CTS
    design features, 109-110
    technology, 105-109
  display methods, 107-109
  excimer photorefractive keratectomy, 115
  future growth, 120
  intraoperative topography, 115
  keratoconus, 113
  keratoplasty, lamellar, post-automated, 115
  keratotomy, post-radial, 113-114
  measurement technique, 105-106
  optometry, 115
  system configuration, 106
PARK, for correction of astigmatism, 255-260
photorefractive keratectomy
  evaluation, STARS maps, 242-245
  for undercorrected RK, 255
Placido-based device, computerized videokeratography, 9
power, cornea, normal, 4-6
PRK. See photorefractive keratectomy

radial keratotomy, corneal topography, 195-199
refractive surgical procedures, corneal topography in, 195-212, 202-203
  astigmatic keratotomy, 199-202
    post cataract surgery, 199-202
    post penetrating keratoplasty, 202
  epikeratophakia, 203-208
  hexagonal keratotomy, 208
  radial keratotomy, 195-199
  refractive surgery enhancements, 202-203

side-by-side image plot, dioptric plot with, EyeMap EH-270, 40
STARS maps, photorefractive keratectomy evaluation, 242-245
symmetrical astigmatism, 26

telocentric method, corneal topography, 47
three-dimensional display, EyeMap EH-270, 40-41
Tomey technology/computed anatomy TMS-1 video-keratoscope, 123-149, 145
    algorithms, 151
    alignment, 125-126, 151
    applications, 140-145
    focus, 125-126, 151
    hardware, 123
    light cone, VKS, 124-125
    map displays
        multiple, 133-140
        single, 128-133
    software, 153
        use of, 127-128
    specifications, 153
    videokeratoscopy, principles of, 123-124
TOPCON computerized mapping system CM-1000, 151-154
topographical maps, evaluation of, 3-4

topography, cornea
    engineering, history of, 90-95
    evaluation
        of corneal transplant patient, 288-306
        excimer procedures, healing patterns, 245-255
    with excimer laser procedures, 242-260
    EyeMap EH-270, 37-52
        telocentric method, 47
    image accuracy, 13
    keratometric measurement, astigmatism, 26-33
    normal, 10-13
    overview, 3-15
    pathology
        characterization of, 159-169
        detection of, 159-169
    qualitative measurement of, 6-13
    in refractive surgical procedures, 195-212

video displays, EyeMap EH-270, 38-45
videokeratography, computerized, 9
    alignment, 17-23, 18-20
        corneal apex, relation to, 21-22
        error, measurement of, 20
        refractive surgery, relation to, 22-23
    applications of, 10-13
    Placido-based device, 9